Nature of Communication Disorders in Culturally and Linguistically Diverse Populations

CONTRIBUTORS

Joan Good Erickson, Ph.D.
University of Illinois at Urbana-Champaign
Department of Speech and Hearing Science
Champaign, IL 61820

Gail Harris, M.S.
University of Arizona
Native American Research and Training Center
c/o Department of Speech and Hearing Science
Tucson, AZ 85721

Aquiles Iglesias, Ph.D.
Temple University
Speech-Language-Hearing Sciences Division
Philadelphia, PA 19122

Kay T. Payne, Ph.D.
Department of Communication Arts and Sciences
Howard University
Washington, DC 20059

Cassandra Peters-Johnson, Ph.D.
Howard University
Montgomery County Public Schools
Silver Spring, MD 20906

Muriel Saville-Troike, Ph.D.
Bureau of Educational Research
College of Education
University of Illinois at Urbana-Champaign
Champaign, IL 61820

Joseph L. Stewart, Ph.D.
Indian Health Service
Albuquerque, NM 87102

Ida J. Stockman, Ph.D.
Department of Audiology and Speech Sciences
Michigan State University
East Lansing, MI 48824-1212

Orlando L. Taylor, Ph.D.
Howard University
School of Communications
Department of Communication Arts and Sciences
Washington, DC 20059

Walt Wolfram, Ph.D.
University of the District of Columbia and Center for Applied Linguistics
Department of Communication Sciences
College of Liberal and Fine Arts
724 9th Street, NW
Washington, DC 20001

NATURE OF COMMUNICATION DISORDERS IN CULTURALLY AND LINGUISTICALLY DIVERSE POPULATIONS

Edited by

Orlando L. Taylor, Ph.D.
Howard University

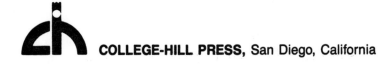

COLLEGE-HILL PRESS, San Diego, California

College-Hill Press, Inc.
4284 41st Street
San Diego, California 92105

Library of Congress Cataloging in Publication Data
Main entry under title:

Nature of communication disorders in culturally
  and linguistically diverse populations.

Companion vol. to Treatment of communication disorders in culturally and linguistically diverse populations.
  Includes indexes.
  1. Communicative disorders. 2. Language disorders.
3. Language and culture. 4. Linguistic minorities.
I. Taylor, Orlando L., 1936-   . II. Treatment of communication disorders in culturally and linguistically diverse populations. III. Title
RC423.N3 1986   616.85'5   85-22426
ISBN 0-88744-185-8

Printed in the United States of America

To LeRoy and Carrie Taylor, my Father and Mother

CONTENTS

PREFACE

The seeds for this book were planted in the late 1960s and early 1970s when the editor of this volume was involved in a number of professional and extraprofessional activities that were designed to help eliminate the social injustices that permeated the American society. In the professions of speech pathology and audiology, these activities were focused within the Black Caucus of the American Speech and Hearing Association and that Association's newly formed Committee on Communication Behaviors and Disorders in Urban and Ethnic Populations.

During this period, there has been considerable discussion — and debate — on many professional issues pertaining to definitions of normal and pathological communicative behaviors in the various cultural and linguistic groups that reside in the United States of America. In addition to the field of communication disorders, much of this discussion has centered on research in such disciplines as sociolinguistics, bilingual education, and cognitive psychology on such diverse topics as (1) social and cultural influences on normal communicative behavior; (2) the nature, validity, and historical characteristics of various languages and dialects spoken by the American people; (3) universals of language and communicative acquisition that cut across all cultures and socioeconomic classes; and (4) the nature and prevalence of communication disorders within various cultural and linguistic groups in the United States.

Most of these disciplines and issues are represented in this volume. Although numerous articles and monographs have been written on the various topics outlined, to date no book has been published that presents a critical, comprehensive review of them as well as proposals for future directions for the discipline of communication disorders in relation to cultural and linguistic diversity.

At the outset, the book was intended to be a single volume on the nature of normal communicative behavior in culturally and linguistically diverse populations, with approaches for valid assessment and management of communication disorders within these populations. Once the project was undertaken in early 1984, it became obvious that the body of literature was too great to be addressed adequately in a single volume. Consequently, two books were written — this volume and a companion volume, *Treatment of Communication Disorders in Culturally and Linguistically Diverse Populations.*

This volume is divided into three parts. Part I, consisting of three chapters, focuses on background issues pertaining to cultural and linguistic diversity. Part II, consisting of two chapters, focuses on language variations within the United States and language acquisition in Black Americans, the largest nonwhite group in the United States. Part III, consisting of four chapters, focuses on the prevalence and nature of communication disorders in Black Americans, Hispanic Americans, Native Americans, and other indigenous peoples of North America.

In Chapter 1, the editor discusses the historical factors associated with the issue of cultural and linguistic diversity within the field of communication disorders and presents a conceptual framework for viewing the issue of diversity. In this chapter, the author describes the positions taken in the late 1960s and early 1970s by scholars and practitioners, during which time the various cultural issues were being framed within the discipline. These descriptions are continued through 1985, when the American Speech-Language-Hearing Association sponsored a National Colloquium on Underserved Populations. The chapter concludes with the presentation of a model for viewing normal and pathological communication from a framework that takes into account the social, cognitive, and communicative norms of the culture from which a person comes.

Chapter 2, written by the editor's colleague, Kay T. Payne, describes some basic concepts pertaining to culture and socioeconomic status. Payne proceeds to a summary discussion on the link between language and culture. The remainder of the chapter contains a somewhat extensive presentation of some of the major descriptive characteristics of white Americans, Black Americans, Hispanics, Asian Americans, and several smaller ethnic groups in Alaska, the Hawaiian Islands, and the Virgin Islands.

Chapter 3, by Muriel Saville-Troike, focuses on anthropological issues to be considered in studying and assessing communication. Drawing heavily from cultural anthropology and the relatively new discipline of ethnography of communication, Saville-Troike defines numerous concepts associated with the study of culture and human communication. She provides excellent examples that show how cultural differences between the communication assessor and the person(s) being assessed can result in serious interferences in the collection and interpretation of communicative data.

Chapter 4, by Walt Wolfram, presents a thorough discussion of general principles pertaining to an understanding of variation within any language, particularly language variation within American English. Wolfram discusses linguistic, social, and cultural parameters that contribute to variation. Several socially significant phonological and grammatical features that constitute major aspects of language variation within the United States are presented and explained.

Chapter 5, by Ida Stockman, is a discussion of the language acquisition in Black Americans, one of the culturally diverse groups of focus in this book. Stockman outlines the relationship of language acquisition research to language disorders and offers several guidelines for evaluating language research. She continues with a summary and critique of a number of language acquisition studies on Black children utilizing these evaluation guidelines. Finally, Stockman presents a set of conclusions pertaining to Black child language, as well as some implications for clinical assessments.

In Chapter 6, the editor and a former colleague, Cassandra Peters-Johnson, review the available research on communication disorders in Black populations in the United States, Africa, and the Caribbean. Particular attention is placed on problems of cultural definitions of communication pathology and culturally sensitive research. In addition, this chapter summarizes the available data on the prevalence and nature of various types of speech, language, and hearing disorders in Blacks. Several questions are raised in the chapter with respect to communicative behaviors and disorders that have been presented heretofore as universals or norms, but which should be reevaluated in view of data obtained from other cultural and linguistic groups.

Chapter 7, by Joan Erickson and Aquiles Iglesias, focuses on speech and language disorders in Hispanic populations. This chapter discusses numerous problems pertaining to culturally and linguistically valid testing of Hispanic persons. Some alternative assessment approaches are presented, together with a review of available data from the research and clinical literature on the prevalence and nature of communication disorders among Hispanics, as well as viable approaches to the delivery of clinical services.

Chapter 8, by Gail Harris, presents a comprehensive discussion of the cultural, linguistic, attitudinal, geographical, and infrastructural barriers facing the speech pathologist in attempting to deliver clinical services to Native Americans. Data on the incidence and prevalence of communication disorders are also summarized. Harris makes several proposals for overcoming the problems in order to address the serious public health and education problems typically faced by this extremely neglected group of Americans — the first Americans.

Chapter 9, by Joseph Stewart, extends the discussion of Native Americans to include a discussion of hearing disorders among several indigenous peoples of North America (American Indians and Eskimos), Asians, and Pacific peoples. Stewart pays particular attention to the problem of otitis media, a major cause of hearing loss among indigenous groups in these regions. He explores various cultural, biological, sociological, environmental, and health care delivery issues that seem to be associated with this problem.

Some may take issue with this book on the grounds that not all cultural and ethnic groups in the United States are sufficiently covered. In a sense, this criticism is valid, especially with respect to the obvious omission of substantial materials on Asian Americans, the nation's fastest growing immigrant population. At the same time, it should be noted that the literature is relatively small for many of these other populations. Moreover, the book is written as a case study on what we know about a select group of the more populous nonwhite populations in the United States. We hope it will serve to stimulate more publications from others on other groups, as well as on the peoples covered herein.

Finally, the reader is encouraged to read the companion volume to this book, *Treatment of Communication Disorders in Culturally and Linguistically Diverse Populations.* This book discusses specific assessment, management, and educational issues pertaining to culturally and linguistically diverse persons. Chapters cover (1) culturally valid and nonstandard approaches to language and cognitive assessment, (2) clinical intervention for language disorders among nonstandard English speaking children, and (3) educational issues involved in teaching standard English as a second dialect.

ACKNOWLEDGMENTS

As editor, I wish to express sincere thanks to my numerous friends and colleagues at Howard University and throughout the country for their support and encouragement during the preparation of this book. Special appreciation is extended to the members of my loyal and dedicated staff for their inspiration and assistance in preparing the final manuscript, and to all of the members of my immediate family for their unequivocal love through the years. Finally, but certainly not least in importance, I wish to acknowledge the stimulation and motivation I have received from many students during the past 20 years at Indiana University, Federal City College (University of the District of Columbia), Stanford University, and particularly Howard University. My scholarship is a reflection of my continuing intellectual commitment to you.

PART I
BACKGROUND

Chapter 1

Historical Perspectives and Conceptual Framework

Orlando L. Taylor

Prior to 1968, little interest was shown within the professions of speech pathology and audiology in addressing the unique clinical needs of individuals with communication disorders from culturally and linguistically diverse populations. With respect to speech-language function, professionals tended to have a poor perception of the distinction between a legitimate linguistic *difference* and a speech–language *disorder*. Moreover, virtually all norms within all subspecialties of communication were based on what we might call a middle class, Euro-American model.

In this introductory chapter, we examine some of the historical events, legal decisions, legislative initiatives, and research findings that have resulted in significant changes in how professionals in communication disorders have come to view the nature of these disorders in culturally and linguistically diverse populations. The chapter concludes with the presentation of a conceptual framework for examining this topic.

THE WINDS OF CHANGE: THE 1968 ASHA CONVENTION

In 1968, a very important event occurred at the Annual Convention of the American Speech and Hearing Association (ASHA) in Denver, Colorado. The ASHA President, John V. Irwin, in a bold change from tradition, decided to forego the annual Presidential Address to permit a debate between Orlando L. Taylor of Indiana University and John Michel of the University of Kansas on "The Role of a Professional Association in a Conflict Society." Irwin's courageous act grew out of severe national discord over the Vietnam war and civil unrest by Blacks in numerous urban centers.

Michel took the position that professional associations should not be involved in social issues.

> It is unwise to jeopardize the purely professional nature of ASHA and the harmony among our Members by introducing current issues outside the realm of speech and hearing. It is both healthy and admirable that individual Members are sensitive to social issues and have the courage to organize opinion against unsatisfactory aspects of our society.
>
> (Michel, 1969, p. 220)

Taylor took an opposite position. He argued, in part, that

> professional organizations should articulate a point of view on the important social and political issues of the day, making it possible for the corporate body to influence decisions . . . . I urge the American Speech and Hearing Association to provide aggressive leadership for moral, ethical, and judicial behavior in areas of significant social significance.
>
> (Taylor, 1969, p. 217)

The Michel-Taylor debate stimulated great discussion and exchange within the professions of speech pathology and audiology. Out of this dialogue came enormous changes, which serve as a backdrop for addressing the topic of communication disorders within culturally and linguistically diverse populations.

THE EMERGENCE OF THE ASHA BLACK CAUCUS

The most immediate and, at the time, the most important outgrowth of the Michel-Taylor debate at the 1968 ASHA Convention was the formation of a Black Caucus. This caucus of the majority of the then minuscule Black membership (probably less than 100 persons) addressed several concerns in a special report (Taylor et al., 1969) to the ASHA membership.

One of the three major objectives of the ASHA Black Caucus was to urge the Association to

> encourage appropriate research and curriculum revisions in the area of urban language behavior, most of which is black language, to the

extent that more intelligent clinical and educational services can be made available to black children.

(Taylor et al., 1969, p. 222)

Speaking to the language objectives more specifically, the ASHA Black Caucus established two related goals:

1. To urge ASHA to require coursework in sociolinguistics (and Black history) for clinical certification.
2. To urge ASHA to organize a committee to generate new ideas on training and research in sociolinguistics, especially as related to Black language.

Addressing the first goal, the ASHA Black Caucus wrote

Unfortunately, far too many speech pathologists view legitimate language differences among Afro-Americans from a pathology model. The result is that a number of black children are receiving speech and language therapy, particularly in urban areas, when they, in fact, have no pathology. Negative psychological effects on the black child are obvious. In order to develop a more intelligent approach to recognizing legitimate linguistic differences and satisfactory methods for second language instruction as a skill, clinicians need training in sociolinguistics (interaction between language and culture) and the historical and cultural roots of black children. All too often clinicians fail to understand the black child's language, as well as the child himself.

(p. 224)

On the second goal, the ASHA Black Caucus asserted

Even if ASHA required institutions to offer a course in sociolinguistics, there is a dearth of knowledge about language, its patterns of acquisition, and viable means for utilizing it for teaching standard English as a skill. Likewise, there is a dearth of qualified teachers in this area. ASHA might assume some leadership in terms of training personnel (clinicians and teachers) for work in this area and stimulating the basic and applied research needed. It is noteworthy that a number of other professionals have already begun serious work in urban language, e.g., linguists, sociologists, and teachers of English. Unless the profession of communication disorders begins to put forth a major thrust in this area, it will lose a great opportunity to catapult itself into an arena of great educational and cultural interest.

(p. 224)

ASHA AND THE PROFESSION RESPOND

Largely in response to the aforementioned Michel-Taylor debate and the advocacy by the ASHA Black Caucus, a number of important actions have been taken within the profession of communication disorders since 1969 to address the needs of clinically and linguistically diverse populations. Among the most important of these actions are the following:

1. ASHA opened an Office of Urban and Ethnic Affairs in 1969 (this office was changed to the Office of Minority Concerns in 1979).
2. ASHA established committees on Communication Behaviors and Problems in Urban Populations in 1969 (now the Committee on Cultural and Linguistic Differences and Disorders of Communication) and on the Status of Racial Minorities in 1973.
3. Several symposia, colloquia, and Continuing Education activities have been presented throughout the United States on normal and clinical issues pertaining to culturally and linguistically diverse populations. ASHA'S 1985 National Colloquium on Underserved Populations is a good example of this type of activity.
4. ASHA has taken official positions on social dialects and on the clinical management of communicatively handicapped minority language populations. (Position papers on each are presented in the Appendix.) The social dialects position recognizes the legitimacy of all dialects of a language, as well as the validity of a linguistic standard. A specific role is outlined for speech pathologists in teaching standard English to *normal* speakers, and the qualifications needed by the professional who engages in this activity are noted. The communicatively handicapped minority language statement outlines national clinical needs in this area, a continuum of language proficiency, professional competencies for bilingual speech pathologists, and strategies for procuring competent personnel to provide clinical services to bilingual persons.
5. Several universities have inaugurated special training projects to address the specific clinical needs of culturally or linguistically diverse populations—for example, University of Arizona (Native Americans); San Diego State University, Temple University, and University of the District of Columbia (Bilingual Populations); Howard University (Black American and Third World Populations).
6. Presentations in professional meetings and publications in professional journals have increased dramatically since 1969 on a myriad of topics pertaining to cultural and linguistic diversity. For example, Cole (1985) reports that at the 1984 ASHA Convention, over 50 sessions focused on minority issues. This percent-

age represented a 100 percent increase over 1982 and a 5,000 percent increase over 1969, when there was only one session on this topic. Regrettably, some of this research on minority issues still contains negative views and invalid assumptions on cultural and linguistic divergence.

LEGAL AND LEGISLATIVE DEVELOPMENTS

Concurrent with the activities within the American Speech-Language-Hearing Association, a number of legal and legislative actions occurred during the 1970s and 1980s that have influenced issues of cultural and linguistic diversity in the field of communication disorders. Some of these actions will be discussed in this section.

The fourteenth amendment to the United States Constitution guarantees, in part, that all citizens are entitled to receive equal protection under the law. This entitlement was defined operationally in Title VI of the Civil Rights Act of 1964. Title VI states

No person in the United States shall, on the ground of race, color, or national origin, be excluded from participation in, be denied benefits of, or be subjected to discrimination under any program or activity receiving federal financial assistance.

Several significant court decisions were made during the 1970s that cited the fourteenth amendment and Title VI as bases for ruling on behalf of plaintiffs in cases that had enormous impact on the field of communication disorders. These decisions have led, in turn, to several important legislative actions (Table 1-4).

Table 1-1. Major Legislative Actions

Bilingual Education Act of 1968, United States Congress.

Public Law 94–142, The Education of All Handicapped Children Act. (November 29, 1975).

Public Law 95-561, The Bilingual Education Act of 1976.

U.S. Code of Federal Regulations, Number 34, Part 300. 532 (a), 1973.

The most important decision was *Lau v. Nichols* (1974). In this landmark case, the U.S. Supreme Court ruled unanimously in favor of the plaintiffs from San Francisco's Chinatown community, who claimed that the absence of programs designed to meet their specific linguistic needs violated their civil rights. The plaintiffs argued further, and the Court agreed, that equality of education goes beyond the provision of the same buildings and books to all students to include intangible factors such as language. Because they could not understand the English language used in the classroom, the Chinese plaintiffs argued, they were deprived of even a minimally adequate, and hardly equal, education. In addition, they asserted that the equal rights provision of the United States Constitution prohibited withholding from them the means of comprehending the language of instruction (Center for Applied Linguistics, 1977).

The importance of *Lau v. Nichols* to the field of communication disorders, and to bilingual education, was that it established unequivocally that the handling of language differences in public facilities, or those receiving Federal funds, fell within the purview of constitutional guarantees pertaining to equal rights and to Civil Rights legislation. *Lau v. Nichols* led to the passage of the Bilingual Education Act of 1976 and to several additional lawsuits pertaining to the rights of persons who speak a language other than English (e.g., *Serna v. Portales Municipal Schools*, 1974 in New Mexico; *Aspira of New York, Inc., v. Board of Education of the City of New York*, 1974).

Citing *Lau v. Nichols* and Section 1703(f) of Title 20 of the United States Code, a United States District Judge in Michigan ruled in 1979 on behalf of nine Black children in Ann Arbor, who claimed that the local school board had denied them their equal rights by failing to take their native Black English into account in the educational process (*Martin Luther King Junior Elementary School Children, et al., v. Ann Arbor School District Board*, 1978). Section 1703(f) of Title 20 states

> No State shall deny equal educational opportunity to an individual on account of his or her race, color, sex, or national origin by . . .
>
> (f) the failure of an educational agency to take appropriate action to overcome language barriers that impede equal participation by its students in its instructional programs.

Since the Ann Arbor School Board did not appeal this ruling, the decision on behalf of the nine children and their parents did not have the effect of federal law. However, it did establish the legitimacy of the claim that dialect variation, like language differences, could not be used to discriminate against children in the implementation of educational programs.

Several other court decisions and legislative actions have spoken even more directly to issues affecting clinical practices in communication disorders. Most have involved issues of assessment procedures used to identify and place children into speech-language therapy and into special and compensatory education classes. It is well documented that children from linguistic and cultural minorities tend to be placed into special education and related services at higher rates than their representation in local school populations. In some cases, however, there is an underrepresentation in these classes and services (Jones and Cartwright, 1981). In either event, inappropriate testing and other assessment procedures are thought to be the cause of the problem.

Three court decisions in state and federal courts have supported the notion that discriminatory testing procedures cannot be used to place children in special education classes and related services. The most celebrated of cases are *Dianna v. Board of Education* (1973) (California); *Larry P. v. Riles* (1977) (California); and *Mattie T. v. Holladay* (1977) (Mississippi).

The Education of All Handicapped Children Act of 1975, Public Law 94–142, and its revision, PL 98–199 provide the most explicit language to date that outlaws the use of discriminatory testing to place children in special education classes and in such related services as speech, language, and hearing therapy. Section 34:300.532(a) of the U.S. Code of Federal Regulations (1983) pertaining to the provisions of PL 94–142 and 98–199 states

State and local educational agencies shall insure, at a minimum, that:

(a) Tests and other evaluation materials:

(1) Are provided and administered in the child's native language or other mode of communication, unless it is clearly not feasible to do so.

These various legal decisions and legislative initiatives in the past two decades have established legitimacy to the claim that a child's native language system has to be considered in the development and implementation of special education programs and in the provision of clinical services to communicatively impaired persons. Moreover, they have provided a basis for advocates of culturally and linguistically diverse populations to couch their claims in legal terms, in addition to academic and intellectual terms.

RESEARCH DEVELOPMENTS

As stated earlier, research issues pertaining to communication disorders in culturally and linguistically diverse populations have increased dramatically since the 1960s. This research, which has come from many disciplines, has provided the underpinnings for the present state of the art with respect to our understanding of the nature of communication disorders in culturally and linguistically diverse populations.

In general, the studies of particular value to the study of this topic have focused on such topics as the following:

1. Cultural preferences of selected populations within the United States
2. The nature and history of various dialects of American English
3. Patterns of first and second language acquisition within several cultural and linguistic groups
4. Ethnographic approaches to the study of language and communication

In subsequent chapters of this book, much of this research will be discussed critically. For now, however, we may state seven conclusions that might be drawn from this research literature to serve as general principles undergirding studies of the nature of communication disorders in culturally and linguistically diverse populations. These conclusions are as follows:

1. Communicative norms within a particular group are a product of cultural values, perceptions, attitudes, and history (Saville-Troike, 1978).
2. All human beings are members of at least one indigenous culture, and they have the capacity to acquire knowledge of other cultures, which may either alter their indigenous cultural norms or permit them to shift from one set of cultural norms to those of some other culture (Penalosa, 1981).
3. All cultural groups in the world tend to have definable characteristics in universal categories of behavior (.e.g., values, family structure, communication, world view, learning styles). However, the specific rules and definitions within these categories tend to be culture specific. Despite the presence of differences among the various groups in the world, numerous overlaps exist, particularly among groups within a given nation state (Saville-Troike, 1978; Banks, 1984).
4. Dialects exist within every language in the world. Contrary to most research reported before the middle 1960s, all dialects are intrinsically valid for the group of persons who speak them. These dialects are products of political, social, cultural, and historical factors. Dialects within a given language typically demonstrate enormous overlaps within all linguistic categories.

These overlaps result in a high degree of mutual intelligibility across the dialects of a given language (Fasold, 1984; Wolfram and Fasold, 1974).

5. General patterns of first language acquisition seem to follow a set of universal principles. However, developmental milestones seem to be influenced by the nature of the language to be acquired (Bowerman, 1980).

6. The acquisition of a second language tends to be influenced by the time at which the second language is introduced and the social circumstances surrounding its introduction. In any event, the acquisition of a second language tends to follow an orderly and predictable process, resulting in various changes of proficiency in the second language (L2), and possibly in the first language (L1) (Cummins, 1981; McCollum, 1981).

7. All language behavior operates within a larger set of communication rules that govern verbal and nonverbal behaviors as a function of cultural rules, which in turn control such factors as the communicative event, participants, shared channels of communication, communicative codes, setting, attitudes and content of messages, and the form of messages (Hymes, 1974).

A CONCEPTUAL FRAMEWORK

Professional, legal, and research developments in communication disorders and related disorders, particularly those since the 1960s, permit us to devise a culturally based framework for studying the nature—and the treatment—of communication disorders in culturally and linguistically diverse populations. The framework devised by this author is schematized in Figure 1–1.

As shown in Figure 1–1, the basic premise of this author's conceptual framework is that the study of normal and pathological communication must be couched in cultural terms. To do otherwise is to run the risk of making claims and judgments about the communicative behaviors of a given group of speakers from an inappropriate or, even worse, an ethnocentric set of assumptions and norms. The omnipresence of culture is demonstrated in Figure 1–1 by virtue of the placement of all four processes and outcomes germane to the study of the nature and treatment of communication pathology within the boundaries of culture.

The four processes and outcomes that operate within the constraints of culture are (1) developmental issues, (2) precursors of communication pathology, (3) assessment and diagnosis, and (4) treat-

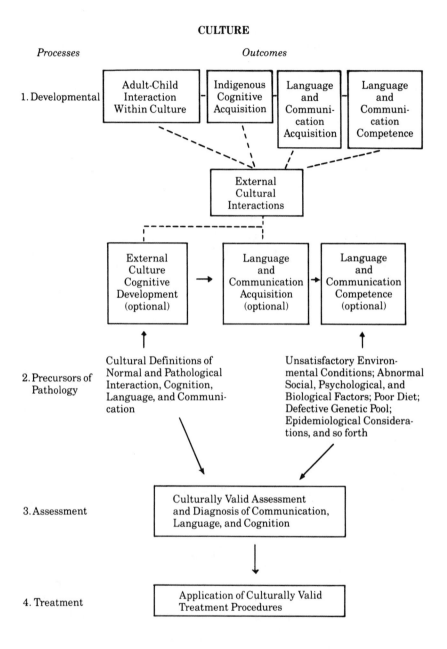

Figure 1-1. Schematic view of a culturally based conceptual framework for studying and treating communication disorders in culturally and linguistically diverse populations.

ment. The first two processes speak to the nature of communication disorders within a given cultural group. Processes three and four speak to clinical issues of diagnosis and management.

These processes are listed hierarchically in terms of their importance in addressing issues in communication disorders. The outcomes, although presented sequentially, are necessarily artificially ordered inasmuch as many components of each process are likely to develop simultaneously with one another.

Process 1 — Developmental Issues

Developmental processes provide the foundation for understanding the nature and treatment of communication disorders within any cultural or linguistic group. Two levels of development are presented: (1) development within the indigenous culture, and, following the likely exposure to outside cultures, (2) optional development of external cultural, cognitive, language, and communicative behaviors. In the model, solid lines denote expected phenomena, whereas dashed lines connote optional phenomena.

The four outcomes of the developmental process *within* the indigenous culture include (1) adult-child interaction within the culture, (2) cognitive acquisition within the framework of a specific culture, (3) the acquisition of indigenous language and communication systems, and (4) the development of adult language communicative competence.

The foundation for all indigenous cultural development is thought to be the adult-child interactions that occur within the sociocultural context of a specified group. These interactions provide a model for the developing child for, among other things, acceptable cognitive, linguistic, and communicative behaviors. Through this early socialization, the child is believed, at least by some, to develop a set of culturally and socially based concepts and thoughts (Vygotsky, 1962). This underlying conceptual development gives rise, in turn, to the acquisition of verbal and nonverbal symbols (language) and rules for using them (communication), within the rules of the indigenous culture. Over time, through practice, increased socialization, and biological maturation, the child is expected to acquire adult language and communication competence within the norms established by the indigenous culture.

Although possible, it is highly unlikely, at least in the economically developed world, for the developing child to be so culture bound that he or she is never exposed to external cultures. If nothing else, modern mass communication systems and compulsory education guarantee some type of external cultural exposure. This optional external cultural interaction is shown through a set of dashed lines emanating from each of the four basic processes of indigenous cultural development. These connections with the box labeled *external cultural interactions* show that the optional (though likely) exposures to other cultures may occur at any stage of the developmental process from infancy through adulthood.

The final stage of developmental outcomes involves *optional* development, which might occur within a person (child or adult) as a result of external cultural interactions. These outcomes, which are schematized in the lower tier of the developmental outcomes in Figure 1-1, may be thought of as *second* cognitive, language, and communicative acquisition. Both the occurrence and the degree of acquisition of these external or second systems are dependent on a number of social, political, and psychological factors (e.g., age of exposure, degree of exposure, relative political and social power of the indigenous and external cultures, motivation for acquiring the external culture, and method of acquiring the second culture). In any case, this second tier of outcomes recognizes the possibility that an individual may acquire, at varying levels of competence, the cognitive, linguistic, and communicative systems of another culture, as a replacement for or addition to his indigenous culture, or as a hybrid of the two. Since language is intimately linked with thought, Figure 1-1 suggests that any type of cognitive acquisition within the external culture will necessarily lead to some level of acquisition of the language and communication of the external culture. As shown by the dashed lines, however, it is not necessarily the case that adult competence will be the result in either area.

Process 2 — Precursors of Pathology

Normal cognitive, linguistic, and communication development may not occur in a given individual even under the best of cultural conditions. There are two major precursors to the emergence of communication pathology, or at least to what individuals consider to be communicatively pathological within a given culture. The first might be called "culturally defined pathological behaviors." The second set of precursors includes the whole array of abnormal or unsatisfactory biological, social, psychological, nutritional, and genetic factors that are known to contribute to the development of communication pathology.

In viewing these precursors of communication pathology, however, the reader is reminded that cultural factors assume an enormously important role in the definition of what is considered pathological. Culture also determines the definition of the quality and *normalcy* of an environment, diet, social condition, psychological state, or even a biological condition.

The role of cultural definitions of communication pathology cannot be overemphasized. Scattered observations from around the world reveal that societies have different perceptions of what they consider pathological communication and, equally important, what to do about it when it does exist. Taylor and Samara (1985) claim that some societies believe that little or nothing should be done about communication disorders, except to keep them hidden from the public. In some cases, these disorders are thought to be acts of God(s) or demons. In Arabic speaking countries, for example, this concept exists and is referred to as "kikmat Rabana."

With this cultural notion in mind, it seems reasonable to argue that based on what is known about the social and cultural dimensions of the form, content, and use of language by people around the world, it is obvious that a communication disorder in any society can only be defined from the vantage point of the speech community of which a given speaker is a member. Therefore, a strong claim can be made that such "standard" definitions of communication disorders, such as the one advanced by Van Riper (1978), should be revised to something like the following:

> Communicative behavior by an individual can only be considered defective if it deviates sufficiently from the norms, expectations, and definitions of his or her indigenous culture (or language group); that is, if it is
>
> (a) considered to be defective by the indigenous culture or language group,
> (b) operates outside the minimal norms of acceptability of that culture or language group,
> (c) interferes with communication *within* the indigenous culture or language group,
> (d) calls attention to itself within the indigenous culture or language group, or
> (e) causes the user to be "maladjusted" as defined by the indigenous culture.

With respect to the standard list of causative factors associated with communication pathology, the point must be reiterated that although the causative factors listed in Figure 1–1 probably exist all over the world, cultural factors influence the values and perceptions that interact with them. For example, a poor diet in one culture may be considered to be a good diet in another culture. Likewise, one culture's view of a satisfactory social environment may be another culture's perception of a completely unacceptable social environment.

Epidemiological considerations as a precursor of communication disorders deserve special attention in this discussion. All too often, the communication disorders specialist determines the relative importance of various diseases and syndromes as etiological factors from within the framework of their prevalence of distribution within his or her given culture. In truth, however, the relative importance of various diseases and syndromes as etiological factors in communication disorders should vary from culture to culture. Thus, within the United States, it is probably appropriate to place considerable attention on such medical conditions as stroke, closed head injuries, and cancer as examples of major causes of communication disorders. In other parts of the world, however, other medical conditions might be considered more important. For example, in much of the Third World, great emphasis might be placed on schistosomiasis* as a disease that contributes to the onset of communication disorders. In Africa, and in countries throughout the world where African descendents now reside, sickle cell disease might be considered to be a major cause of hearing loss and, therefore, the recipient of considerable professional attention.

Process 3 — Assessment

The third conceptual notion of the model in Figure 1–1 addresses the need for culturally and linguistically valid testing and other assessment procedures for determining communication pathology in individuals from a specified culture or language group. As stated earlier in this chapter, culturally valid procedures are required by federal law and conform with what many would consider ethical practice in the field of communication disorders.

Culturally valid assessment, by definition, includes the use of test instruments and other formal and informal procedures for collecting linguistic and communicative data from an individual or for determining his or her level of development or the presence of abnor-

---

*Petersdorf and colleagues (1983) describe schistosomiasis as a water-carried parasitic disorder that affects the gastrointestinal system, the liver, and the vascular system and causes central nervous system (CNS) damage. Over 200 million persons are thought to be afflicted with this disease in more than 71 countries, virtually all in the developing world, although the disorder is probably being brought to Europe and North America by immigrant populations. There are no reports in the literature on the effects of schistosomiasis on speech, language, or hearing function, despite its capacity to cause vascular obstructions and CNS damage.

mality. These assessments must be conducted from the vantage point of the indigenous or preferred system of communication of the person being assessed. If group comparisons are to be made, they must be made in the context of standards or norms derived from comparable individuals from the same cultural or linguistic group as the client.

The entire Spring, 1983, edition of *Topics in Language Disorders* provides an excellent discussion of nonbiased assessments of communicative behaviors. In that volume, Taylor and Payne (1983) observe, quite accurately, that when a researcher wishes to construct culturally valid assessment instruments and procedures, controls must be carefully chosen to prevent the emergence of several sources of potential bias: linguistic, format, situational, examiner, values, and directions.

Finally, Taylor (1985) has argued that culturally valid assessment procedures should

1. Recognize that clients may perform differentially under differing clinical conditions because of their cultural and language backgrounds.
2. Recognize that different modes, channels, and functions of communication events in which individuals are expected to participate in a clinical setting may result in differing levels of linguistic or communicative performance.
3. Use ethnographic techniques for evaluating communicative behavior and establishing cultural norms for determining the presence or absence of communication disorders.

Process 4 — Treatment

Finally, the conceptual framework schematized in Figure 1–1 suggests that when it has been validly determined that an individual from a given culture has a communication disorder, culturally and linguistically valid therapy may ensue. Given the cultural orientation of the model, it goes almost without saying that treatment must be in the context of the values, attitudes, and wishes of the indigenous culture relative to communication disorders and what to do about them. Treatment should also take into account the preferred learning style of the client and the rules of social and communicative interaction as defined by the client's indigenous cultural or linguistic group.

Taylor (1985) claims that all clinical encounters are cultural events and, as such, the clinician should develop an ethnological approach to all clinical practice. In addition to the principles mentioned in Process 3, he claims that clinicians should

1. View each clinical encounter as a socially situated communicative event that is subject to the cultural rules governing such events by both the clinician and the client.
2. Recognize possible sources of conflicts in cultural assumptions and communicative norms in clients prior to clinical encounters, and take steps to prevent them from occurring during service delivery.
3. Recognize that learning and culture are on-going processes that should result in a constant reassessment and revision of ideas and greater sensitivity to cultural diversity.

Finally, culturally valid clinical treatment uses culturally appropriate materials, activities, and subject matters of high interest, which are packaged within intervention strategies compatible with the preferred learning styles of the client's culture.

SUMMARY

In this chapter, we presented an overview of some of the major historical, legal, legislative, and research issues that undergird the study of the nature of communication disorders in culturally and linguistically diverse populations. A culturally based conceptual framework was also presented for viewing developmental, etiological, assessment, and treatment issues for these same populations.

This conceptual framework forms the basis for much of this volume and should be referred to often as the reader addresses various issues pertaining to the nature of communication disorders within culturally and linguistically diverse populations.

REFERENCES

Aspira of New York, Inc., v. Board of Education of the City of New York, 72 Civ. 4002 (S.D.N.Y. August 29, 1974) (unreported consent decree).

Banks, J. (1984). *Teaching strategies for ethnic studies*. Boston: Allyn and Bacon.

Bowerman, M. (1980). Language development. In H. C. Trinandis and A. Heron (Eds.), *Handbook of cross-cultural psychology: Developmental psychology* (Vol. 4). Boston: Allyn and Bacon.

Center for Applied Linguistics (1977). *Bilingual Education: Current perspectives (law)*. Washington, DC: Author.

Cole, L. (1985). ASHA Interviews. *ASHA, 27,* 23–25.

Cummins, J. (1981). *Role of primary language development in promoting educational success for language minority students.* Paper prepared for the California State Department of Education Compendium on Bilingual-Bicultural Education, Sacramento.

Dianna v. State Board of Education, C.A. 70 RFT (N.D. Cal., Feb. 3, 1970).

Fasold, R. (1984). *The sociolinguistics of society.* London: Basil Blackwell.

Hymes, D. (1974). *Foundations in sociolinguistics: An ethnographic approach.* Philadelphia: University of Pennsylvania Press.

Jones, R.R., and Cartwright, L.R. (1981). *National survey: Foreign speakers in speech and hearing clinics.* Paper presented at the Annual Convention of the American Speech and Hearing Association, Los Angeles.

Larry P. v. Wilson Riles, Civil Action No. 0-71-2270, 343 F. Supp. 1306 (N.D. Cal., 1972).

Lau v. Nichols, 411 U.S. 563 (1974).

Mattie T. v. Holladay, 522 F. Supp. 72 (N.D. Miss., 1977).

Martin Luther King Junior Elementary School Children, et al., v. Ann Arbor School District Board, Civil Action No. 7-71861, 451 F. Supp. 1324 (1978), 463 F. Supp. 1027 (1978) and 473 F. Supp. 1371 (1979) Detroit, Michigan (1979).

McCollum, P.A. (1981). Concepts in bilingualism and their relationship to language assessment. In J. Erickson and D. Omark (Eds.), *Communication assessment of the bilingual bicultural child.* Baltimore: University Park Press.

Michel, J.F. (1969). The role of ASHA in social, political, and moral activities. *ASHA, 11,* 219–220.

Penalosa, F. (1981). *Introduction to the sociology of language.* Rowley, MA: Newbury Publishers.

Petersdorf, R.G., Adams, R.D., Braunwald, E., Isselbacher, K. J., Martin, J.B., and Wilson, J.D. (1983). *Harrison's principles of internal medicine.* New York: McGraw-Hill.

Saville-Troike, M. (1978). *A guide to culture in the classroom.* Rosslyn, VA: National Clearinghouse for Bilingual Education.

Serna v. Portales Municipal Schools, 351 F. Supp. 1279 (N.D. Mex. 1972) aff'd, 499 F. 2d 1147, 1154 (10th Cir. 1974).

Taylor, O. (1969). Social and political involvement of the American Speech and Hearing Association. *ASHA, 11,* 216–218.

Taylor, O., Stroud, R., Hurst, G., Moore, E., and Williams, R. (1969). Philosophies and goals of the ASHA Black Caucus. *ASHA, 11,* 221–225.

Taylor, O., and Payne, K. (1983). Culturally valid testing: A proactive approach. *Topics in Language Disorders 3,* 8–20.

Taylor, O., and Samara, R. (1985). *Communication disorders in underserved populations: Developing nations.* Paper presented at the National Colloquium on Underserved Populations, American Speech and Hearing Association, Washington, DC.

Taylor, O. (in press). Clinical practice as a social occasion: An ethnographic model. *ASHA Reports.*

Van Riper, C. (1978). *Speech corrections.* Englewood Cliffs, NJ: Prentice-Hall.

Vygotsky, L.V. (1962) *Thought and language.* Ed. and Tr. by E. Hanfmann and G. Vakar. Cambridge, MA: MIT Press.

Wolfram, W., and Fasold, R. (1974). *The study of social dialects in American English.* Englewood Cliffs, NJ: Prentice-Hall.

Chapter 2

Cultural and Linguistic Groups in the United States

Kay T. Payne

A FRAME OF REFERENCE FOR VIEWING CULTURAL AND LINGUISTIC DIFFERENCES

Cultural Pluralism

The United States has often been referred to as a "melting pot" of cultural groups and nationalities from throughout the world. This thesis suggests a process whereby people of various racial, social, cultural, economic, linguistic, and historical backgrounds amalgamate and produce a new and homogeneous society. It is evident throughout the history of America that the melting pot phenomenon has never become a reality. In their widely acclaimed book, *Beyond the Melting Pot*, Glazer and Moynihan (1970) concede the futility of maintaining the melting pot theory, maintaining, however, that the American culture is still forming, with the final smelting being continuously passed to the next generation. Banks (1979) posits that to ignore cultural difference in America or to contend that ethnic groups have melted into one is intellectually indefensible and represents a gross misinterpretation of American life.

Modern social scientists typically characterize the present sociological condition of the United States as "culturally pluralistic." The concept of cultural pluralism is based on the recognition that American society is made up of a number of diverse and distinct ethnic subsocieties that retain a high degree of group identity. Furthermore, the concept of cultural pluralism recognizes that ethnicity is an integral and salient feature of general American culture.

Principles of cultural pluralism refute some of the popular myths about ethnicity in American society. One popular myth is that the term ethnic group is synonymous with minority group. Although these terms are commonly used synonymously in the media and by the general public, an important distinction is required. A minority group is specifically defined in terms of its quantitative representation within the society or in relation to whatever larger group is used as a referent. For example, women are sometimes referred to as a minority group in certain milieus in which they are disproportionately represented according to their actual numbers in the population.

A second widely held misconception is the notion that white Anglo-Saxon Protestants do not constitute an ethnic group. The mention of ethnic foods, ethnic dress, or the ethnic vote usually evokes images of pizza, tacos, a kimono, Black or Jewish political organizations, and so forth. Rarely are hot dogs and hamburgers referred to as ethnic food or blue jeans and sneakers as ethnic dress. The point is made that Anglo-Americans, although the dominant cultural group within American society, nonetheless meet all the requisite criteria for classification as an ethnic group.

At this juncture, it is appropriate to define ethnicity in the context of culture. Saville-Troike provides a definition of culture in Chapter 3. It should be added that culture is learned through direct teaching, observation, or socialization. Therefore, culture may operate within an individual at varying levels of conscious or subconscious awareness. Aspects of culture may also vary within the group. Finally, it should be noted that culture is dynamic. Thus, making accurate observations and generalizations about cultures must not be approached in a cavalier manner. Although culture and ethnicity are often used interchangeably, culture is a broader and more abstract concept than ethnicity. Ethnicity refers to the more concrete and identifiable aspects of culture, such as national or racial origin, food, dress, customs, and so forth. The National Council on Social Studies Task Force on Ethnic Studies (1976) outlines six characteristics common to "ethnic groups":

1. Origins that precede the creation of the nation or state or that were external to the state (e.g., American Indians and immigrant groups).
2. Group membership that is involuntary (although identification with the group is sometimes optional).

3. Ancestral tradition and sharing of a sense of peoplehood and interdependence of fate.
4. Distinctive value orientations, behavioral patterns, and interests.
5. Influence of the group on the lives of its members.
6. Group membership that is influenced by how members define themselves and how they are defined by others.

A third myth about American society is the belief that ethnic groups aspire to, and will eventually assimilate into, the dominant culture. To the contrary, Gordon (1964) asserts that ethnic groups develop a "sense of peoplehood" that is exceedingly resistant to change or eradication. Also, American society is highly dynamic. Rather than a one-way process wherein ethnic groups partially or totally assimilate into general American society, there is a reciprocal exchange wherein the society also adopts characteristics of the various ethnic groups of which it is composed. For example, American culture has been greatly influenced by foods from the world over, Black American musical style, Asian philosophy, and so forth. Even American English contains many "borrowed" words from other languages, which have typically become Anglicized (e.g., kindergarten, cuisine, rapping, villa, kosher).

To demonstrate this concept, Figure 2–1 shows the relationship of four ethnic subsocieties within the United States to the general American culture. The central shaded area (A) represents human traits that are common to all groups in the United States regardless of culture (e.g., self-preservation and desire for freedom). The cross-hatched area is a conceptualization of general American culture that is common to, and influenced by, all of the various subsocieties of which it is composed. The influences of the four subsocieties, Anglo-American, Black American, Mexican-American, and Jewish-American, are represented as overlapping circles to denote their relationship to each other, as well as to the general American culture.

Culture Versus Socioeconomic Class

The distinctions between culture and socioeconomic class are often confused and misrepresented. Regrettably, there are too many methodologically unsound studies on human behavior in which the variables of culture and socioeconomic class are confounded. There is no doubt that some cultural differences are class derived. Similarly, there are class differences that cut across all ethnic and cultural groups.

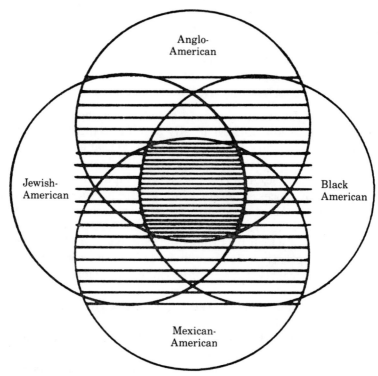

Figure 2-1.   Relationship of ethnic subsocieties to the general American culture.

According to Rossides (1976), the socioeconomic class system in the United States exhibits distinctions not only in income but also in property ownership, occupation, education, personal and family life, and education of children. Five socioeconomic class distinctions are noted, along with their percentages within the society: lower class (20 to 25 percent), working class (40 to 45 percent), lower middle class (30 to 35 percent), upper middle class (10 to 15 percent) and upper class (1 to 3 percent). What is typically "middle class" in the United States is defined as having a modest to high income; accumulation of savings and property; occupation status representative of clerical service; small business ownerships and professional positions; education including college and graduate school; better physical and mental health with longer life expectancy; and attainment of college education by descendants.

It is important to note that although it is highly correlated, "middle-classness" is not defined only by income level and material or personal possessions. In fact, middle class status typically entails a specific ideology. For example, the general American middle class is marked by a particular set of values, a distinctive life-style associated with "conspicuous consumption" of goods and services and material acquisitions, and specific leisure activities. An example of a value of the general American middle class that may not necessarily be shared by working class or lower class individuals is the emphasis placed on education. Some members of the working class or lower class may value vocational education or even stress work as opposed to the typical middle class value placed on high school or college education.

Despite the income level needed for identification with the middle class, many working class and lower class individuals may share middle-class ideologies. A value often shared by all socioeconomic classes relates to the acquisition of material possessions. It is also important to note that there can be cultural variation in "middle classness." For example, leisure time activities and what is considered fun often vary greatly among ethnic groups, even those of similar income levels who share other typical middle class values.

The ideologies associated with the general American middle class are not entirely arbitrary. In most cases, these ideologies represent the values and traditions that will perpetuate the quality of life enjoyed by the economically privileged. It is also no accident that in the United States, middle class ideologies are overwhelmingly synonymous with those of Anglo-Americans. By virtue of their economic power, Anglo-Americans also achieve social prestige. Together, their total representation within the population, their economic power, and their social prestige establish Anglo-Americans as the dominant culture within the society. Other ethnic groups have the option of adopting the ideologies of the middle class Anglo-American or holding to those of their own group. The degree to which other ethnic groups adopt Anglo-American middle class ideologies depends, in part, on (1) the degree of association with Anglo-American middle class individuals, (2) the strength of the individual's ethnic identification, and, (3) the individual's preference for his or her own ethnic ideologies.

Herein lies a major reason why socioeconomic class and culture are often not distinguished. Although it is evident that the middle class is made up of Anglo-Americans to an overwhelming extent, both economically and in ideology, there is no doubt that members of other ethnic groups are also represented. Since a disproportionate number of non-Anglo-Americans are relegated to the working and lower classes owing to the unavailability of economic opportunities, behaviors or values exhibited by individuals in these groups are often misinterpreted as having origins in their ethnicity when the behavior is actually attributable to socioeconomic class.

Cultural Stereotyping

In any discussion of culture, a word about stereotyping is warranted. Stereotyping exists when an uncritical judgment is made about an entire group based on the actions of a few members. Sometimes stereotyping is the result of a misinterpretation or exaggeration of an actual cultural behavior, either intentionally or unintentionally. For example, a cultural group that places high value on physical closeness and touching—even across gender lines—may be erroneously stereotyped as being promiscuous by a group that prefers physical distance and disdains touching.

To avoid stereotyping, it is necessary to understand three critical influences on human behavior. Two of these influences—culture and social class—were discussed previously. A third influence is individual choices within the intrapersonal realm.

Many human behaviors are indeed idiosyncratic, stemming neither from ethnic nor from social class influences. Also included in the intrapersonal realm are family, gender, and peer group influences, since identification with these groups is more readily amenable to conscious selection. Therefore, generalizations about cultures or ethnic groups are valid only when influences of class and personality can be factored out or when historical evidence is unquestionable.

Language and Culture

Having gained a general understanding of culture, we may now consider the phenomenon of linguistic differences. There is no doubt that language shares an intimate relationship with culture. This relationship may be demonstrated by comparing two accepted definitions of these terms. Goodenough (1957) defines culture as, "whatever one has to know or believe in order to operate in a manner acceptable to [the society's] members." He further elaborates that culture is not objects, people, behavior, or emotions, but an organization of these things. Language is defined by Sapir (1921) as "a purely human and non-instinctive method of communicating ideas, emotions and desires by means of a system of voluntarily produced symbols." By analogy, if culture is an organization (system) of objects, behaviors, and emotions, and language is a system (organization) of symbols representing ideas, emotions, and desires, it must be concluded that language is a part of culture, albeit a very important part. The intimacy of language and culture is epitomized in the example of how idioms of one language are often not easily translated and, in fact, may lose some meaning when translated to other languages.

The depth of the relationship of language and culture is further demonstrated in the recognition that language is acquired only in a cultural context. Although the human brain is uniquely organized to acquire language, studies of children reared by wolves show that devoid of the human social context, language does not emerge. Studies of language acquisition also show that language is acquired through active social participation (Bloom and Lahey, 1978). Thus, the expectation that children will learn language through passive listening to radio and television is a serious misconception.

Understanding of the relationship of language and culture is a prime requisite in both the educational and therapeutic contexts. Many teachers and speech-language therapists have been perplexed as to why certain elements of language in linguistic minority groups have been highly resistant to change. The explanation lies in the fact that the linguistic system used by any group is directly and intricately related to the indigenous culture. For any group, language is the most important means through which the culture is communicated. Consequently, there is a strong cultural allegiance to the indigenous language. In addition, language is an important vehicle for cultural identification and solidarity. Some cultures resist any change in their language or dialect. Consider, for example, France's Academie Française, a government sanctioned institution that exists to preserve the purity of the French national language.

Given that the roots of language are deeply embedded in culture, it is logical, therefore, to state that language cannot be studied properly except in its cultural context. For linguists, the basic entity for language study is the speech community. Speech community has been variously defined by linguists and sociolinguists. Bauman (1972) follows Hymes in defining a speech community as "a social group sharing both rules for the conduct and interpretation of acts of speech and rules for the interpretation of at least one linguistic code." Fishman (1968) asserts that a speech community is ultimately defined in terms of its set of shared norms, rather than agreement in the use of language elements. That is, speech communities are not merely identifiable as groups producing a particular language variety or sharing the same geographical region, ethnicity, or social class. Rather, a speech community is defined by its particular set of shared attitudes, values, and beliefs concerning speech and language, as well as the norms for speech and language use.

Properly conceived, these definitions set up the possibility for the existence of an infinite number of speech communities for any given society. In addition, speech communities may have any number of sociological factors as the basis for their existence (e.g., region, ethnicity, social class, gender, and age). One individual, therefore, may be a member of several speech communities concurrently, consciously or unconsciously using the language of each as appropriate for the social context.

It must be noted that there is much overlap in the linguistic patterns of speech communities, such that no speech community within the same language nation is completely autonomous. The linguistic patterns, together with the norms and rules for language usage, that are germane to separate speech communities are known as dialects. Although a single language may consist of many dialects, which have varying degrees of similarities and differences, linguists view all dialects as equal, to the extent that each codifies and communicates the cultural experience of the speech community. Much in the sense that no culture is superior to another, different languages and dialects are not arranged hierarchically.

Nonetheless, for most languages, one dialect tends to emerge as a normative exemplar for the language nation. This variety is known as the linguistic standard. There are several observations about the standard variety of American English. Bloomfield (1933) observed that standard English is generally spoken by those born into homes of privilege, wealth, or education. He also observed that standard English is that which receives institutional support and endorsement through use in schools, churches, and other formal situations, as well as being the only form of English acceptable for written communication.

Quirk (1968) discussed why standard English emerged as the normative variety of American English, stating that its preeminence is not achieved through its esthetic qualities, though these may be sincerely believed in by its speakers. Rather, standard English became the norm for American society because of the prestige of its representative speakers—that is, middle and upper class individuals. Thus, standard English achieved its preeminence through a socially constructed reality rather than through factors inherent in its linguistic structure.

There are two basic characteristics of standard varieties of any language that help to preserve its status. First, as Garvin and Mathiot (1960) stated, the standard variety of language is characteristically less free to vary than other language varieties, owing to the fact that it is the written language variety, and that rules of grammar and pronunciation are explicitly stated. Second, the standard variety enjoys the privilege of "language loyalty" or that attitude which leads its speakers to defend its "purity" against "corruption."

Through concepts such as the speech community and recognition of the equality of dialects, sociolinguists have modified the general notion of the linguistic standard. Standard English, as it is generally known, is recognized as formal language and the language of education. In the modified notion, standard English is given freedom of variation in terms of spoken patterns. Therefore, it is possible to recognize other standard varieties of language. For example, Taylor (1974) calls for the recognition of an ethnic variety of standard English to accommodate the dialect that is spoken by educated Black Americans and which reflects a uniquely Black influence on general American standard English. Likewise, McDavid (1968) discusses regional varieties of standard English. Hence, Southern English is no longer stigmatized as a nonstandard variety of English.

Although the linguistic notions discussed in this chapter reflect novel exceptions to traditional views of language, all are consistent with, and indeed crucial to, the concept of cultural pluralism. For disciplines such as communication disorders, in which the study of language is a major component, it is untenable for us to operate from a conceptual framework that ignores the principles of cultural pluralism.

MAJOR CULTURAL GROUPS IN THE UNITED STATES

The culturally pluralistic character of the United States was largely developed through territorial acquisitions and immigration policies. In addition, the slave trade prior to 1864 was mainly responsible for the presence of the majority of the Black population in America.

At present, the United States is the protectorate of several acquired territories, including Puerto Rico and the Virgin Islands in the Caribbean; Guam, Samoa, Mariana, Midway, Wake, Canton, and Endenbury Islands in the Pacific; and Panama Canal Zone. Inhabitants of these territories are citizens of the United States but possess distinct cultural or language characteristics, or both.

Within the 50 states, diverse indigenous cultural groups exist, including American Indians, Eskimos, and Hawaiians. Also, by immigration, the United States is composed of representatives from cultures and nationalities from throughout the world. In many cases, settlement patterns have produced distinct cultural and linguistic communities.

Settlement patterns of the immigrants were influenced by proximity to the nation of origin, industrial opportunities, agricultural opportunities, and the slave trade. For example, the industrial revolution in the Northeastern and Midwestern states attracted many immigrants from Western Europe. Thus, New York, Illinois, and Michigan contain many cultural communities of Western European origin (see Fig. 2–2). Similarly, the Asian populations of the Western states, the Mexican-American population of the Southwest, and the Black American population of the Southern states all reflect these settlement trends. It is no surprise, therefore, that California, New York, and Texas, for example, are among the most culturally diverse states within the nation, owing to their unique features such as portal entries and agricultural or industrial economies.

Inevitably, the pattern of settlement and cultural mix resulted in the development of various linguistic communities and distinct dialects. The most prominent regional dialects of the United States are Southern, New York City, New England, Appalachian, and Midwestern. In addition, some social dialects emerged as a result of historical factors within a cultural group. Black English is one example of a social dialect that has been shown to have deep historical roots and many survivals from African languages (Turner, 1949).

American Indians

It is rumored that when Christopher Columbus "discovered" America, he called the inhabitants "Indians" since he thought he had reached India. Whether they are called Indians, American Indians, or Native Americans, it is undeniable that this cultural group is the one true indigenous culture of the United States.

According to the 1980 census, the population of American Indians numbered 1,420,000. However, these figures are often disputed since many American Indians do not cooperate in the census count, and there is no established definition that identifies a person as American Indian. Indeed, Alaskan Aleuts and Eskimos are sometimes counted as "Indian" because of their racial features, although they did not inhabit the continental United States at the inception of the nation. Since Native Alaskans have had a different historical

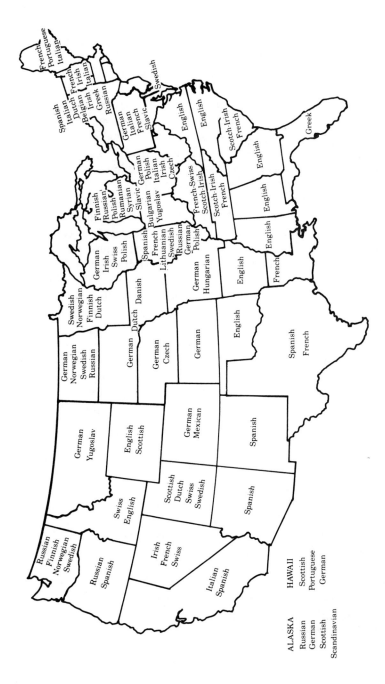

Figure 2-2.   Map of the major white ethnic groups in the United States.   After Stround, D. M. (1973). *The major minority.* Minneapolis, Winston Press.

experience from American Indians, for purposes of this chapter they will be dealt with as separate cultural groups.

Racially, American Indians represent a distinct and homogeneous population. Yet, culturally there is a high degree of diversity. Although there is controversy over the definition of the word "tribe," the Bureau of Indian Affairs identifies some 260 to 280 American Indian nations in existence.

According to Highwater (1975), the usual anthropological method of classifying American Indians was based on how they sought food (i.e., hunters, fishers, gatherers) or by shelter, religious conviction, or language. Eight major linguistic groups are identified by Highwater: Algonquinian, Iroquoian, Caddoan, Muskogean, Siuan, Penutian, Athapaskan, and Uto-Aztecan.

Today American Indians are overwhelmingly concentrated in the West and Southeastern states. Previously, the greatest number of American Indians resided in Oklahoma as a result of the forced migration from the East after 1830 and resettlement on reservations. In recent years, however, American Indians who have migrated from reservations to cities have made California the state with the largest American Indian concentration, with Oklahoma being the state with the second largest concentration of American Indians.

The state with the third largest population density of American Indians is Arizona, the home of the Navajo nation. The Navajo nation occupies the largest reservation, and is the fastest growing Indian nation in the United States. In addition, substantial numbers of American Indians may be found in New York, Minnesota, North Dakota, South Dakota, North Carolina, Montana, New Mexico, Washington, and Oregon.

Today, almost all American Indians speak English or a variety of English that has been influenced by Indian language. In addition, many older persons may speak one of the 50 to 100 Indian languages still in existence. Highwater (1975) states further that American Indians possess a great admiration of words, oration, and proper form. Yet elements of what others call friendliness is often perceived as invasion of privacy, to which American Indians react with a deep, uncomfortable silence.

Although there is a great diversity among American Indian nations, there are other cultural generalities that are important to note in cross-cultural relations. For example, Highwater states that paternalism is the most repulsive condition in the relationship between Anglo-Americans and American Indians. He further elaborates that racist terms such as "chief," "squaw," and "redskin," and beating the hand against the mouth while making a "wow-wow" sound, are highly offensive to American Indians since they, as other groups, feel a great sense of cultural pride.

In general, American Indians feel a kinship with nature, a world view which Highwater (1981) characterizes as the "primal mind." Individual identity, a highly valued aspect of American culture, is virtually nonexistent in traditional Indian cultures. Instead, American Indians tend to value the concept of "communal homogeneity," in which each member of the nation is related in some unique way to the community. Thus, it is sometimes astonishing to non-Indians that handicapping conditions are so easily accepted. Harris (1982) in a published interview provides a unique insight into perceptions of handicapping conditions by American Indians.

There is no doubt that American Indian cultures are as complex as any other. Subsequent chapters provide a more in-depth view of American Indian cultures as they relate to the nature, diagnosis, and treatment of communication disorders.

Whites

Approximately 83 percent of the population of the United States is classified as "white." However, within this group there are many cultural variations. Based on nationality of ancestry, the following major "white ethnic groups" and percentages within the population are recorded in the 1980 census data: Italian (13 percent), German (11 percent), English (7 percent), Polish (7 percent), Russian (5 percent), and Irish (4 percent). Other groups, particularly from other Western European nations, Canadians, and Jewish-Americans contribute to the total percentage of whites within the population.

There are many similarities and differences in the cultural tendencies of white ethnic groups. Ethnic identification, the number of post-European generations, and patterns of intermarriage contribute to whether or not individuals operate according to ethnic and cultural standards.

Although whites reside in large numbers in all of the states, there are particular regions in which specific ethnic communities other than Anglo-Americans may be found. Northern states, particularly those east of the Mississippi, and states surrounding the Great Lakes exhibit the greatest diversity among white ethnic groups. Southern states exhibit the least amount of diversity, being composed largely of persons of Anglo-Saxon descent. Cities, such as New

York City, Chicago, Milwaukee, Boston, Detroit, and Baltimore, contain many white ethnic communities that maintain a high degree of cultural identification and allegiance.

White ethnic groups of non-English speaking heritage may also maintain their native language. In fact, recent census reports show that more than 600,000 Americans speak European languages other than Spanish. Among these groups, 36.8 percent of those who speak Portuguese have difficulty speaking English, as do 29 percent of Greek speakers, 18.9 percent of those who speak Italian, 16.5 percent of Polish speakers, 6.4 percent of French speakers, and 5 percent of German speakers.

Even when keeping native dress, foods, holidays, and other overt aspects of culture, white ethnic groups are generally able to assimilate with ease into general American society. However, the development to this stage has been difficult for some groups. In 1899, Ripley published a treatise, *The Races of Europe*, which popularized the notion that the Teutonic race of northern Europe was genetically superior to other white races of southern and eastern nations. In the United States, laws such as the Alien and Sedition Acts, the nativist era of the 1800s, and the Know-Nothing movement of the 1850s reflected bigotry and intolerance. Tests containing cultural bias are not a recent phenomenon; heavily biased literacy tests were used extensively during the period of greatest immigration from southern Europe to discourage and prohibit immigrants from entering the United States.

Among white ethnic groups, Jewish-Americans of European ancestry are a highly visible cultural-religious group. Cutting across many nationalities, and several races, the Jewish people possess a unique historical experience. For centuries, Jewish peoples were scattered throughout the world and severely persecuted; the establishment of the State of Israel in 1948 was an attempt to provide a Jewish homeland.

At present, approximately 6 million Jews reside in the United States, constituting about 3 percent of the nation's population. Jews have lived in this nation since the original 13 colonies, settling predominantly in the Dutch colony of New Amsterdam. A great influx of Jews from Germany occurred from 1820 to 1880. Most German Jews settled in the Ohio and Mississippi valleys, establishing themselves as merchants and traders. From 1881 to 1924, more than 2 million Jews immigrated from Eastern Europe, settling mainly in the Northeastern port cities of New York, Boston, Philadelphia, and Baltimore.

Many Jews have moved away from the traditions of Orthodox religion. This has produced three separate movements within the religion. Those who remain faithful to ancestral traditions are known as Orthodox Jews. Those who do not conform totally to traditional practices, yet wish to retain some aspects of the religion, adopt the principles of either Conservative or Reform Judaism.

Yiddish is the native language of Eastern European Jews, although almost all Jews in the United States speak English. Another common language, Hebrew, is reserved for prayer and religious activities (Hebrew is the official language of Israel, however). Both of these languages have greatly influenced American English.

The Jewish culture places high value on education. On the whole, Jews represent one of the best educated groups in American society. Achievement is also valued highly, and Jews have made tremendous contributions to medicine, science, and technology.

Black Americans

There is perhaps no cultural group with greater diversity than Black Americans. Indeed, Black Americans cut across all socioeconomic classes; religions; educational backgrounds; skin colors; political persuasions; and social beliefs and traditions. Therefore, any discussion of Black Americans must be qualified by specific descriptors, such as urban Blacks, rural Blacks, Southern Blacks, and working-class Blacks. A typical error of much of the past and current research, as well as of many media accounts today, is the failure to provide such descriptors. Regardless of the accuracy of such reports for the specific group of Blacks in question, if the results are applied to all Black Americans they amount to no more than stereotypes.

A particular cultural tendency of Black Americans is their public sense of social solidarity. For example, middle class Blacks, although they have achieved success, often align themselves with the struggles of less fortunate members of the group. Words such as "brother" and "blood" used in reference to other group members denote this solidarity. This cultural trait also leads some non-Blacks to the misperception of Blacks as separatists and helps to fuel stereotypes.

Black Americans constitute approximately 11 percent of the population of the United States, numbering about 26.5 million persons. More than one half of the Black American population resides in Southern states. In addition, about one third of all Blacks reside in urban centers of the Midwest and Northeast, particularly Chicago, Detroit, Baltimore, Washington DC, New York, and Philadelphia.

It should be noted that the Black American population includes not only direct descendants of the African slaves in America but also other immigrants from Caribbean nations. Though similar in heritage and some structural aspects of language, these groups present somewhat different cultural tendencies. For example, Glazer and Moynihan (1970) observed that, on the whole, Blacks from Caribbean nations achieve more education and higher social status than do Blacks whose ancestral roots are in American soil. However, the cause of this phenomenon is not known, stemming perhaps from selective migration from Caribbean nations of those who wish to better their lives in general. Nonetheless, the language, foods, traditions, and some values differ between native American Blacks and Caribbean immigrants.

As a race, Blacks have endured severe bigotry and intolerance in the United States. Physical features and overt cultural tendencies that are at maximal contrast to those of the dominant American society have made assimilation more difficult. As a result, Black Americans have developed strong in-group defenses, cultural allegiances, and a tremendous sense of cultural pride. In addition, Black Americans, irrespective of socioeconomic status, tend to possess a strong sense of justice, especially on racial issues, sometimes appearing to others as overly defensive. Much like the Jewish dedication to preserving the memory of the Holocaust, Blacks are always wary of possible inequalities or violations of their civil rights.

Among many urban and working-class Blacks, the language is an element of culture that is used to denote solidarity. Many educated and middle class Blacks consider themselves to be bidialectal, using standard English as required for formal situations or communication with non-Blacks and Black English vernacular as an in-group linguistic code. One reason why Black English vernacular has been so resistant to eradication is its function within the culture as a unifying device.

Few would argue that Black Americans should be proficient in standard English for use when required. Yet, issues of language loyalty, as previously defined, if not afforded to all cultures will hinder progression in education as well as social achievement. The language of Black Americans will be discussed in more detail in a later chapter.

The basic unit of Black American culture is the family. In 1971, the National Urban League issued a monograph entitled *The Strengths of Black Families*. Five attributes were cited that characterize Black families, including (1) strong kinship bonds, (2) strong work orientation, (3) flexibility of family rules, (4) strong achievement, and (5) strong religious orientation. Flexibility of family roles should be particularly noted because recent statistics show that 47.1 percent of Black families exist in female headed households.

As in many cultures worldwide, the traditional American model is a family structure headed by a male. It is necessary for a family unit to have some strong authority figure regardless of that person's sex. In many urban and working-class Black families, authority is relegated to mothers or even grandmothers. It is not uncommon, however, to have males within the household (e.g., brothers, uncles) who assume nonauthoritative roles. The full implication of what it means to have female dominated families is not known. It is known, however, that these families tend to have lower incomes than those in which males are heads of households.

In addition to other cultural tendencies, Black Americans possess distinct communication styles, both verbal and nonverbal. These styles, however, vary according to social class, gender, age, region, and so forth. Many descriptions, especially Thomas Kochman's *Black and White Styles in Conflict*, purport to describe Black-white relations in general, yet they fail to present an accurate account since they compare working class Black styles, particularly those of young Black males, to the styles of middle class whites.

On the basis of a review of available literature and anecdotal reports, Taylor (1985) listed some general verbal and nonverbal communication styles of working class Black Americans and Anglo-Americans. Some of these differences, and some similar differences between Hispanic and Asian Americans and working class Anglo-Americans, are presented in Table 2–1.

Hispanics

Hispanic refers to any person of Spanish, Mexican, Puerto Rican, Cuban, Central or South American, or other Spanish culture or origin, regardless of race. Needless to say, Hispanics include a broad representation of cultures bound together by one language. In the United States, major Hispanic populations include Puerto Ricans, Mexican-Americans, and Cuban-Americans. It is estimated that there are 15 million persons of Hispanic origin in the United States. The 1980 census figures also indicate that Spanish is the major home language of approximately 8.7 million persons. About 48 percent of those persons, primarily adults, reportedly have difficulty with English.

Much like American English, British English, and Australian English, the language spoken by Hispanics of various nationalities is minimally variable. Except for a few phonological, lexical, and idi-

Table 2-1. Some Verbal and Nonverbal Communication Styles of Various Ethnic Groups

Black Americans

Hats and sunglasses are sometimes considered as adornments much like jewelry, to be worn inside.

Agreement and approval are given through gestures such as "giving skin."

Touching one's hair by another person is often considered offensive.

Direct eye contact in conversation ("rolling one's eyes") is considered offensive.

Public behavior (e.g., at a play or concert) is emotionally intense, dynamic, and demonstrative, as in laughter, shouts, and so forth.

"Signifying" as a form of verbal insults is common among men.

Asking personal questions of someone one has met for the first time is seen as improper and intrusive.

Use of direct questions is sometimes seen as harrassment (e.g., asking when something will be finished is seen as rushing that person to finish).

"Breaking in" during conversation is usually tolerated. Competition for the floor is granted to the person who is most assertive.

Conversations are regarded as private between the recognized participants; "butting in" is seen as eavesdropping and is not tolerated.

Use of "you people" is seen as pejorative and racist.

Anglo-Americans

Hats and sunglasses are considered utilitarian, and as outerwear and are to be removed indoors.

No gestural counterpart for agreement or approval exists.

Touching of one's hair by another person is a sign of affection.

Direct eye contact is considered a sign of attentiveness and respect.

Public behavior is modest and emotionally restrained; outward displays are seen as irresponsible or in bad taste.

No engagement of verbal insults as an extended activity.

Inquiring about jobs, family, and so forth of someone one has met for the first time is seen as friendly.

Use of direct questions for personal information is permissible.

Rules on turn-taking in conversation dictate that one person has the floor at a time until all of his or her points are made.

Adding points of information or insights to a conversation in which one is not engaged is sometimes seen as being helpful.

Use of "you people" is tolerated.

Hispanic Cultures

Hissing to gain attention is acceptable.

Booing and hissing at a play or concert indicated extreme approval.

Anglo-Americans

Hissing is considered impolite and indicates contempt.

Booing and hissing at a concert are signs of disapproval and bad manners.

Table continues on opposite page

Table 2-1 (continued)

Touching is often observed between two people in conversation.	Touching is usually unacceptable and often carries sexual overtones.
Avoidance of direct eye contact is a sign of attentiveness and respect; direct eye contact is regarded as an insult.	Direct eye contact is a sign of attentiveness and respect.
Relative distance between two speakers in conversation is closer.	Relative distance between two speakers in conversation is farther apart.
Telling a woman that she is getting fat is considered as a compliment.	Commenting about a person's weight is considered as an insult.

Asian Americans	*Anglo-Americans*
Touching or hand-holding between members of the same sex is acceptable.	Touching or hand-holding between members of the same sex may be considered a sign of homosexuality.
Hand-holding, hugging, kissing between men and woman in public looks ridiculous.	Hand-holding, hugging, kissing between men and women in public is acceptable to some groups.
A slap on the back is insulting.	A slap on the back denotes friendliness.
It is not customary to shake hands with persons of the opposite sex.	It is customary to shake hands with persons of the opposite sex.
Waving motions are used only by adults to call little children and not vice-versa.	Waving motions are often used to call people.

Anglo-Americans	*Others*
Symbols of the old South, such as confederate flags, Black lamppost lawn ornaments are acceptable to some groups.	Blacks view confederate flags and Black lamppost ornaments as offensive and racist.
Using cultural in-group gestures such as "giving skin" and bowing is seen as acceptable.	Using cultural in-group gestures is seen as patronizing.
Including a minority person in group activities is seen as democratic.	Purposely including a minority person in group activities is seen as tokenism.
Adopting the dance pattern or music styles of other cultural groups is seen as free exchange.	Adopting the dance patterns or music styles of other cultural groups is offensive.
Maintaining eye contact in conversation is regarded as respectful or as a sign of sincerity.	Maintaining eye contact is conversation is regarded as staring or a sign of condescension.

omatic differences, the language of Spain, Mexico, Cuba, and Puerto Rico is virtually the same. There is no doubt, however, that despite the similarities in the language, the cultures of these groups are very distinct.

The island of Puerto Rico has been a United States territory since 1898. Although Puerto Rico is not a state, its residents have been citizens of the United States since 1917. Since this time, there has been a constant influx of Puerto Ricans to the mainland, especially to the Northeastern states of New York, New Jersey, and Pennsylvania. At present, there are more than two million Puerto Ricans residing on the mainland, of which approximately 1.3 million reside in the three Northeastern states cited.

Puerto Ricans share a mixed racial heritage of Indian, African, and Spanish ancestry. On the island, racial differences and color distinctions are noted, albeit much less than on the mainland. In Puerto Rico, although it is preferable to be white rather than Black, social class status is more important than race. This phenomenon causes some problems for Puerto Ricans who migrate to the mainland, because Puerto Ricans, as a group, are subjected to prejudice and discrimination. In addition, some Puerto Ricans face identity problems as they try to adjust to life in the general society.

In general, Puerto Rico is a monolingual society. When immigrants arrive in the States, Spanish is usually their only means of communication. After residing on the mainland for some time, they may achieve various levels of English proficiency. Because Spanish is the official language of the community, homes, churches, and most institutions, the school is the major vehicle for learning English for new arrivals from Puerto Rico. Thus, bilingual education is important for these children. Adults, however, face many problems in adjusting to the language difference.

Mexican-Americans compose the second largest Hispanic cultural group in the United States. In 1980, about 8.7 million Mexican-Americans lived within United States boundaries. It is important to note that not all Mexican-Americans are immigrants. Indeed, Mexicans inhabited the land that is now the state of Texas prior to its annexation in 1845. Today, Texas still maintains the second largest Mexican-American population among the states.

California contains by far the largest Mexican-American community. Substantial numbers of Mexican-Americans also reside in Colorado, New Mexico, and Arizona. Smaller pockets of Mexican-Americans are to be found in all the states, including Alaska and Hawaii. Racially, most Mexicans are a mixture of Spanish and Indian ancestry. Also, through Spanish contact with the Moors and a small slave trade in Mexico, there is an African strain present in some Mexicans.

Prior to 1924, the border between the United States and Mexico was a "free border." During the gold rush of 1849, many Mexicans immigrated to work the mines of California. Also, during the early settlement of the Southwest, Mexicans were needed to develop the agricultural economy. The Mexican Revolution of 1910 forced many persons across the border seeking refuge from the war. By the beginning of World War II, Mexicans were again recruited to fill the labor demands created by the war. At this time, anti-Mexican sentiment was already high in the United States. In addition, seasonal workers were frequently brought into the states on a temporary basis to perform unskilled work as needed, and to return to Mexico when the work season ended.

Mexican laborers have always been exploited. Yet many prefer this exploitation to the poverty conditions in their own nation. As a result, many undocumented aliens continue to flock across the border from Mexico. Most recent immigration laws permit 20,000 persons per year to legally emigrate to the United States from Mexico.

As in other Hispanic cultures, the family is the center of Mexican culture. An extended family, including grandparents, uncles, aunts, and cousins, may reside under the same roof. Ironically, American homes are not constructed to accommodate the extended family, so by American standards, Mexican-American dwellings seem to be overcrowded. Although there are distinct roles, the Mexican-American families are closely intertwined and involved in almost all aspects of each individual's life. It is not unusual for family members to accompany each other to the market, to the clinic, for a stroll, and so forth.

Although many Mexican-Americans are bilingual, most maintain a special allegiance to their native language of Spanish. There is a growing number of Mexican-American newspapers and radio and television programs broadcasting in Spanish. Even among third and fourth generation Mexican-Americans, bilingual programs within the schools may be necessary.

A third major Hispanic group within the United States is Cuban-Americans. Although there is a sizable difference in the number of Cuban-Americans compared with Puerto Ricans and Mexican-Americans, this group is highly visible. Of the 803,000 Cuban-Americans presently residing within the United States, more than half are found in Florida, particularly Miami. The second largest concentration of Cuban-Americans is in New York City. However, in all of New York State, there are only 39,000 Cuban-American residents. Cuban-Americans represent a distinct racial group, in comparison with Puerto Ricans and Mexican-Americans. For the most part, Cuban-Americans are of direct European ancestry.

Unlike most other immigrants who entered the United States for economic promise, Cuban-Americans overwhelmingly came from the middle and upper classes, who were threatened by the political regime of Fidel Castro. Since the revolution of 1959, there have been four stages of Cuban immigration to the United States. Between 1959 and 1962, Cuban immigrants were given preferred status. In 1962, the Cuban missile crisis ended commercial airflights between the United States and Cuba, forcing immigrants to employ more clandestine means of entry. The third stage of immigration was known as the Cuban Refugee Airlift, whereby the United States government sponsored flights to Miami. This program was terminated in 1973. Finally, during the Carter administration in 1979, Cubans were again permitted to enter the United States in large numbers. Immigrants entering during this recent stage have faced greater adjustment problems, because it is alleged that Castro exported many undesirable citizens, such as those in prisons and mental hospitals.

Because of their socioeconomic status, Cuban-Americans have generally been easily accepted into American society because they brought with them cultural values that are similar to the dominant society in the United States. Teachers report that Cuban-American students are highly motivated. As in the general American culture, education, hard work, and personal accomplishments are valued highly in Cuban-American culture. Yet, the adjustment of many Cuban-Americans to American culture has not been easy. The refugee situation has fostered separation of families. Many customs, such as chaperoned dating, which is virtually unknown in American society, frequently pose adjustment problems, especially for second generation Cuban-Americans.

Asian Americans

The term Asian American, as commonly used today, refers to all people of Chinese, Japanese, Filipino, Korean, Burmese, Vietnamese, Laotian, Malasian, Cambodian, and Thai descent. This term replaces the term "oriental" which is less preferred by Asian Americans. Even Asian American is a somewhat loose title, because the groups differ in physical and cultural characteristics as well as in the languages spoken. According to the 1980 census, the three most populous groups of Asian Americans include those of Chinese (806,000), Filipino (775,000), and Japanese (701,000) descent. The overwhelming proportion of each of these three major groups resides in Western states, particularly California and Hawaii, although there is a substantial representation of Chinese-Americans in New York.

The gold rush of 1848 attracted many Chinese immigrants to California. By 1862, many Chinese were employed to develop the Central Pacific Railroad. As a result, there was a migration of Chinese people inward toward the Eastern states. During their initial immigration, Chinese people suffered severe exploitation and racial prejudice. From 1882 until 1965, the Chinese Exclusion Act and other subsequent revisions were passed, which limited Chinese immigration. The Geary Act of 1892 not only excluded Chinese laborers from entering the United States but also abolished immigrants' legal rights as well. It was not until 1965 that the new immigration law eliminated the national origins quota system and established fair immigration policies for all foreign nations.

Despite the racism they experienced, Chinese-Americans have made many contributions to American life, having made a great number of achievements in education, sciences, and the arts. Although many Chinese-Americans still reside in Chinatowns, many upwardly mobile descendents of the first immigrants have moved into other communities. Almost one third of Chinese-American workers are employed in professional and technical occupations, of which only 4 percent work as laborers. Moreover, the median income of Chinese-Americans is higher than that of the general population.

Almost half of Chinese-Americans have some difficulty with the English language, including about 11 percent of the school age population. Thus, bilingual education programs are of extreme importance. In fact, it was the celebrated case of *Lau v. Nichols* in 1974 that became the legal basis for bilingual education in the United States. In this case, the Supreme Court ruled that the San Francisco School District was denying Chinese students who did not speak English their constitutional right by not giving them the opportunity for a meaningful education in their native language.

Perhaps more than any other group, Chinese-Americans still adhere to the traditions of their homeland. Many Chinese-Americans maintain their native food, dress, attitudes, holidays, and customs. The family is tremendously influential in individual lives. Thus, Chinese-Americans rarely take advantage of social services, with exception to those within the community. The Chinese-American family is a male-dominated organization. Traditionally, women, regardless of age, are subservient. Several generations of married sons may still live with their parents. Chinese-Americans tend to give tremendous respect to age and authority.

Japanese immigration into the United States was much like that of the Chinese. Curiously, during the years when the Chinese Exclusion Act was in effect, many Japanese persons entered the United States to fill the void left by Chinese workers. Japanese farm workers arrived in California and Hawaii. The racism that the Chinese immigrants experienced was soon extended to the Japanese. Immigration restrictions were imposed through the Gentlemen's Agreement of 1908 and the Immigration Act of 1924. Other laws were passed, as in the case of Chinese immigrants, to limit Japanese citizenship, land ownership, and upward mobility.

The most blatant violation of Japanese civil rights was the internment of 1942. Because of a prevalent and an irrational fear that they would remain loyal to Japan and turn against the United States during World War II, Japanese-Americans were removed from their homes and placed in concentration camps. Since World War II, racism against Japanese has still been pervasive, however subtle.

Japanese-Americans have made tremendous adjustments to American life. On most social indicators they are found above the norms for the general society. The internment caused a serious disruption of traditional Japanese cultural life. In addition, a growing rate of intermarriages within the community has contributed to the discontinuity of cultural traditions. Among Japanese-Americans who remain faithful to their cultural traditions, factors such as family, strong group orientation, and strong moral training may dictate individual behavior.

Slightly more than one fourth of Japanese-Americans have difficulty with English. This difficulty lies overwhelmingly among adults. Educational achievement is a major priority among Japanese-Americans. As a result, Japanese-Americans represent one of the most highly educated groups within the United States.

Regardless of their adherence to cultural tradition, most Japanese-Americans place great value on hard work. Perseverance and resilience are also cultural traits. Another cultural trait that makes Japanese-Americans easily accepted into general American society is their polite and respectful style of communication. Japanese-Americans are seen as agreeable, nonaggressive, loyal, and devoted.

OTHER CULTURAL GROUPS

Within the United States, there are many other cultural groups with lesser visibility than those discussed previously. Some are immigrant groups who have entered in fewer numbers. Other immigrants, such as Filipinos, may be present in large numbers but are more widely dispersed throughout the nation. Still other groups are citizens of the United States but live in remote or isolated locations. Among the latter, there are three distinct cultural groups that deserve consideration. These are Eskimos, Native Hawaiians, and Virgin Islanders.

Eskimos

Eskimos represent one of the three native Alaskan groups that together total one sixth of the state's population. Eskimos represent over half of this total. Also represented are Indians and Aleuts.

In a land that is one of the richest reserves in the world, nearly all Eskimos live in dire poverty. Previously, Eskimos were a migratory people. More recently, however, many small permanent villages have been established, varying in size from a few families to 1,000 persons. Eskimo villages are distributed throughout the state, usually along coastal areas and far from the state's population centers.

Although many Eskimos still depend on the land and fishing for subsistence, there is a growing interest in the cash-based economy of American culture. Poor educational opportunities and high unemployment are the rule in Eskimo villages. Thus, many people are dependent on public assistance. Because of harsh weather conditions for most of the year, there are many health problems among Eskimos. As discussed in a later chapter, the incidence of otitis media is higher than for the general population. Respiratory diseases, tuberculosis, influenza, pneumonia, and enteric diseases are among the principal causes of death in Eskimo villages.

Language is a major barrier to education. The Eskimo language has a number of dialects. The dialects most commonly spoken are Inupiaq and Yupik, both of which are written languages. Most Eskimos in the remote villages do not speak English; thus English is learned primarily in the schools. On the average, however, Eskimos complete 7.9 years of school.

The future for Eskimos can be improved. Eskimo people are known to be a very diplomatic and peace-loving people. Although they hold to many of their cultural traditions, they have begun to participate in the general society. Moreover, improved bilingual educational programs and better health care can be expected to facilitate their economic continued development.

Native Hawaiians

Until the arrival of Captain Cook in 1788, Hawaiians existed virtually in splendid isolation. Whereas some 300,000 Hawaiians inhabited the islands at the time of his arrival, today only 152,000 Native Hawaiians remain, constituting a minority group in their own land. Diseases introduced by contact with Westerners were responsible for the tragic decline in the Hawaiian population. Even this population has been diffused so much through intermarriage that very few pure Hawaiians currently remain.

At present, very little remains of the highly structured culture that existed prior to contact with the European sailors and American missionaries from New England. The Hawaiian language, which is a branch of the Polynesian family, is currently spoken only in remote and rural enclaves. Of the cultural tendencies that remain, Native Hawaiians continue to place strong emphasis on group-oriented values and deemphasize individual achievement. Contrary to the values of general American society, Native Hawaiians tend to be extremely noncompetitive. Peace and harmony are preferred, and Native Hawaiians chose to invest resources in social relationships rather than accumulate material wealth.

In a state that has tremendous resources, Native Hawaiians share very little of the wealth. In general, the incomes of Native Hawaiians are 15 percent below those of other residents, and approximately one fifth of Native Hawaiians are below the poverty level. Native Hawaiians also have a disproportionately higher incidence of health conditions such as cancer, diabetes, heart disease, prematurity, infant mortality, and congenital birth defects.

Virgin Islanders

Composed of three main islands—St. Croix, St. Thomas, and St. John—the Virgin Islands lie in the Caribbean Sea, approximately 990 miles from Miami. Although these islands were transferred to the United States from Denmark in 1917, very little evidence of Danish influence on the people remains.

Native Virgin Islanders are of mixed African and European descent. Natives make up at least 60 percent of the population of St. Thomas and 40 percent of the population of St. Croix. Natives of both of these islands possess their own dialect variations of American English.

Because the islands are territorial possessions of the United States, many of the sociological conditions are similar to those of the mainland, with some exceptions. The availability of health care is considered to be a serious problem because there is a shortage of physicians in the specialty areas. The major health problems of the islands are heart disease, diabetes, hypertension, and obesity, and the incidence of cancer is noted to be on the increase. In addition, the infant mortality rate is above that for the general American population.

Because of government subsidies, economic conditions on the islands are fair, although they are below the levels for most states. There are distinct class differences among natives and non-natives, and even among natives themselves. The average income of native Virgin Islanders is substantially less than that of their non-native counterparts. In addition, the class distinctions have created two separate educational systems. The higher status population tends to prefer private schools, whereas people of lower social status send their children to lesser quality public schools.

The culture of native Virgin Islanders is similar to that of other African descendents in the United States and Caribbean nations. Within the family, children tend to be revered and protected. Each successive generation is encouraged to raise itself by education and personal achievement. However, a cultural "brain drain" is created as many individuals prefer to leave the islands for better economic and social opportunities on the mainland.

CONCLUSION

There is no argument that American society is culturally pluralistic. The concept of cultural diversity gives recognition to the fact that all cultures can maintain their identity while making unique and valuable contributions to the improvement of the quality of life for the general society. In this chapter we have seen that there are more similarities among cultures than differences. The family is always the central unifying force. This concept extended, the most perfect society is a family of mankind.

46 Communication Disorders in Culturally Diverse Populations

REFERENCES

Banks, J. (1979). *Teaching strategies for ethnic studies*. Boston: Allyn and Bacon.

Bauman, R. (1972). Ethnographic framework for investigation of communicative behaviors in R. Abrahams and R. Troike (Eds.), *Language and cultural diversity in American education*. Englewood Cliffs, NJ: Prentice-Hall.

Bloom, L., and Lahey, M. (1978). Language development as an active process. In *Language development and language disorders* (pp. 266–285). New York: John Wiley and Sons.

Bloomfield, L. (1933). *Language*. New York: Henry Holt.

Fishman, J. (1968). Varieties of ethnicity and varieties of language. In O'Brien, R., *Selected papers on linguistics*. Georgetown University Roundtable Conference. Washington, DC: Georgetown University Press.

Garvin, P., and Mathiot, M. (1960) The urbanization of the Guarani language: A problem of language and culture. In *Men and Cultures*. Selected Papers, of the Fifth International Congress. Philadelphia: University of Pennsylvania Press.

Glazer, N., and Moynihan, D. (1970). *Beyond the melting pot*. Cambridge, MA: The MIT Press.

Gordon, M.M. (1964). *Assimilation in American Life*. New York: Oxford University Press.

Goodenough, W. (1957). Cultural anthropology and linguistics. In P. Garvin, Report of the Seventh Annual Roundtable Meeting on Linguistics and Language Study. *Georgetown University Monograph Series on Language and Linguistics No. 9*. Washington, DC: Georgetown University Press.

Harris, G. (1982). Gail Harris: Indian advocate. *ASHA, 24*(6), 392–394.

Highwater, J. (1975). *Indian America*. New York: David McKay Company, Inc.

Highwater, J. (1981). *The primal mind*. New York: Harper and Row.

Kochman, T. (1981). *Black and white styles in conflict*. Chicago: University of Chicago Press.

McDavid, R. (1968). Variations in standard American English. *Elementary English, 45*, 561–564, 608.

National Council on Social Studies. Task force on ethnic studies (1976). *Curriculum guidelines for multiethnic education* (pp. 9–10). Arlington, VA: Author.

National Urban League (1971). *The state of Black America: The Strengths of Black Families*. New York: Author.

Quirk, O. (1968). Standard dialect. In A. Edwards, *Language in culture and class*. London: Heinemann Educational Books, Ltd.

Rossides, D. (1976). *The American class system: An introduction to social stratification*. Atlanta: Houghton-Mifflin.

Sapir, E. (1921). *Language: An introduction to the study of speech*. New York: Harcourt, Brace and World.

Taylor, O. (1974). Black language: the research dimension. In J. Daniel, *Black communication: Dimensions of research and instruction*. New York: Speech Communication Association.

Taylor, O. (1985). *Communication styles of some ethnic groups*. Unpublished manuscript.

Turner, L. (1949). *Africanisms in the Gullah dialect*. Chicago: University of Chicago Press.

Chapter 3

Anthropological Considerations in the Study of Communication

Muriel Saville-Troike

The study of communicative behavior has been enlightened both by the primary organizing concept that guides much anthropological research and thought and the set of tools that practitioners in that discipline use for discovery, description, and analysis. The organizing concept is *culture,* and the tool set consists of the subdiscipline of *ethnography.*

In this chapter we (1) provide some examples of research questions that illustrate anthropological considerations in the study of communication; (2) discuss the orientation and methodology of the field of anthropology; and (3) present certain results and problems that have emerged, particularly as they bear on the study of communication in relation to language assessment and educational issues. Reference will be made to the author's work with the Navajo culture and children's second language acquisition, as well as findings from other sources.

CULTURE

The term "culture" as it will be used in this chapter requires some clarification at the outset, because it may represent different things to persons with training and experience in different fields. To anthropologists, culture encompasses all of the shared rules for appropriate behavior that are learned by individuals as a consequence of being members of the same group or community, as well as the values and beliefs that underlie overt behaviors and are themselves shared products of group membership. In other words, culture is what individuals need to know to be functional members of a community and to regulate interaction with other members of the community and with individuals from cultural backgrounds different from their own.

Because knowledge, perception, and behavior are so strongly influenced by culture, members of different cultural groups can never live in exactly the same "real" world. Nor can terms ever be assumed to have exact correspondences across cultural boundaries. It is unlikely that the concepts labeled in English as *good, family,* or even *blue* can ever be equated exactly with categories in other cultures. Although this is also true to some extent even for individuals within any group, it is nevertheless essential to recognize that there are sharply different modes of thinking, feeling, perceiving, and behaving, which are not merely idiosyncratic but are characteristic of whole groups as such and are learned by virtue of being a member of a given group.

Whether we realize it or not (and usually we do not, until we encounter a cross-cultural experience which makes us reflect on it), each of us sees the world from a culturally conditioned perspective that we share with other members of our group. Indeed, our very concept of "normal" is culturally defined and may differ radically among different cultures. An anthropological orientation, then, is essential in sensitizing the speech professional or educator to the potential existence of cross-cultural differences in communication and in pointing to ways to discover and work with these when they exist.

The process by which an individual acquires his or her native culture is termed *enculturation.* Much of culture learning is informal and even unconscious, although some of it may be arranged by deliberate instruction. Hall (1959) has distinguished three levels of culture learning (and teaching): *formal, informal,* and *technical.*

Formal learning takes place through precept and admonition, and transmits those aspects of culture that are not to be questioned. This often includes the expression of the traditional wisdom of a group in the form of proverbs or other aphorisms, or such positional appeals as the following (Bernstein, 1972):

> You should be able to do that by now (age status rule).
> Little boys don't cry (sex status rule).
> People like us don't behave like that (subcultural rule).
> Daddy doesn't expect to be spoken to like that (age relation rule).

Informal learning takes place primarily through nonverbal channels of communication, with the chief agent being a model used for imitation. This process is often "out of awareness," with knowledge and rules formulated unconsciously on the basis of informal observation.

Technical learning occurs at an explicitly formulated, conscious level; rules are explained and reasons given.

All cultures make use of all three of these modes of enculturation to some degree. Formal learning tends to be prominent, however, when authority in the family is strictly ordered in a hierarchy, in cultures in which attitudes about the supernatural exert a pervasive control on behavior, and when there is a great respect for tradition. Children are more likely to be taught on a technical level in a knowledge-oriented society that values information and cognitive skills, and in which the mental capacities of youth are accorded great respect.

LANGUAGE AND COMMUNICATION

Definitions of *language* usually refer to its verbal features (vocabulary, grammar, and phonology or orthography) and to its uniquely human character, but the study of communication requires a much deeper understanding of its complex nature and use. The most important consideration from an anthropological perspective is that language is a key component of culture. It is the primary medium for transmitting much of culture; therefore, children learning their native language are also learning their own culture. Thus, the process of language learning in children is, in part, a process of enculturation. Learning a second language or a second dialect often involves learning a second culture to varying degrees, which may lead to acculturation and have very profound psychological and social consequences for both children and adults.

The Navajo people and their children provide good illustrations on the role of language in both processes and the conflict which may be generated by contact between two different systems of communication. At the same time, precisely because of the radical differences between Navajo culture and that of the dominant Euro-American society in the United States, the example helps throw into relief cultural features that influence education and communication, which might otherwise be taken for granted.

A NAVAJO EXAMPLE

Today, the Navajo people represent the largest extant group of American Indians in the United States. The Navajo refer to themselves as *Diné*, which means simply "the people" (i.e., human beings). Although many Navajos now reside in urban areas, such as Dallas and Los Angeles, nearly 100,000 live on or near the large Navajo Reservation in the Southwestern United States. Many adults who were educated in English-only boarding schools are not fluent in the Navajo language, but there are still many who are, and the language remains a vital and viable medium for cultural transmission and communication. Approximately one fourth of all Navajo children on the reservation are still learning Navajo as their mother tongue, with English as their second language. Even many of the Navajo parents and grandparents who themselves dominantly use English continue to transmit traditional lore to their children and continue to socialize them into the beliefs and values that constitute what the people call "The Navajo Way." This "way" sometimes comes into conflict with formal schooling as acculturation takes place.

For Navajo children, cultural conflict in the classroom often begins on the first day of school. The setting is strange, the buildings and furnishings unlike any they have known. Often they do not understand English, and even if they understand the surface structures of the language, they may not be familiar with the way it is used. In the first place, the strange teacher talks to them immediately, and it is Navajo custom to keep silence initially upon encountering unfamiliar people and situations. When children, following the social rules they have learned, do not respond verbally in this context, they earn the teachers' stereotype of "shy" and "unresponsive."

When this author first started collecting data for research on the language of Navajo children, she, too, received no response when attempts were made to interview children. Assuming her attempts to speak Navajo were incomprehensible to the children, the author asked a Navajo friend to correct her grammar and pronunciation. Instead, her entire communicative approach was corrected. When the author sat by a child silently for an appropriate period of time before asking questions, fluent and willing responses were then obtained. The same thing happens with others who understand Navajo culture.

When the first question that teachers ask a child or parent is, "What is your name?", an additional dimension of cultural conflict is created. Traditional Navajos do not believe in revealing their names, and the teacher is asking the person to violate a sociolinguistic constraint at best, and at worst a religious taboo. Unfortunately for the understanding of non-Navajos, Navajo children (and most adults) do not tell them when they are violating acceptable practices. It is the responsibility of anyone who works with the Navajo to be sensitive and informed.

The standard box of eight color crayons presents another hurdle in the classroom. Perception of experience, including the color spectrum, is categorized differently in different languages, and the "basic" colors in English do not correspond to the basic color divisions in Navajo. The blue and green crayons are placed in a single category, labeled *dott'izh*, whereas English "black" corresponds to two distinct Navajo colors. In Choctaw (an unrelated language), a single term signifying "earth color" covers the range of both English brown and yellow. A teacher in Oklahoma reported she had thought a Choctaw child was stupid for coloring a duck *brown* when he had been instructed (in English) to color it *yellow*, until she learned that the two belong to the same color in Choctaw.

The symbolic significance attached to colors may differ also. Whereas Anglo-American culture attributes primarily psychoaesthetic values to colors (yellow is cheerful, black is depressing, white represents purity, etc.), the significance and evaluation of colors in Navajo is radically different. Colors are often associated with the cardinal directions in sandpaintings and songs, the more frequent association being the following:

> white: east
> yellow: west
> black: north
> blue or green: south

Four is the basic number in Navajo religion, and may ritual associations with the four directions and the four colors, including the order in which they are given, occur in songs and sacred accounts. The religious meanings with which color becomes thus imbued are also reflected in various ways in sandpaintings and to some extent in the handwoven rugs for which Navajo craftsmen are rightly famous. In addition, blue or green is often associated with femaleness and white with maleness, virtually the opposite of associations in Anglo culture.

A similar problem is encountered in dealing with shapes. The basic shape categories expressed in Navajo do not correspond to the basic shapes taught in English. Introducing the concept *triangle* in a

Navajo bilingual program presented a problem, for example, because no single term for it existed in the language, and it was not referred to commonly. Six Navajo teachers chose four different descriptive phrases to translate it. On the other hand, the hexagon is a common shape in Navajo culture, and children know the Navajo term for this by the time they enter kindergarten, whereas in most Anglo-American curricula the hexagon is not introduced until the intermediate grades. Navajo children building with blocks are likely to erect six-sided houses rather than four-sided ones, replicating the shape of most Navajo hogans.

Religious taboos also constitute a potentially serious conflict in classroom language use. The bear, for example, is not to be talked about or depicted in any Navajo instructional materials, and stories about most other hibernating animals should be told or read only during the months the animals are sleeping. A Navajo teacher was to help this author adapt some coyote stories to a controlled Navajo vocabulary sequence for children to begin reading at the appropriate time of year, and our production schedule had not adequately considered the strength of this taboo. Even though she denied believing in it herself, my colleague was so disturbed by the prospects of beginning work on the books "too soon" that she was unable to actually start on them before winter.

OTHER CULTURES, OTHER MEANINGS

As we have seen, the vocabulary of a language provides an interesting reflection of the culture of the people who speak it. It is a catalogue of things of import to a society, an index of the way speakers categorize experience, and often a record of past contacts and cultural borrowings. The grammar, on the other hand may reveal the way time is segmented and organized, beliefs about animacy and the relative power of beings, and salient social categories in the culture (cf. Whorf, 1940; Witherspoon, 1977). It would be completely impossible to separate language from culture, even if it were desirable to do so. Cultural information is solidly embedded in language use and interpretation.

Many examples could be cited to demonstrate the way language may reflect a world view, but a few will suffice. Greek and some varieties of Quechua (the language of the Inca empire still spoken in Peru and Bolivia) consider the future tense to refer to events "behind" the speaker and the past tense to refer to events that are "ahead," the reverse of the way they are thought of in English. According to Nida (1975), Quechua speakers point out that we can "see" the past, since it has happened, but not the future. Therefore, the past must be in front of our eyes, whereas the future that we cannot "see" must be behind us. As this illustrates, the meaning of any word or grammatical category is purely arbitrary and depends upon the agreement of a group of speakers as to its symbolic value.

A great deal of cross-cultural misunderstanding occurs when the "meanings" of words or grammatical structures in two languages are assumed to be the same but actually reflect differing cultural patterns. Some may seem humorous, as when a Turkish visitor to the United States refused to consume a "hot dog" because he inferred that it was made of dog meat, which it was against his Muslim beliefs to eat, or when some students from the Dominican Republic precipitated an argument on a Texas college campus by referring to the Texas students as "Yankees." Some are much more serious, as when Navajo parents gave up their children for "adoption," not realizing that this meant they would not return to their families at the end of the school year.

Speakers of a variety of Asian languages, despite their unrelatedness, share an interpretation of the passive formation in sentences which could cause serious misunderstanding in English. The passive is used in English for a number of purposes, including emphasizing the object, deemphasizing the agent, focusing on the completed state of the action, or merely stylistic variation. For example,

Miro's assistant painted the picture.
The picture was painted by Miro's assistant.

To speakers of many Asian languages, however, the two sentences have different meanings, since the subject of a passive sentence is understood to be the "victim" of the action. Thus, the first sentence would be merely a statement of fact, while the second would imply that the agent did a bad job. Even fluent English speakers from Chinese and Japanese backgrounds continue to make this interpretation.

Many cases of cross-cultural differences in meaning are never recognized as such, but merely add to negative stereotypes of other cultural groups. Spanish speakers sometimes encounter negative attitudes from English speakers for their use of the common expletive *Dios mío*, since the English translation "My God" is much stronger than the Spanish and is socially disapproved for use in many contexts. The common use of the name *Jesús* in Spanish is regarded as bordering on the blasphemous by some English-speakers, who consider it taboo (and usually change it to *Jesse* at school).

STEREOTYPING

Making judgments about people according to linguistic features is a common form of stereotyping; it is possible because of the highly "visible" nature of the markers, which are often correlated with categories of race, sex, age, region, social class, religion, and ethnicity. The social categories, in turn, carry with them traditional attitudes and expectations that may strongly affect communication.

Social "typing" or categorization is probably a necessary part of our procedures for coping with the outside world. It allows us to quickly define our orientation to other individuals, and is a basis for our cultural sense of manners and other conventions of interpersonal relations. It provides an efficient means for establishing preliminary relationships (Abrahams, 1972). If we did not "know" how to relate appropriately to different groups of people before we were acquainted with them personally, we would be socially ineffective to say the least, and perhaps even unable to function normally in a society.

Social typing should be seen, therefore, as potentially positive, and in any case as inevitable. Typing may assume negative aspects, however, and then it ceases to be just an aid to facilitate social interaction and interpretation. It may become a means of disaffiliation or rejection or of rationalizing prejudice, and it is this negative connotation that is usually associated with the term "stereotyping."

Stereotypic expectations may well become self-fulfilling prophecies. Our preconceptions of how a physician "should talk," for instance, are usually met; if not, patients may be suspicious of the doctor's credentials or professional competence. Such expectations have negative educational consequences when children are characterized as "good" or "bad," at least partly, in terms of their language use, not only in terms of the employment of politeness rules and "proper" (i.e., middle class) vocabulary, but even in features of pronunciation (Fischer, 1958). Negative consequences may also ensue when teachers make use of vocal features attributed to ethnic or social class categories to prejudge children's likely achievement (Williams, 1973).

Recognition of the stereotypes that are held by and about groups of people are relevant for the study of communication in three respects: (1) as a dimension of the attitudes and values that are part of culture, (2) as part of the framework of sociocultural expectations within which communicative behavior must be interpreted, and (3) as a check on the objectivity of a person's own perceptions.

THE ETHNOGRAPHY OF COMMUNICATION

The intrinsic relationship of language and culture has long been acknowledged, particularly by anthropologists. Despite this recognition, however, the results of ethnographic and linguistic research until recently have tended to show little connection. It was Hymes' definition (1962) of the *ethnography of communication* as a distinctive new subdiscipline that revolutionized the study of the interpenetration of language and culture. That perspective is continuing today to produce new and important insights in the study of communication.

The ethnography of communication, not surprisingly, takes its fundamental direction from its parent field, ethnography. Its basic orientation is descriptive, and although it may be (and often is) focused on a particular type of activity, it attempts to be as open-ended as possible throughout. This open-endedness is its particular hallmark, implying that new issues, hypotheses, and solutions are sought throughout the course of data collection and are expected to arise from the data themselves and from the interaction of the data and various interpretive frameworks. It is also frequently characteristic of this type of work that the phenomenological perspective of the actors involved is sought as much as possible to provide an additional vantage point on the action and to serve as a corrective to the external observations and interpretations of the investigator.

The ethnography of communication provides a synthesizing focus that concentrates on *the patterning of communicative behavior* as it constitutes one of the subsystems of culture, as it functions within the holistic context of the culture of a group, and as it relates to patterns in other component systems. This perspective first and foremost takes *language as a socially situated cultural form,* while at the same time recognizing the necessity of analyzing the linguistic code itself and the cognitive processes of its speakers and hearers. To accept a lesser scope for the study of communication is to risk reducing it to triviality and to abandon any possibility of understanding how language actually functions in the lives of individuals and cultural groups.

As with any science, the ethnography of communication is both particularistic and generalizing. On the one hand, it is directed at the discovery and description of communicative behavior in specific cultural settings, but it is also directed toward the formulation of concepts and theories on which to build a global metatheory of human communication. Its basic approach does not involve a list of facts to be learned so much as questions to be asked and means for finding out answers.

There is no single best method for collecting information on the patterns of language use within a speech community, although the most common method of collecting ethnographic data in any domain of culture is participant-observation. Appropriate procedures depend to a great extent on the relationship of the ethnographer and the speech community, the type of data being collected, and the particular situation in which the study is being conducted. The essential defining characteristics of ethnographic procedures are that they are designed to get around the recorder's biased perceptions and that they are grounded in the study of communication in natural contexts.

The subject matter of the ethnograpy of communication is best illustrated by one of its most general questions: What does a speaker need to know to communicate appropriately within a particular speech community, and how does he or she acquire this knowledge? Such knowledge, together with whatever skills are needed to make use of it, is termed *communicative competence* (Hymes, 1966). The requisite knowledge includes not only rules for communication (both lingustic and sociolinguistic) and shared rules for interaction but also the cultural rules and knowledge that are the basis for the context and content of communicative events and interaction processes. A primary aim of this approach is to guide the collection and analysis of descriptive data about the ways in which social meaning is conveyed, constructed, and negotiated.

The communicative competence of speakers is a body of knowledge and skills that involves not only the language code that they use but also what they can say to whom, how they should say it appropriately in any given situation, and even when they should say nothing at all. It involves interaction skills such as knowing how to develop conversations, and how to avoid becoming involved in a conversation if you prefer to be engaged in some other activity. It involves receptive as well as productive facility, written as well as oral modes of communication, and nonverbal as well as verbal behaviors. Communicative competence further involves having appropriate sociocultural *schemata,* that is, the social and cultural *knowledge and expectations* that speakers, hearers, readers, and writers are presumed to have that enable them to use and interpret communicative forms. The concept of communicative competence must be embedded, therefore, in a larger notion of *cultural competence*; interpreting the meaning of linguistic behavior requires knowing the cultural meaning of the context within which it occurs.

The following outline (from Saville-Troike, 1982) summarizes the broad range of shared knowledge and skills that speakers must have to communicate appropriately. These are essentially the components of communicative competence:

1. Linguistic knowledge
   a. Verbal elements
   b. Nonverbal elements
   c. Patterns of elements in particular speech events
   d. Range of possible variants (in all elements and their organization)
   e. Meaning of variants in particular situations
2. Interaction skills
   a. Perception of salient features in communicative situations
   b. Selection and interpretation of forms appropriate to specific situations, roles, and relationships (rules for the use of speech)
   c. Norms of interaction and interpretation
   d. Strategies for achieving goals
3. Cultural knowledge
   a. Social structure
   b. Values and attitudes
   c. Cognitive map or schema
   d. Enculturation processes (how knowledge and skills are transmitted).

COMMUNICATIVE COMPETENCE AND ASSESSMENT

One important application of the concept of communicative competence is to the assessment of communicative skills, especially as they relate to requirements of the educative process. Traditional language proficiency tests that measure pronunciation, grammar, and vocabulary do not reveal all of the communicative requirements necessary for success in school (Troike, 1983). Although the full potential in this area of application has not yet been realized, much progress has been made (e.g., Rivera, 1983). Such efforts are vital to questions of entry and exit in special educational programs designed for speakers of other languages, such as Bilingual Education and English as a Second Language, and to questions of the identification and remediation of abnormal speech.

The first factor to consider is that testing is itself a socially situated communicative event, and students may perform differentially in differing testing conditions because of their language and cultural background. Evaluation instruments can seldom be considered neutral in these respects, no matter how "objective" their format. The reliability of tests is affected not only by the ethnicity of the tester and the experience that students have had taking tests but also by the type of questions (e.g., true-false questions are not widely used in Latin America), the modality of the test (written versus oral), and the language code used (a Spanish test developed in Puerto Rico is not valid in California or Texas, and perhaps not even in New York).

The task of determining and testing for the specific linguistic knowledge and skills required by the education process is made even more complex by the fact that "competence" (as language itself) must be considered a variable phenomenon in at least two basic respects. First, since communicative competence as a cultural construct refers to knowledge and skills for contextually appropriate use and interpretation of language in a community, it refers to the communicative knowledge and skills shared by the group; but these, by their very nature, must reside variably in its individual members. Problems arise when individual competence is judged in relation to a presumed ideal speech community, as it often is, or assessed with tests given in a limited subset of situations that do not represent the true range of an individual's verbal ability. The problems are particularly serious when such invalid judgments result in some form of social discrimination against the individual, such as unequal or inappropriate educational treatment.

Different modes, channels, and functions represent a second kind of variability. The relatively decontextualized nature of written texts may well require a different subset of skills for successful expression and interpretation than does face-to-face communication through an oral medium, for instance. The same may be true for the use of language in some types of cognitive processing. This may account in part for the fact that individual students may sometimes appear to have a very high level of communicative competence, at least in some contexts, yet not perform well in school (Cummins, 1981). The problem in this case may well be that some researchers are inappropriately (in terms of Hymes' original definition) restricting their use of the term "communicative" to apply only to direct personal interaction, rather than to all uses of language and other symbolic systems.

From an anthropological perspective, children develop communicative competence as an integral part of their enculturation process in three ways. First, language is part of culture, and thus part of the body of knowledge, attitudes, and skills that is transmitted from one generation to the next. Second, language is a primary medium through which other aspects of culture are transmitted. Third, language is a tool that children may use to explore (and sometimes manipulate—e.g., Bauman, 1977; Corsaro, 1978) the social environment and establish their status and role-relationships within it.

Ethnographic modes of investigation are of particular value in the study of both first and second language acquisition and development. This is particularly true now that the primary focus of research attention in the field has shifted from phonology and grammar to such topics a the functions language serves for children, the communicative strategies they use, how these are developed, and how input is structured in the process of social interaction. We can begin to understand how language is learned only if we examine the process within its immediate social and cultural setting and in the context of conscious or unconscious socialization. We must ask about the nature of linguistic input and sociolinguistic training, how and for what purposes children acquire particular communicative strategies, and how language is related to the definition of stages in the life cycle. We must seek to identify the differential influences of family, peers, and formal education, and we must consider such matters as the beliefs that the community itself (including its children) holds about the nature of language origin and development.

One of the greatest influences the peer group has on the acquisition of communicative competence comes through various kinds of speech play. This aspect of child communication can yield information on a far broader scope of socialization processes than just language development, and it provides insights into the culture that is being acquired and the social structure of which the children are a part. According to Bernstein, this is so because children's speech play influences organization of experience and behavior. It makes "the child sensitive to role and status and also to the customary relationships connecting and legitimizing the social positions within his peer group" (1960, p. 180). Adult ways of speaking may be practiced in make-believe roles, such as giving tea parties and offering "One lump or two," or playing school and assuming the mannerisms and speech of teacher and principal.

Verbal contests yields particularly valuable cultural information, because a comment on a cultural value is always one of their defining features. Abrahams (1973) describes one of their general functions as "trying on" mature roles within the safe confines of the peer group while arming the children with verbal weapons that will be useful in adult life. Among Black males, these contests include categories labeled *rapping* (often competitive repartee between male and female), *shucking* and *jiving* (flattering or cajoling), and *signify-ing* (goading) (see Kochman, 1972, especially pp. 241–264, for descriptions and illustrations of these categories).

A verbal contest unique to young (8 to 11 year old) Black girls is *stepping* (organized competitive "spelling," foot stepping, and hand clapping), in which the body is used to iconically represent the shape of letters, following the spelling *M I Crooked Letter Crooked Letter I Crooked Letter Crooked Letter I Hump Back Hump Back I* for "Mississippi." Skilled performers are called *kookalaters* (crooked letter). Gilmore (1981) reports that *stepping* was banned from public schools in Philadelphia because of its frequent sexual explicitness.

One final example comes from Venezuela (although analogues could probably be found in the United States), where preschool children are taught a game called *Matare.* The game begins when two children choose a name to call another child. They start by calling out an "ugly" name, which other children sing that they won't accept, and continue in this manner until a "good" name is picked and accepted by the group. Conveyed are cultural notions of the status of different occupations and appropriate sex roles: for example, only boys can be called a name like "shoemaker" and "carpenter," and only girls a name like "servant" and "cook."

One of the most complete ethnographic studies of language development yet conducted is by Heath (1983), who describes how children from three culturally different communities in the Piedmont Carolinas learn to use language. Their differential socialization experiences yield differential "readiness" for school, even though all three groups acquire full competence in the language patterns of their home and community. Heath goes further beyond description to suggest ways in which educators can make us of knowledge from ethnographies of communication to build bridges between communities and schools and accommodate group differences in language and culture.

Ultimately, all aspects of culture are relevant to communication, but those that have the most direct bearing on communicative forms and processes are the social structure, the values and attitudes held about language and way of speaking, the network of conceptual categories that results from shared experiences, and the ways knowledge and skills (including language) are transmitted from one generation to the next and to new members of the group. Shared cultural knowledge is also essential to explain the shared presuppositions and judgments of truth value that are the essential undergirdings of language structures as well as of contextually appropriate usage and interpretation.

FINDING PATTERNS IN COMMUNICATION

Understanding that overt behavior is a manifestation of underlying "rules" requires recognizing that it follows regular patterns and constraints. (Note: "Rule" as used herein refers to *unconscious* constraints on behavior, *not* explicitly formulated prescriptions.) Concern for pattern has long been basic for anthropology (cf. Benedict, 1934; Kroeber, 1935, 1944), with interpretations of underlying meaning dependent on the discovery and description of normative structure or design. More recent emphasis on processes of interaction in generating behavioral patterns (cf. Barth, 1966) extends this concern to both explanation and description. With respect to language, ethnographers are concerned with how communicative units are organized and how they pattern in the sense of "ways of speaking" (cf. Bauman and Sherzer, 1974, 1975), as well as with how these patterns interrelate in a systematic way with and derive meaning from other aspects of culture.

At a societal level, this patterning generally occurs along dimensions of social organization and community attitudes. Communication patterns vary according to particular roles and groups within a society, such as sex, age, social status, and occupation: for example, a teacher has different ways of speaking from a lawyer, a doctor, or an insurance salesman. Ways of speaking also pattern according to educational level, rural or urban residence, ethnicity, and geographical region.

When studying communication from an anthropological perspective, function has primacy over form in description and analysis, although an integration of function and form is ultimately required. Societal macrofunctions include social control, maintenance of homeostatic relations with the supernatural, and establishing or reinforcing group identity. Another societal function of language is creating or reinforcing boundaries, unifying its speakers as members of a single speech community, and excluding outsiders from intragroup communication. Many languages are made to serve a social identification function within a society by providing linguistic indicators that may be used to reinforce social stratification. At the level of individuals and groups interacting with one another, the functions of communication are directly related to the participants' purposes and needs (Blom and Gumperz, 1972).

To the extent emotional factors such as nervousness have an unintentional reflexive effect on the vocal mechanism, they are usually not considered part of "communication," unless they receive a standardized interpretation within the culture. However, there are many conventional symbols of emotional attitude that are part of patterned communication. An example of conventional expression of emotion in English speakers is the increased vocal volume that signals "anger." To express anger, a Navajo does not raise the volume of his or her voice, but instead uses specific words or suffixes that serve as emotion markers. A friendly greeting on the street between Chinese speakers may have surface manifestations that would be interpreted erroneously as anger by speakers of English. Similarly, American Indian students often interpret Anglo-American teachers' "normal" classroom projection level as markers of anger and hostility, whereas teachers conversely interpret students' softer level (intended to imply respect) as indicative of shyness or unfriendliness. Clearly, we cannot make the assumption that even "universal" emotions will be uniformly expressed in all cultures, or that the expression used in our own language or cultural group is "natural" or "instinctive."

Most instances of conflict in school settings are charged with emotion, and understanding the culturally different ways in which emotions may be expressed and interpreted are vital to the classroom climate for learning. Gilmore (1984), for instance, focuses on the displays of "stylized silent sulking" that characterize clashes of will between teachers and students in a low-income, black urban community which she studied. Teachers identify students exhibiting such behaviors as having a "bad attitude," which often results in tracking them out of academic programs. Close examination of the behavior, however, shows a great deal of variation in its form and meaning and relates the mode of expression to community norms of appropriate demeanor. In this case, better mutual understanding of different patterns of communication might well contribute to improvement in the quality of learning and teaching.

Classroom interaction is also affected by other aspects of language diversity, including rules regarding who should talk and when. The school generally supports the convention of one person speaking at a time (after raising a hand and being called on) and not interrupting; other cultures would consider that rude, a sure sign that no one was interested in what the primary speaker was saying (cf. Gay and Abrahams, 1972). Mitigation techniques also differ, and students encounter many problems in school when they come from cultures that do not use the same ones that are accepted there. A middle-class student from the dominant culture has typically learned to avoid unpleasant assignments with such indirect excuses as "I'm tired. Can't I do that later?" or with nonverbal dawdling or daydreaming until time is up. Although the attempt is often unsuccessful, it brings no serious reproof. If a student has not learned these cultural strategies and says, "No, I won't," or just "No"—which have essentially the same meaning—he or she may be considered belligerent or rude.

It seems clear that training in language or linguistics, although necessary, is not sufficient for understanding the study of communication. Ethnography provides an important additional set of tools that are essential for achieving an understanding of the patterns of language use in the communication systems of different cultures.

UNITS OF DESCRIPTION AND ANALYSIS

The ethnography of communication takes the *speech community*, and the way in which communication is patterned and organized within that unit, as being of central importance. Many definitions of "community" have been proposed (cf. Hudson, 1980, pp. 25–30), but all of those used in the social sciences include the dimension of shared knowledge, possessions, or behaviors, derived form Latin *communitas* ("held in common"). Identification of this unit for the study of communication generally includes such criteria as shared language use (Lyons, 1970), frequency of interaction by a group of people (Bloomfield, 1933; Hockett, 1958; Gumperz, 1962), shared rules of speaking and interpretations of speech performance (Hymes, 1972), shared attitudes and values regarding language forms and use (Labov, 1972), and shared sociocultural understandings and presuppositions with regard to speech (Sherzer, 1975).

Speech communities may be recognized at different levels of abstraction; virtually any grouping of people in a complex society might be considered part of another, larger group or subdivided into smaller groups. A study of communication might focus on a single neighborhood (e.g., Attinasi, Pedraza, Poplack, and Pousada, 1982), a single school, or even members of a single occupation, but an integrated ethnographic approach would require relating such subgroups to the social and cultural whole, with its full complement of roles. Small-scale studies, dubbed "microethnography," are common in studies of classroom communication but often provide detail of interactional analysis at the expense of contextual or "ecological" validity.

A speech community need not be linguistically homogeneous, but as a collectivity it may include a range of language varieties (and even different languages) that will pattern in relation to the salient social and cultural dimensions of communication. The variety of language codes and ways of speaking available to members of a community is called its *communicative repertoire*. This includes "all varieties, dialects or styles used in a particular socially-defined population, and the constraints which govern the choice among them" (Gumperz, 1977). Any one speaker also has a variety of codes and styles from which to choose, but it is very unlikely that any individual is able to produce the full range. Different subgroups of the community may understand and use different subsets of its available codes.

Individuals typically belong to more than one speech community (which may be discrete or overlapping), just as they participate in a variety of social settings. Which one or ones a person orients himself or herself to at any given moment — which set of social and communicative *rules* he or she uses — is part of the strategy of communication. To understand this phenomenon, it is necessary to recognize that each member of a community has a repertoire of social identities, and each identity in a given context is associated with a number of appropriate verbal and nonverbal forms of expression. Knowing the alternatives and the rules for appropriate choice from among them are part of speakers' communicative competence.

Accounting for the rules or system for such decision-making is part of the task of describing communication within any group and of explaining communication more generally. These may include the general subject area under discussion (e.g., family, health, schoolwork), the role-relations between the participants (e.g., mother-daughter, doctor-patient, teacher-student), and the setting of the interaction (e.g., home, doctor's office, school). All of these dimensions contribute to the concept of *domain* (cf. Fishman, 1964, 1966, 1971, 1972), which is important for describing and explaining the distribution of patterns of communication. (Consider, for example, the differences involved if a doctor is talking to her mother at home or is taking an evening course on computer programming from a patient.)

The *communicative units* (i.e., communicative activities with recognizable boundaries) that are frequently used in ethnographic studies (following Hymes, 1972) are *situation, event,* and *act.*

The *communicative situation* is the context within which communication occurs. Typically, terms exist in the language by which to label situations, such as (in English) a church service, a trial, a cocktail party, or a class in school. A single situation maintains a consistent general configuration of activities and the same overall ecology within which communication takes place, although there may be great diversity in the kinds of interaction that occur there and, in some cases, even discontinuity of interaction. For example, the author observed and videotaped a group of non–English-speaking children each week over the course of an entire school year in a single communicative situation that occurred when these children were "pulled out" of their regular English-medium classrooms for 30 minutes each day for a common class in English as a Second Language (ESL) (Saville-Troike, 1984; Saville-Troike, McClure, and Fritz, 1984). Although the composition of the group changed with illness and family trips or migrations, and the specific activities changed with seasonal interests and the students' developing English language proficiency, the overall structure and purpose of the sessions remained the same.

The *communicative event* is the basic unit for descriptive purposes. A single event is defined by a unified set of components throughout, beginning with the same general purpose of communication, the same general topic, and the same participants, generally using the same language variety, maintaining the same tone or key, and using the same rules for interaction, in the same setting. An event terminates whenever there is a change in the major participants, their role-relationships, or the focus of attention. If there is no change in major participants and setting, the boundary between events is often marked by a period of silence, and perhaps, a change of body position.

In the pull-out ESL situation referred to earlier, for instance, the sessions were found to divide into a regular sequence of recurring events: (1) unstructured play, (2) claiming a seat, (3) opening routines, (4) teacher-directed lesson, (5) follow-up activity, and (6) closing routines. Each event in this situation involved different ways of speaking and different rules for interaction. On many occasions, a shift in language occurred at event boundaries.

The event as a unit for analysis is important in part so that observations made at different times will be comparable, and so that generalizations can be made about patterns of communication within a constant *frame* or context. In the situation just described, for instance, patterns and forms for communication varied greatly from event to event, and yet they stayed constant for each type of event throughout the year. The author was able, therefore, to analyze the development of children's competence in English, and the strategies that they used to achieve different communicative functions within each event. However, any comparison of child or teacher language forms and rules for language use at different points of the lesson (or in other situations) would have been quite misleading without taking these units into account.

For example, the word *is* in the sentence, "This is a pencil," which was used consistently in the ESL opening routines and teacher-directed lessons beginning in the first week of school, was still absent in the speech of many children in all other events (and in other situations) after weeks and even months of English instruction. Without reference to different event structures, it might appear that this grammatical form occurred randomly, rather than as part of memorized patterns that were used only during teacher-child interaction when focus was on the form, rather than the content, of communication. Children and teacher also (unconsciously) recognized that organizational rules, such as raising hands and talking one at a time, operated only during certain segments of the class.

The *communicative act* is generally coterminous with a single interactional function, such as a referential statement, a request, or a command, and may be either verbal or nonverbal. For example, not only may a request take several verbal forms ("I'd like a piece of candy," "Do you have a piece of candy?" or "May I please have a piece of candy?"), but it may be expressed by raised eyebrows and a "questioning" look or by a longing sigh. In the context of a communicative event, even silence may be an intentional and conventional communicative act used to question, promise, deny, warn, insult, request, or command. Just as "One can utter words without saying anything" (Searle, 1969), we can say something without uttering words (cf. Tannen and Saville-Troike, 1985).

Within the ESL teacher-directed lesson event mentioned earlier, each question or request from the teacher is a single communicative act, as is each bid for attention or response from a child. In classroom discourse, these often cycle in a regular triadic pattern: question from the teacher, response from a student, and evaluation of the response from the teacher (cf. Johnson, 1979; Sinclair and Colthard, 1975). This is illustrated by the following exchange:

Teacher (question): What is the date?
Student (response): Today is October the tenth.
Teacher (evaluation): Good.

Other cycles of speech acts occur in other recurring communicative events, including greetings, telephone calls (e.g., Schegloff, 1968), and sales transactions (e.g., Tsuda, 1984).

DISCOURSE ANALYSIS

In analyzing a communicative event, it is important to note features that constitute the "frame"—the salient context. As discussed earlier, a change in any of these elements is likely to indicate that the boundary has been crossed into a different event, and that different rules for interaction may be in effect. Even a very detailed description of situations and events is likely to be static in nature, however, and fall short of accounting for the dynamic processes involved in communication. This situation is likely to be true unless the descriptions are supplemented with analysis at the level of discourse, and frames are considered in an interactive model as dynamic "schemata" or "structures of expectation" (Tannen, 1979). Meaning itself is not static, after all, but negotiated in the process of human interaction (Gumperz, 1977; Tannen, 1984).

In naturally occurring communication, meaning is derived not just from speech forms but also from such factors as the information or presuppositions the communicants bring to the task, the extralinguistic context, and nonverbal cues. Perception and interpretation of these factors are strongly dependent on cultural experience and account for much of the miscommunication between individuals from different cultural backgrounds — even when they are speaking the same language.

These underlying cultural bases for communication are easiest to recognize, perhaps, in cross-cultural contexts. In such cases the "meaning" that emerges may not be the same for all participants. For example, the author observed the following (mis)communicative event in a kindergarten classroom on the Navajo Reservation:

A Navajo man opened the door to the classroom and stood silently, looking at the floor.
The Anglo-American teacher said, "Good morning," and waited expectantly. The man did not respond.
The teacher said, "My name is Mrs. Jones," and again waited for a response. There was none.
In the meantime, a child in the room put away his crayons and got his coat from the rack.
The teacher, noting this, said to the man, "Oh, are you taking Billy now?"
The man said, "Yes."
The teacher continued to talk to him while Billy got ready to leave, saying, "Billy is such a good boy, I'm so happy to have him in class," and continuing in a similar vein.
Billy walked toward the man (his father), stopping to turn around and wave at the teacher on his way out and saying "Bye-bye."
The teacher responded, "Bye-bye."
The man remained silent as he left.

From a Navajo perspective, the man's silence was appropriate and respectful. The teacher, on the other hand, expected not only to have the man return her greeting, but to identify himself and state his reason for being there. Although such an expectation is quite reasonable and appropriate from an Anglo-American perspective, it required the man to break not only Navajo rules of politeness but also the traditional religious taboo that prohibits an individual from saying his or her own name. The teacher interpreted the contextual cues correctly in answer to her own question ("Are you taking Billy?") and then engaged in small talk in an attempt to be friendly and to cover her own discomfort in the situation. The man continued to maintain appropriate silence. Billy, who was more acculturated than his father to Anglo-American ways, broke the Navajo rule to follow the Anglo-American one in leave-taking.

This encounter undoubtedly reinforced the teacher's stereotype that Navajos are "impolite" and "unresponsive," and the man's stereotype that Anglo-Americans are "impolite" and "talk too much." Although this was a single event, it illustrates systematic differences in communicative rules used in the Anglo-American and Navajo speech communities, and it helps explain why language-based stereotypes exist.

A more subtle example of miscommunication at a discourse level is described by Michaels (1981) in her analysis of "sharing time" in a racially integrated first grade classroom. The white children's discourse style generally matched the white teacher's own style and expectations, and she provided collaborative enrichment experiences that were designed to prepare them for literacy. The black children's narrative strategies and prosodic conventions, on the other hand, were at variance with her expectations, and her efforts at collaboration were unsuccessful and even disruptive to communication. The different styles of communication that the children bring to school thus give them differential access to the "oral preparation for literacy" that is offered there, and these are likely to have a long-range effect on school performance and evaluation.

Understanding what the speakers' frames are, what processes they are using to relate these expectations to the production and interpretation of language, and how the schemata and interaction processes relate to their cultural experiences is the ultimate goal in explaining communicative competence. Methods developed to collect and analyze data at this level have included the showing of a film to subjects from different cultures and the eliciting of narratives describing its content. Speakers' culturally determined structures of expectation are then inferred from the way objects and events are organized and changed in the retelling (Chafe, 1980; Tannen, 1981). Other methods that have proved useful are (1) *playback* (Fanshel and Moss, 1971; Labov and Fanshel, 1977), in which participants are interviewed in depth about the meaning of their own utterances in the process of microanalysis, and (2) the study of institutionalized speakers who are judged by psychiatrists to exhibit communicative behavior that is "inappropriate in the situation" (Goffman, 1963). Such procedures may be profitably integrated with more traditional ethnographic methods to assist in the study of communication.

APPLIED CONSIDERATIONS

Appropriate identification and remediation of communicative "disorder" must be based on full understanding of communicative "order," or normal patterns of communication. For culturally and linguistically diverse populations, this requires a definition of "normal" in terms of the speech community to which an individual belongs, not in terms of deviations from the sociolinguistic and linguistic norms of another group—even if the other group is the Anglo-American majority in this society. An anthropological perspective provides both an organizing concept and methodology for the holistic study of communication in its social and cultural context, which in turn provides the basis for recognizing legitimate differences in patterns of communication and distinguishing them from genuinely handicapping conditions.

Additional applications of the ethnography of communication potentially include more effective and efficient interventions in those cases in which handicapping conditions do exist, by enabling practitioners to adapt their instructional programming to fit the cultural and linguistic characteristics and competence of learners. A further benefit would undoubtedly be the improvement of communication with home and community, leading to closer and more effective collaboration in advancing opportunities for children or older clients. Both as part of a prevention strategy for reducing the numbers of individuals erroneously referred for special treatment, and as part of an intervention strategy for enhancing the quality and effectiveness of treatment given, the ethnography of communication has a significant contribution to make to the education of minority students — indeed, all students — in our schools.

REFERENCES

Abrahams, R. D. (1972). Stereotyping and beyond. In R. D. Abrahams and R. C. Troike (Eds.), *Language and culture in American education* (pp. 19–29). Englewood Cliffs, NJ: Prentice-Hall.

Abrahams, R. D. (1973). Toward a Black rhetoric: Being a survey of Afro-American communication styles and role-relationships. Texas Working Papers in Sociolinguistics No. 15.

Attinasi, J., Pedraza, P. Poplack, S., and Pousada, A. (1982). *Intergenerational perspectives on bilingualism.* New York: Center for Puerto Rican Studies.

Barth, F. (1966). *Models of social organization.* Occasional Papers of the Royal Anthropological Institute of Great Britain and Ireland No. 23.

Bauman, R. (1977). Linguistics, anthropology, and verbal art: Toward a unified perspective with a special discussion of children's folklore. In M. Saville-Troike (Ed.), *Linguistics and anthropology* (pp. 13–36). Washington, DC: Georgetown University Press.

Bauman, R., and Sherzer, J. (Eds.). (1974) *Explorations in the ethnography of speaking.* Cambridge: Cambridge University Press.

Bauman, R., and Sherzer, J. (1975). The ethnography of speaking. *Annual Review of Anthropology, 4,* 95–119.

Benedict, R. (1934). *Patterns of culture.* Boston: Houghton Mifflin.

Bernstein, B., (1960. Review of "The lore and language of school children" by Opie Iona and Opie Peter. *British Journal of Sociology, 11,* 178–181.

Bernstein, B. (1972). A sociolinguistic approach to socialization; with some references to educability. In J. J. Gumperz and D. Hymes (Eds.), *Directions in sociolinguistics: The ethnography of communication* (pp. 465–497). New York: Holt, Rinehart and Winston.

Blom. J.-P., and Gumperz, J. J. (1972). Social meaning in linguistic structure: Code-switching in Norway. In J. J. Gumperz and D. Hymes (Eds.), *Directions in sociolinguistics: The ethnography of communication* (pp. 407–434). New York: Holt, Rinehart and Winston.

Bloomfield, L. (1933). *Language.* New York: Holt.

Chafe, W. L. (1980). *The pear stories: Cognitive, cultural and linguistic aspects of narrative production.* Norwood, NJ: Ablex.

Corsaro, W. A. (1978). "We're friends, right?": Children's use of access rituals in a nursery school. Texas Working Papers in Sociolinguistics No. 43.

Cummins, J. (1981). The role of primary language development in promoting educational success for language minority students. In *Schooling and language minority students: A theoretical framework* (pp. 3–49). Los Angeles: California State University.

Fanshel, D., and Moss, F. (1971). *Playback: A marriage in jeopardy examined.* New York: Columbia University Press.

Fischer, J. L. (1958). Social influence in the choice of a linguistic variant. *Word, 14,* 47–56.

Fishman, J. A. (1964). Language maintenance and language shift as fields of inquiry. *Linguistics, 9,* 32–70.

Fishman, J. A. (1966). *Language loyalty in the United States.* The Hague, Netherlands: Mouton.

Fishman, J. A. (1971). The links between micro- and macrosociolinguistics in the study of who speaks what language to whom and when. In J. A. Fishman, R. L. Cooper, and R. Ma, *Bilingualism in the barrio* (pp. 583–604). Bloomington: Indiana University Press.

Fishman, J. A. (1972). Domains and the relationship between micro- and macrosociolinguistics. In J. J. Gumperz and D. Hymes (Eds.), *Directions in sociolinguistics: The ethnography of communication* (pp. 435–453). New York: Holt, Rinehart and Winston.

Gay, G., and Abrahams, R. D. (1972). Black culture in the classroom. In R. D. Abrahams and R. C. Troike (Eds.), *Language and cultural diversity in American education* (pp. 67–84). Englewood Cliffs, NJ: Prentice-Hall.

Gilmore, P. (1981). Spelling "Mississippi": Recontextualizing a literacy-related speech event. Paper presented at the Second Annual University of Pennsylvania Ethnography in Education Research Forum, Philadelphia.

Gilmore, P. (1984). Silence and sulking: Emotional displays in the classroom. In D. Tannen and M. Saville-Troike (Eds.), *Perspectives on silence* (pp. 139–162). Norwood, NJ: Ablex.

Goffman, E. (1963). *Behavior in public places: Notes on the social organization of gatherings.* New York: Free Press.

Gumperz, J. J. (1962). Types of linguistic communities. *Anthropological Linguistics, 4* (1), 28–40.

Gumperz, J. J. (1977). Sociocultural knowledge in conversational inference. In M. Saville-Troike (Ed.), *Linguisitcs and anthropology* (pp. 191–212). Washington, DC: Georgetown University Press.

Hall, E. T. (1959). *The silent language.* Garden City, NY: Doubleday.

Heath, S. B. (1983). *Ways with words: Language, life, and work in communities and classrooms.* Cambridge: Cambridge University Press.

Hockett, C. F. (1958). *A course in modern linguistics.* New York: Macmillan

Hudson, R. A. (1980). *Sociolinguistics.* Cambridge: Cambridge University Press.

Hymes, D. (1962). The ethnography of speaking. In T. Gladwin and W. C. Sturtevant (Eds.), *Anthropology and human behavior* (pp. 13–53). Washington, DC: Anthropological Society of Washington.

Hymes, D. (1966). On communicative competence. Paper presented at the Research Planning Conference on Language Development among Disadvantaged Children, Yeshiva University.

Hymes, D. (1972). Models of the interaction of language and social life. In J. J. Gumperz and D. Hymes (Eds.), *Directions in sociolinguistics: The ethnography of communication* (pp 35–71). New York: Holt, Rinehart and Winston.

Johnson, M. C. (1979). *Discussion dynamics: An analysis of classroom teaching.* Rowley, MA: Newbury House.

Kochman, T. (Ed.). (1972). *Rappin' and stylin' out: Communication in urban Black America.* Urbana: University of Illinois Press.

Kroeber, A. L. (1935). History and science in anthropology. *American Anthropologist, 37,* 539–569.

Kroeber, A. L. (1944). *Configurations of culture growth.* Berkeley: University of California Press.

Labov, W. (1972). On the mechanism of linguistic change. In J. J. Gumperz and D. Hymes (Eds.), *Directions in sociolinguistics: The ethnography of communication* (pp. 512–538). New York: Holt, Rinehart and Winston.

Labov, W., and Fanshel, D. (1977). *Therapeutic discourse: Psychotherapy as conversation.* New York: Academic Press.

Lyons, J. (Ed.). (1970). *New horizons in linguistics.* Harmondsworth, England: Penguin.

Michaels, S. (1981). "Sharing time": Children's narrative styles and differential access to literacy. *Language in Society, 10,* 423–442.

Nida, E. A. (1975). *Language structure and translation.* Stanford, CA: Stanford University Press.

Rivera, C. (Ed.) (1983). *An ethnographic/sociolinguistic approach to language proficiency assessment.* Clevedon, England: Multilingual Matters, Ltd.

Saville-Troike, M. (1982). *The ethnography of communication: An introduction.* Oxford: Basil Blackwell Publisher.

Saville-Troike, M. (1984). What REALLY matters in second language learning for academic achievement? *TESOL Quarterly, 18*(2), 199–219.

Saville-Troike, M., McClure, E., and Fritz, M. (1984). Communicative tactics in children's second language acquisition. In F. Eckman, L. H. Bell, and D. D. Nelson (Eds.), *Universals of second language acquisition* (pp. 60–71). Rowley, MA: Newbury House.

Schegloff, E. A. (1968). Sequencing in conversational openings. *American Anthropologist, 70,* 1075–1095.

Searle, J. (1969). *Speech acts.* Cambridge: Cambridge University Press.

Sherzer, J. (1975). Ethnography of speaking. Manuscript, University of Texas at Austin.

Sinclair, J., and Coulthard, M. (1975). *Towards an analysis of discourse: The language of teachers and pupils.* Oxford: Oxford University Press.

Tannen, D. (1979). What's in a frame? Surface evidence for underlying expectations. In R. Freedle (Ed.), *New directions in discourse processing* (pp. 137–181). Norwood, NJ: Ablex.

Tannen, D. (1981). Indirectness in discourse: Ethnicity as conversational style. *Discourse Processes, 4*(3), 221–238.

Tannen, D. (1984). *Conversational style: Analyzing talk among friends.* Norwood, NJ: Ablex.

Tannen, D., and Saville-Troike, M. (Eds.) (1985). *Perspectives on silence.* Norwood, NJ: Ablex.

Troike, R. C. (1983). Can language be tested? *Journal of Education, 165*(2), 209–216.

Tsuda, A. (1984). *Sales talk in Japan and the United States: An ethnographic analysis of contrastive speech events.* Washington, DC: Georgetown University Press.

Whorf, B. L. (1940). Science and linguistics. *Technological Review, 42,* 229–231, 247–248.

Williams, F. (1973). Some research notes on dialect attitudes and stereotypes. In R. W. Shuy and R. W. Fasold (Eds.). *Language attitudes: Current trends and prospects* (pp. 113–128). Washington, DC: Georgetown University Press.

Witherspoon, G. (1977). *Language and art in the Navajo universe.* Ann Arbor: University of Michigan Press.

PART II
LINGUISTIC AND CULTURAL DIVERSITY IN NORMAL COMMUNICATIVE PROCESSES AND BEHAVIOR

Chapter 4

Language Variation in the United States

Walt Wolfram

The existence of dialect variation within the English spoken in the United States is hardly a matter in dispute. It takes little linguistic sophistication to recognize of a range of American English varieties, and such variation is a frequent topic of popular social comment. Furthermore, the observation of dialect variation in the United States is hardly a recent phenomenon, for as long as English has been spoken in the New World, there has been some recognition of different dialects. Along with this recognition has come a persistent debate over the social role of the respective varieties and their symbolic significance. The recent emergence of the field of sociolinguistics may have brought the social significance of dialect variation into sharper research focus, but the recognition of dialect diversity will persist long after the faddish sociolinguistic debates of the current generation. Sociolinguistic diversity seems to be one of the inalienable manifestations of human behavioral differences.

Given the persistence of sociolinguistic diversity as a human language characteristic and the delicate faddishness with which particular social and educational "issues" rise and fall, it is valuable to understand some of the enduring principles that account for variation within language in general, and within the English language in particular. This chapter focuses, therefore, on explicating some of the primary social and linguistic parameters that help account for the continuing and persistent state of diversity, and it presents some models of variation that help account for the systematic nature of this diversity. In the process, it should be apparent that some of the popular myths surrounding the nature of diversity are unreasonable and unjustified, and that this phenomenon of variation, so readily recognizable on the surface, is indeed the manifestation of an intricate human adaptation process in a complex society.

WHY DIALECTS?

In the final analysis, dialects reflect basic behavioral differences between groups of individuals within a society and should be considered as natural as any other cultural manifestation of group differences. The same variables that account for differences in other dimensions of culture thus are typically relevant to the understanding of linguistic differences in society. However, the precise contribution of various variables to the overall configuration of dialect difference may be worked out somewhat differently from some other cultural phenomena, so that it is necessary to survey the major and minor factors that are operative in the definition of variation in the English of the United States. In addition, there are some important constraints that are placed on language diversity by the internal structure of *language* organization itself. In the following sections, we shall attempt to identify some of these variables and illustrate how they are manifested in representative dialects of English in the United States. It is hoped that this will give us a profile that can help us understand the systematic ways in which dialects are united and differentiated.

LINGUISTIC EXPLANATION

It is sometimes assumed that dialects of a language may differ in multifarious, random ways. This is not true. In fact, all of the accumulated evidence suggests that there exist some higher-order language principles that determine, to a large extent, the ways in which dialects of a language will differ from each other. Interestingly enough, these are the same principles that help us account for internal language change within a given variety over time, generalized adaptation strategies in second language learning, and certain first language adaptation strategies as well. It is not accidental that a common set of structures in English keeps recurring in the inventory of items characteristic of language variation across a number of different language situations. For example, aspects of subject-verb agreement, plural formation, verb phrase formation, and negative structures, among others, appear particularly susceptible to modification in the different language situations identified earlier. Why is it that these same structures are so susceptible to language variation, given the fact that the situations may be quite removed from one another in terms of language contact? The answer lies within the internal structure of language itself, the cognitive basis of its organization, and the pressures that the system places upon the modification of its structures.

As a starting point, we must understand that language is a dynamic system that is constantly in a state of change. The only unchanging language is a "dead" language. Some of the pressure to change comes from within the system, as the organizational patterns themselves exert pressure to adjust other items within the system on the basis of certain principles of organization, and some of the pressure comes from outside the system, as communities of language speakers come into contact with other communities of speakers using different patterns. Along the way, certain items fall prey to the pressure, often because of their inherent status within the system. In the following paragraphs we briefly present some of these linguistic principles that account for the high susceptibility of particular items to change and show how they are operative in the dialects of English.

Generalization

Other things being equal, there is natural pressure within a language to become more general in the application of its rules. A rule may naturally extend the parameters of its operation from a more specific to a more general linguistic environment, or it may extend the range of items included within the operation of a rule. For example, consider the current rule of negation in English and how the boundaries of this rule might be extended. The current standard English rule restricts the negative element to only one item within a sentence. With indefinites, the rule becomes somewhat selective, for the negative may be placed on the indefinite (preceding the verb) as in *Nobody went to school* or remain in the verb phrase (following the verb), as in *He didn't like anybody*. A further complication is added by the fact that an indefinite following the verb may take the negative instead of the verb under certain stylistic conditions, as in *He did nothing*. A rule for negative placement that slightly adjusts its parameters so that that it automatically negates the verb phrase and the indefinite is thus a more general version of the rule than one that selectively places it on one element only. Thus, in the following sentences, example 2 shows a more generalized version for negative placement than those in example 1, in which the sentences restrictively mark negation at one point only.

(1) a. The dog *didn't* like *anybody.*
     b. *Nobody* was there.
(2) a. The dog *didn't* like *nobody.*
     b. *Nobody wasn't* there.

In examples 1a and 1b, the negative element appears only at one point in the sentence, whereas in the examples 2a and 2b, the negative element appears without this restriction. Hence, we say that example 2 is a more general version of the rule of negation than example 1, and the kind of rule we might expect the English language to adopt as it changes over time or across varieties. In fact, we know that rules like those exemplified in example 2 are found in a number of vernacular varieties of English, the interlanguage of speakers learning English as a second language, and first language learners of English in their acquisitional process.* All of these language situations might be quite independent of each other in terms of language contact, but they fall subject to the same organizing principle of language patterning in its pressure to move toward more general language rules.

Similar cases of rule generalization can be found in the phonology of a language, as rules found in a restricted context in one language variety are generalized in other varities. For example, there is a restricted rule in standard English that operates to delete the unstressed initial [w] in the modal *will* or *would* (e.g., *I'll, I'd*). A more general version of this rule extends the deletion to other classes of words beginning in [w], so that items such as *was* or *ones* (in *they's* for *they was* or *young 'uns* for *young ones*) are produced by a more general version of the same rule affecting the initial [w] of *will* or *would,* which is lost in the "contraction" of modals.

The important point is that all languages prefer more general versions of rules, and there are inherent pressures from the language system to move in this direction. It is thus only natural that rule generalization would be a major linguistic cause standing behind the development of dialects within a language, as some varieties accept these natural changes and others reject them for one reason or another.

---

*The term "vernacular" is used to refer to nonstandard English varieties spoken typically by socially subordinate groups. In previous publications, terms such as "nonstandard" or "nonmainstream" have been used.

Regularization

Another natural pressure on language systems from within is the tendency toward regularization. Language systems tolerate irregularities, but they do not prefer them, and, over the course of time, they are predisposed to make irregular patterns conform to the dominant, productive patterns. Today's version of standard English has, of course, regularized many of yesterday's irregularities, and it is only reasonable to expect that some current varieties of English would differ from others in the application of this natural linguistic predisposition. For example, each of the sentences in example 3 typifies a regularization of some type.

(3) a. He *knowed* the man.
     b. They pulled the *oxes*.
     c. *Mines* is here.
     d. That is *badder* than this.

Example 3a illustrates regularization of an irregular verb form, 3b the regularization of an irregular plural, 3c the regularization of the possessive suffix form, and 3d the regularization of the comparative form. Students of the history of the English language know, of course, that many of our present-day regular forms resulted exactly from this process. It is natural, expected, and predictable that a language should be modified in this way, and language variation will often manifest this principle. And the observer of dialect diversity in American English will readily recognize that each of the forms illustrated in example 3 is typical of representative vernacular varieties and the interlanguage in some stages of L_2 learners of English as well, as it is subject to the same principle.

Redundancy Reduction

All languages contain considerable redundancy in their structure, that is, they mark at more than one point a particular grammatical function. Although a certain amount of redundancy appears necessary within language to maintain its communicative efficiency, there exists pressure within systems to eliminate some of the structural redundancy. Common examples of redundant marking in English are the third person singular present tense form, which co-occurs with a third person subject noun or pronoun (e.g., *She* likes the story) and the plural form, which often co-occurs with a quantifier of some type (e.g., *many* boys, *four* inches). Given the inherent pressures of language systems to reduce structural redundancy, we might reasonably expect it to be one of the natural ways in which varieties of a language will differ from each other. The sentences in example 4, to be found in some vernacular varieties of English, reflect this natural process.

(4) a. She like ___ the class.
     b. The pole is four inch ___ long.
     c. John ___ hat is on the floor.

The sentences in example 4 illustrate that the three structural functions of the -s or -es suffix — third person singular (4a), plural (4b), and possessive (4c), are, to some extent, redundant structural markers, since other structural factors may also signal the structural information. Similarly, a construction such as the copula verb in present tense may be a redundant form in many types of predication, as in constructions such as *He's ugly* and *He's the man*. No information is lost, and the relationships of predication are indicated just as adequately in structures such as *He ugly* and *He the man*. Historically, we again see parallels in the development of modern standard English. For example, English lost many of the case endings of Latin as it developed more strict ordering of elements to indicate grammatical relationships such as subject, object, and so forth. The case endings became vulnerable when other structural details marked the same function as well. The essential point is that redundantly marked structures are particularly susceptible to modification, and they are a natural way in which dialects of a language would thus differ.

Analogy

In analogy, patterns of language are remodeled on the basis of existing patterns. In most cases, the analogy operates to create conformity to majority patterns, as in the case of regularization cited earlier. Regularization is, in fact, one kind of analogy. However, patterns may also be remodeled on the basis of minority patterns, in which case some of the irregular patterns may be enhanced. In current standard English, the past and participle forms of *ring, rang*, and *rung* developed by analogy with the minority irregular pattern *sing, sang*, and *sung*. In some vernacular dialects, we see shifts toward some of the irregular paradigms that coexist with regularization. For example, the vernacular formation of *bring, brang, brung* (e.g., *He brang them a present* or *He has brung them a present*) conforms to a minority pattern of *sing, sang*, and *sung* by analogy. Shifting of subclasses in this manner is not an uncommon change in language and is found in a number of different dialects of English. For example, the undifferentiation of present and past tense forms in *come* and *run* (e.g., *Yesterday he come to my house; Yesterday he run to my house*), as found in some vernacular dialects, may be seen as a shift that aligns these items with an existent class of irregular verbs in standard English, including *put* and *set* (e.g., *Yesterday he put it up; Yesterday he set it up*). In fact, the only difference is that the one class of items has become socially stigmatized and the other has not. Analogy toward majority and minority patterns in language is a natural process in language and must be expected as language progresses through time. As mentioned earlier, many of our current standard English forms developed in this way, and there is no reason to expect that the situation should be any different in vernacular varieties. The social judgments that rendered some changes by analogy socially acceptable and others socially stigmatized has nothing to do with the natural course of language itself, but instead relates to the social status of particular groups in society in which these changes were manifested.

Although the principles presented here are neither exhaustive nor mutually exclusive, they illustrate the essential dynamics of language variation that originate from the internal structure of language itself. Perhaps more importantly, they illustrate the naturalness of the changes that result in different varieties. So long as language is spoken, it will continue to develop and change, and dialect difference is just one of the ways in which the different stages and rates of change are captured. In fact, the major difference between standard and vernacular dialects is not in the principles of change, for they are universal, but in the social parameters that deem some changes socially acceptable and others socially stigmatized.

THE SOCIAL PARAMETER*

As repeatedly seen in the preceding discussion, the changes in language that result in different dialects are both natural and inevitable. What gives such natural change social significance is not the structure of language but the structure of society and the various social factors that take on significance within a given society. In complex, heterogeneous societies, there can be a number of different variables that interact with each other in the constitution of dialectal entities. We shall discuss some of the major social factors that have

---

*The discussion of the social parameter and sociolinguistic models of variation is a revised and updated version of sections found in Wolfram (1981).

contributed to the current configuration of American English dialects. Again, the inventory of identified variables is not exhaustive, and they do not work in isolation. It is, however, convenient to discuss these factors separately, with the understanding that it is an artifice of our description rather than a reflection of social reality.

Region

Historically, probably more attention has been given to geographically correlated variation in American English than to any other type; in fact, it has only been within the last two decades that other factors have been given any primary consideration at all. The correlation of varieties of English with geographical location is, of course, a reflection of underlying historical patterns that have led to the present-day pattern of variation. In some cases, regional variation can be traced to different patterns of settlement history in which the migration of early settlers is still reflected in the language. For the Anglo-American population, some of the regional differences reflect the fact that settlers came from different regions of England where regionally based variation was already existent; others may reflect the influences of another language, as when settlers came from non–English-speaking lands, or from creole-speaking contexts, as hypothesized for the Black population historically (cf. Dillard, 1972; Stewart, 1970).

Patterns of population movement within the United States are also reflected in regional differences. Thus, a major shift in the Anglo-American population has been from east to west, and a number of dialect differences parallel this movement. For the Black population, the major dialect boundaries run from south to north, in line with the major migratory routes of the population historically within the United States.

When considering the regional aspects of variation in American English, the role of physical geography cannot be overlooked, since it, too, has exerted its historical influence on language differences. Although transportational obstacles are not generally considered to be a serious handicap with modern technological advances, separation of areas by rivers, mountains, and other natural boundaries has inhibited the spread of language in the past, because it restricted the mobility necessary for the diffusion of linguistic forms from one location to another. For the Anglo-American population, the case of "Appalachian" and "Ozark" English is such an instance, in which the highland isolation is cited as the physical basis for the resistance to some changes that occurred elsewhere in the development of

American English. A similar case of physical isolation is often cited for the historical maintenance of Gullah (or "Geechee"), a creole-based variety found among Blacks in the South Sea Isles off the coast of South Carolina and Georgia. In this case, of course, the physical boundary is the island status.

Traditionally, the geographical distribution of differences in American English was traced by plotting particular linguistic items on maps. It is possible to draw *isoglosses* on a map (i.e., lines separating areas that use a particular item from those that do not) demarking the boundaries of usage regionally. These differences can be identified on any level of language organization, including phonological (e.g., the pronunciation of *father* with or without a final *r*), morphological (e.g., the use of *hisself* for *himself* as the third person masculine reflexive), syntactic (e.g., forming indirect questions as *He asked could he go to the movies* versus *He asked if he could go to the movies*), lexical (the use of the term *pop* versus *soda*), or pragmatic (e.g., the different use of respect terms such as *sir* and *ma'am* by children to parents in the North and South). Most of the traditional studies in dialect geography focused on phonological and lexical differences in their surveys of regional patterns, although significant differences may exist on all of these levels. Major regional areas are defined, then, on the basis of a number of isoglosses that cluster in approximately the same way. An example of one type of map delimiting some major regional varieties of English for the Anglo-American, Black, and Hispanic populations is illustrated in Figure 4-1.

Although such a map is useful in an approximative way, some qualification is necessary. Lines on a map such as this make it appear that the dialects are discrete entities exclusively possessing the territories in the area demarked by the lines. More detailed examination would reveal that dialect boundaries most often do not coincide in a precise way. In many cases, differences between varieties are not discrete, but are relative in terms of a continuum of differences. Furthermore, some of the differences between varieties may be quantitative rather than qualitative. That is, two or more varieties may share a particular feature, but its relative frequency in one variety may distinguish it from another one. In addition, there is often a transitional area between dialects where forms may be in considerable fluctuation.

When we examine the nature of regional variation, we find that it most frequently is the result of the spread of language changes through geographical space over time. By analogy, this is likened to the effect of a pebble that is dropped into a pool of water. A particu-

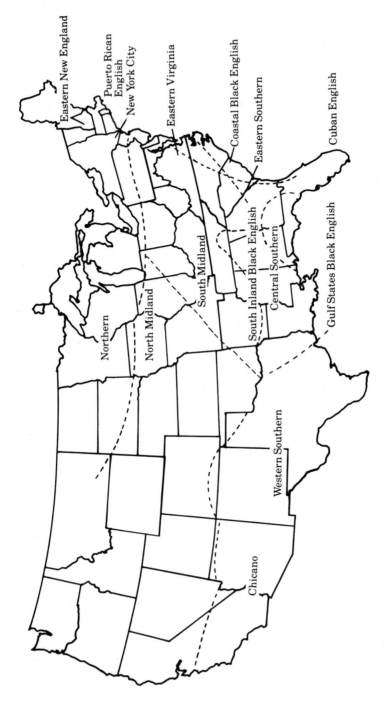

Figure 4-1. Map of major dialect areas for Anglo-American, Black, and Hispanic English.

lar change takes place at a given point in time and space and spreads from that point in successive waves or stages. The most concentrated existence of the linguistic item will be in the area where it was first introduced, and the outer periphery of the diffusion will evidence less concentration, because the change came later to the area. The outer boundaries, however, are not static but dynamic, constantly undergoing change., which makes the rigorous delimitation of geographically related boundaries a relative rather than an absolute thing.

Finally, there are other social factors, such as those to be discussed later, that complicate the examination of differences in simple terms of geographical space. Variables such as social status, ethnicity, gender, and so forth, clearly transcend the simple geographical distribution of items. Regional differences, then, are an important first step in examining the social variables affecting language, but they cannot be discussed in isolation from other social variables. In the last two decades, sociolinguists have shown that other factors may be just as important, if not more important, in arriving at a realistic picture of variation in American English. If the multiple dimensions of diversity in American English are to be understood, it is necessary to describe and analyze language variation as it co-occurs and intersects with as many of these dimensions as possible.

Social Status

In a society in which social status is such an obvious dimension of its structure, it can be expected that essential aspects of variation will correlate with social status differentiation. Naturally, this variable does not operate independently of other considerations, including the regional dimension just discussed. We can speak of social status dialects of American English so long as we realize that they do not exist in isolation from other social variables, including region, ethnicity, and style, among others. As it turns out, there are some aspects of variation in American English that have social significance only within a given regional context, whereas others have a much broader geographical significance. For example, the absence of the upgliding of the vowel in items such as *time* and *ride* (i.e., [tam] and [rad]) or the lack of contrast between the vowels in *pin* and *pen* (i.e., both occurring as [pIn]) may not be particularly significant in some Southern contexts, whereas its use in a Northern context may hold social significance. On the other hand, the absence of a third person singular -*s* and possessive -*s* as in *She go* for *She goes* or *the boy coat* for *the boy's coat* are socially significant regardless of the particular locale. Although there are exceptions, phonological features tend to be more regionally constrained than grammatical ones in their status differentiation.

Socially diagnostic items (i.e., items that distinguish social groups from one another) may be either *prestigious* or *stigmatized*; prestigious items are those used by high status groups as linguistic manifestations of social status, whereas socially stigmatized items are associated with low status groups. In some varieties of English, the slight raising quality of the vowel in items like *pass* or *fact* and the pronunciation of *either* as [ayðɚ] have a prestige function. On the other hand, the pronunciation of the word-initial *th* as a stop in *they* (i.e., [dey]) and the the pronunciation of *th* as *f* in *tooth* (i.e., [tuf]) are stigmatized, as is the the use of so-called double negative in *They didn't do nothing*. It is important to understand that the absence of a prestige feature does not necessarily imply that the alternative is stigmatized; nor does absence of a stigmatized feature imply that the alternative is prestigious. For example, the absence of the raised quality in the vowels of *pass* or *fact* or the pronunciation of *either* as [iðɚ] is not stigmatized. Conversely, the use of single negatives as *He didn't do anything* or the use of an interdental fricative in *they* is not particularly prestigious; it is simply not stigmatized. It is further important to understand that the social significance of particular items changes over time, for one reason or another. For example, in the history of the English language, double negatives were well within the standard dialect in earlier centuries, and the use of *ain't* was socially acceptable well into the eighteenth century in England. In New York City speech, the absence of postvocalic *r* (e.g., [fo] for *four*) was the prestigious pronunciation until the 1940s but has since reversed its social significance (i.e., it is now stigmatized) among the younger generation of New Yorkers.

Among the dialects of American English, contrasts between stigmatized and nonstigmatized variants are much more typical than constrasts between prestige and nonprestige variants. This observation tends to match the subjective reaction that most Americans have to the varieties of American English: they tend to react more in terms of negative responses to socially stigmatized linguistic items than they do in terms of positive responses to socially prestigious forms. On an informal level, mainstream or standard dialects of English are most practically defined in terms of the absence of socially stigmatized variants rather than in terms of the presence of prestige items. Clearly, the importance of the stigmatized or nonstigmatized dimension on an overt level is much more dramatic in differentiating social status than the prestige or nonprestige dimension.

Socially diagnostic items in American English may differ considerably in how they correlate with social status. There are some features that correlate with more finely differentiated social status groupings, whereas there are others that reveal a much more discrete break between groups. For example, within the different social groups of the Black community in Detroit there are quite different distributions for the absence of postvocalic *r* in items like *father* or *four* and the absence of third-person singular *-s* as in *He go*. The contrast for four social status groups of Black speakers, taken from Wolfram (1969), is given in Figures 4–2 and 4–3.

For the most part, socially diagnostic grammatical items tend to stratify more sharply than phonological ones. Sharp stratification refers to a clearcut demarcation of linguistic features between adjacent social classes so that the middle class would be clearly differentiated from the working class in the use of the features. Phonological features tend to stratify gradiently. Gradient stratification refers to a more graded progressive increase in the use of the features. This probably reflects the relative significance of phonological and grammatical items in defining the differences between the vernacular and standard dialects of English. The more rigid the social boundaries in a society, the more sharply we expect the linguistic features to stratify the population. In a sense, the operation of both gradient and sharp linguistic stratification in American society reflects the

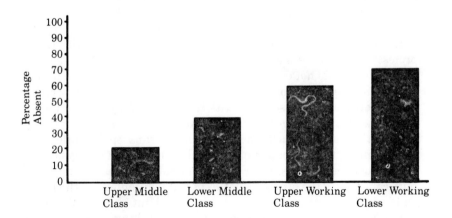

Figure 4-2. Postvocalic *r* absence in four social status groups of Blacks in Detroit, as an example of gradient stratification.

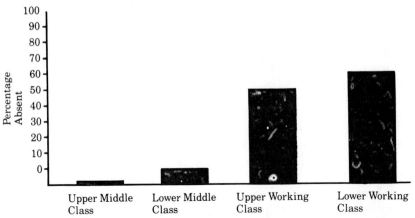

Figure 4-3. Third person singular -*s* in four social status groups of Blacks in Detroit, as an example of sharp stratification.

complexities of the system, in which both a social status continuum and a class system have been operative historically.

Ethnicity

Without a doubt, the most emotionally laden topic in the discussion of variation in American English is that relating to ethnicity and language differences. The essential debate here is whether varieties of American English correlate in a unique way with America's different ethnic groups, be they Black, Hispanic, American Indian, Jewish, Vietnamese, or any other group. Issues surrounding language and ethnicity have become highly charged for both lay and professional observers alike, and there are few social discussions of this topic that do not evoke strong feelings on the part of the participants. For the layperson, the possibility of distinct ethnic varieties has sometimes been associated with the supposed physical or mental attributes of the particular ethnic group. If, for example, it were admitted that some Black and Anglo-Americans spoke differently, then it might be a reflection of some inherent mental or physical difference between the groups. For the professional researcher, the dispute concerning the ethnic varieties of English centers on the historical origin of varieties used within the United States and the dynamics of the social patterns that affect language. Language scholars take as axiomatic that a language variety acquired by a given ethnic group has no inherent relation to the physical or mental characteristics of that group. The supposed physical or mental basis of such a correlation is readily disproved by those situations in which a person from one ethnic group is isolated from that particular ethnic group. In these situations, we find the individual's speech indistinguishable from persons of the immediate community. Thus, a Black who is socialized in an exclusively Anglo-American group will speak as the others in the group, and vice versa. Similarly, a Vietnamese child raised exclusively in an Anglo-American group will speak no differently from the other members of the group.

In recent years, the most hotly debated issue on ethnicity and language is the relationship between Black and white vernacular dialects. In Northern urban areas, it is quite apparent that working-class Blacks often use a variety of English that is much different from their white working-class counterparts, but the issue is more hotly contested when comparable socioeconomic groups are compared in the rural South, since most vernacular varieties of Black speech have had their origin within the United States in rural Southern environments.

Although some data are still necessary, recent analyses of available evidence (e.g., Fasold, 1981) indicate that even in the rural South, where the vernacular varieties are much more similar, they are not identical. The dialects in the rural South are not as dissimilar as sometimes alleged (e.g., Dillard, 1972; Stewart, 1970), and a number of the structures thought to be unique have been found in both varieties (e.g., Bailey, 1985). Still, they are not identical. As with other varieties of English (for example, "Appalachian English" as defined by Wolfram and Christian, 1976), the uniqueness of vernacular Black English may rest not in the establishment of unique structures per se but in the combination of items that make up the variety. Reinforcement of the objective evidence comes from various identification tasks in which listeners are asked to identify the ethnicity of a speaker on the basis of an audio-recording. In most structured research of this type (Giles and Powesland, 1976), the accuracy of ethnic identification exceeds 80 percent.

In most instances, the extent to which ethnicity correlates with language diversity is a function of the social distance between particular ethnic groups. With the increased assimilation of ethnic members into the mainstream culture, we may expect the factor of ethnicity to be reduced, but with ethnic isolation of one type or another, the variable will take on major significance. In reality, ethnic isolation occurs in varying degrees, depending on the social roles of various groups in American society. We may expect, for example, that a relatively homogeneous Jewish community will reveal some linguistic differences in comparison with other groups (Gold, 1981), but we would predict that the differences will not be nearly as striking as those revealed by the Black community because of the relative social segregation of these groups historically within the United States.

When an ethnic group speaks another language, the influence of this language may be incorporated into the differential basis of the English variety as well. Given the influence of German in southeastern Pennsylvania, it is not surprising to find structures such as *The soup is all* or *Are you going with* as ongoing English remnants of this historical German language background. Similar kinds of influence in terms of a creole language predecessor have frequently been cited to account for vernacular Black English forms such as *she nice* or *He been known that*. Varieties of Hispanic English (Ornstein-Galicia, 1984; Penalosa, 1980) and American Indian English (Leap, 1977; Wolfram, 1984) also reveal such substratal influence in the stabilizing English varieties. In examining structures attributable to ancestral language background, it is necessary to distinguish "interlanguage" forms, which result as an intermediate stage in the transitory process of acquiring English as a second language, and to identify those structures that become integrated and maintained by successive generations of speakers as a part of the ethnic variety of English. Some of the perpetuated structures may be evidenced in quite indirect and subtle ways (cf. Baugh, 1983), thus making the factor of ethnicity and language much more complex than it appears on the surface.

Gender

Although we do not typically think of American English as being differentiated in terms of male and female varieties, there are certainly aspects of language selection and usage that correlate with the sex of the speaker or hearer. If asked to identify the sex of the speaker who utters a sentence such as *Oh my, you shouldn't have done that, but you are a dear*, or *What an adorable package*, most of us would have little difficulty identifying the speaker as female. This is because the selection of vocabulary items, such as expletives and descriptive adjectives, in certain domains typically correlates with the sex of the speaker.

In the last decade, the topic of language and gender has gained popular notoriety, and it has now become one of the major areas of focus for some sociolinguists. Many articles, anthologies, and textbooks have recently appeared on this topic (cf. Frank and Anshen, 1984; Smith, 1985), but it is still difficult to ascertain some of the definitive conclusions of such studies. For levels of language organization such as phonology and grammar, gender does not appear to be a major variable; it tends to be a moderating variable that intersects with other major variables, such as region, status, and ethnicity. Various studies have, for example, indicated that males show a higher incidence of socially stigmatized phonological and grammatical variants than their female counterparts, but that the differences are quantitative rather than qualitative. For example, both working-class males and females may use multiple negatives (e.g., *He didn't like nothing*) or "*g*-dropping" (e.g., *sittin'*), but males tend to use these structures more frequently.

The tendency of males to use more stigmatized variants than females in their speech is probably best seen as a reflection of different socialized behavioral roles for men and women. There are clearly positive values of masculinity associated with vernacular speech for males, although in some cases these are more covert than overt (Trudgill, 1972). Conversely, we expect females to have a higher incidence of prestige features than their male counterparts of comparable socioeconomic class within a given region. Thus, if a raised quality of the vowel in *bat* and *rack* takes on a prestige value, we would expect higher frequency levels of its usage among middle-class women. The socialized sensitivity of women to prestige norms makes them prime candidates for linguistic change, and studies of change across the United States (Labov, Yaeger, and Steiner, 1972) indicate that women are often responsible for the initial adoption of new prestige variants in a given locale undergoing change.

Many of the more recent studies of gender-related differences in English have focused on the higher levels of language usage, including pragmatics, discourse, and conversational analysis. Although some of the evidence is still preliminary, it appears that these levels of language usage may reveal some of the more significant language differences between the sexes (e.g., Kramarae, 1981, indicates that women are much more likely to be interrupted in turn-taking than men). Future studies may reveal that some of the subtle, but significant, differences between male and female language usage reside in *how* language is used rather than *what* is used in terms of linguistic items per se.

Age

Two aspects of age differences are relevant to the understanding of dialect diversity in English. One aspect of age differences relates to the changes taking place in American English that differentiate successive generations. Typically, a change taking place in a younger generation will not affect the older generation of speakers, whose language system has been firmly stabilized. For example, older residents of Appalachia and the Ozarks use a prefix on certain *-ing* participial forms as in *He was a-hunting and a-fishing* or *He was busy a-fixing the meal.* The current generation of speakers learning English, however, does not use this form nearly as frequently as older speakers (Christian, Wolfram, and Dube, 1984). This is a function of the language change taking place in these highland dialects as the forms are undergoing change or being eliminated. From this perspective, successive generations within the population may be viewed as representing the English language in its varying stages of evolution. Apart from the contact situations that have brought about change (and there are a number of such situations), the difference between the English brought to the New World by the original English-speaking settlers and the varieties of English extant today is thus a summation of changes exhibited by different generations of speakers.

The other aspect of age differences relates to the life cycle of an individual speaker. Within this cycle, there are certain behavioral patterns considered appropriate for various stages of life. The most stereotyped of these is the case of so-called teen-aged slang, in which particular vocabulary items are correlated with a particular phase of the life cycle. For the most part, vocabulary items of this type (e.g., *gig* for *job*, *smooth* for *nice*, etc.) have a rapid life cycle, so that the expressions of today's youth will not be carried over to the next generation; subsequent generations will come up with their own items. Although the particular items will change, the selection of a slang unique to each generation's youth will be perpetuated.

The most stereotypical aspects of age-graded language differences in American English are certainly found in certain vocabulary items, but there are also differences on other levels of language as well. It is quite possible that certain phases of adolescence, influenced heavily by peer pressure, will show more socially stigmatized language variants than adult speech in the community. It is also possible that linguistic influences from other communities will be maximized during certain age periods. For example, in East Harlem, New York, adolescent and teen-aged Puerto Rican boys may be directly and indirectly influenced by the vernacular Black English (Wolfram, 1974) of the surrounding community. As the life cycle of these speakers proceeds, however, many of the vernacular Black English features will be leveled or eliminated. Although this manifestation of life cycle differences in language variety is a bit more extreme than that found in other communities, moderate adaptations of language during the earlier stages of the life cycle are quite typical within American society.

Language Style

Style is one of those dimensions of language that intersects in an important way with all of the preceding variables we have discussed. Virtually every speaker of the English language has some range of style along a continuum of formality. The range of styles used by individual speakers and the conditions for adjusting along this continuum, however, vary considerably. In earlier sociolinguistic studies, the critical variable defining the dimension of formality and informality in language style was reduced to a single "principle of attention" paid to speech (Labov, 1972): the more attention paid to speech, the more formal the style. Formal styles were thus defined as those used in situations in which speech is the primary focus, whereas informal styles were defined in terms of those used in situations in which there is the least amount of speaker audio-monitoring.

More recent focus on the parameter of style (Bell, 1984; Romaine, 1980) has shown that the reduction of stylistic formality to a single principle such as the attention to speech is oversimplified and unjustified. Bell claims that considerations such as the language variety of the interlocutors and accommodation of the addressee audience seem to supersede the simple principle of attention paid to speech. It seems essential to recognize that there are other social dimensions that may be responsible for stylistic shifts, and these may or may not work in tandem with the "attention" paid to speech. It is also erroneous simply to equate formality with the standard-vernacular continuum (Baugh, 1983), although there is an obvious interactional effect between formality-informality and standard-nonstandard forms.

In many cases, the relative usage of particular features is clearly related to style, regardless of the social or regional definition of the variety. For example, the use of -in' for -ing in unstressed syllables (e.g., swimmin', nothin') is found to some extent in all varieties of English, but is found more frequently in informal styles by all groups. We thus expect that a stigmatized variant will show reduced usage and a prestige variant increased usage as we move from informal to more formal styles. The ideal situation for -in' usage is illustrated in Table 4–1 (adapted from Wolfram and Fasold, 1974).

Some variants, such as taboo terms and certain socially stigmatized features, may be totally absent from more formal styles while persisting in more informal styles. It has also been shown that some

Table 4-1. Frequency Patterns for -*in'* Usage in Different Social Classes and Styles

Social Class	Style	
	Informal	*Formal*
Middle	Intermediate frequency	Low frequency
Working	High frequency	Low frequency

Adapted from Wolfram, W., and Fashold, R.W. (1974). *The study of social dialects in American English.* Englewood Cliffs, NJ: Prentice-Hall. Reprinted with permission.

older forms of a language variety undergoing change may be retained as symbolic, stylistic indicators of indigenous speech. Feagin (1979) has identified such a function for the Appalachian English a-prefix mentioned earlier.

The dimension of style has different significance at various periods in the life cycle of an individual and may take on differing roles in different communities. For example, stylistic variation may be maximized during those stages of life when young adults are establishing their own role and status in American society vis-à-vis their parents, as they are caught between "where they come from and where they are going." Older speakers, particularly men, are more likely to be resigned to their particular status and role in American society and less likely to shift styles in any significant way. Different groups may also show different tendencies in terms of the range of stylistic repertoires. For example, Blacks tend to have greater stylistic flexibility than whites, although particular individuals within respective communities may certainly defy this pattern.

An essential point to remember in examining the variable of style is that all varieties of English are subject to this constraint, and that the collection of dialect data may be highly sensitive to the conditions under which it is gathered. For this reason, quite different pictures of an English variety may emerge when the focus is on single item responses collected by an outsider in the context of some formal institution, rather than on the natural flow of spontaneous conversation among peers in an informal community setting.

MODELS OF DIALECT RELATIONSHIPS

In the previous sections, we attempted to set forth some of the linguistic principles that account for the natural language change resulting in different dialects and the social parameters that are essential to the definition of English varieties. At this point, we want to turn to the nature of the linguistic relations among these variations. As a preface to this discussion, we must recognize that there exists a large core of structures common to all varieties of English. The clear majority of patterns on all levels of language are common to all varieties of English. Granted this common base, we still want to know the nature and extent to which the varieties of English differ from each other. On the basis of our previous discussion of linguistic principles accounting for diversity, we expect the varieties to show structured, systematic relations to each other. Although the interpretation of linguistic patterning found in recent "variation theory" takes us beyond some of the traditional notions of patterning in traditional linguistics, it can be demonstrated that there are sometimes intricate and subtle aspects of patterning to be found among the varieties of American English.

Systematic Variability

First of all, we must point out that differences between varieties may be either qualitative or quantitative, and often varieties are differentiated on the basis of both types of patterns. In qualitative differences, linguistic forms found in one variety are categorically absent in another variety. For example, the so-called "habitual *be*" found in vernacular Black English (e.g., *He usually be upstairs*) is completely absent from the systems of many other varieties of English, as is the use of *a*-prefixing found in Appalachian English (e.g., *He was a-huntin'*). Similarly, regionally defined constructions such as *The house needs painted* or so-called "positive *anymore*" (with a meaning approximate to "nowadays") in constructions such as *She goes to the movies alot anymore* are found in some varieties but never in others. Hence, we may say that these forms show a qualitative dimension in their distribution.

At the same time, there are a number of structures that show a quantitative dimension. That is, varieties are differentiated from each other not on the basis of discrete sets of features, but by variations in the frequencies with which certain forms or rules occur. This discovery by sociolinguists over the past two decades is in some ways at variance with popular perceptions of how the varieties of English are differentiated, because it is commonly held that particular low status groups always use a particular socially stigmatized variant and high status groups never do. Thus, it may be thought that vernacular dialects always use *-in'* for unstressed *-ing* and middle-class varieties never do, or that the respective groups differ categorically in their use of the stop for *th* as in *dis* for *this* or *dey* for *they*. In these cases, however, the varieties are more typically differentiated by the extent to which the process is applied rather than the qualitative absence or presence.

Table 4–2 below shows the actual frequency levels of *-in'* for *-ing*, a phonological variable, and pronominal apposition (e.g., *My mother she's coming to school* as opposed to *My mother's coming to school*) in four different social status groups of Detroit speakers. In this table, adapted from Wolfram (1969), the percentage represents the number of times the item was actually used in relation to the number of times it could have been used. For example, every time an unstressed form of *-ing* occurs, as in *He went fishing*, the item was transcribed as [ŋ] or [n], and the percentage represents the incidence of [n] out of the total of unstressed *-ing* forms transcribed for each social status group. Although the figures represent the mean for each group, all of the individual speakers exhibit this variability in *-ing* and *-in'*. A similar pattern of variation between forms like *My mother, she's coming to school* and *My mother's coming to school* is found.

Table 4–2. Relative Frequency of a Variable Phonological and Grammatical Feature in Four Social Status Groups in Detroit

	Upper Middle Class	Lower Middle Class	Upper Working Class	Lower Working Class
Percentage of *-in'* Forms	19.4	39.1	50.5	78.9
Percentage of Pronominal Apposition	4.5	13.6	25.4	23.8

That we can observe variation between alternate forms such as *-ing* and *-in'* does not necessarily mean that the fluctuation is completely random or haphazard. Although we cannot predict which variant might be used in a given instance, there are factors that increase or decrease the likelihood that certain variants will occur. For example, the various social factors cited previously can all be important influences that affect the relative frequency of *-in'* occurrence. Not all of the systematic effectson variability, however, can be accounted for simply by appealing to social factors. There are also aspects of the linguistic system itself that may systematically affect the variability of particular forms. Particular types of linguistic contexts, such as structure of surrounding forms, may also influence the relative frequency with which these forms occur.

The systematic effect of independent linguistic factors on the relative frequency of particular forms can best be understood by way of illustration. Consider the case of word-final consonant cluster reduction as it affects sound sequences such as *st*, *nd*, *ld*, *kt*, and so forth. In this rule, items such as *west*, *wind*, *cold*, and *act* may be reduced to *wes'*, *win'*, *col'*, and *ac'*, respectively. It is observed that the incidence of reduction is quite variable, but certain linguistic factors systematically influence its reduction. The linguistic factors include whether the following word begins with a consonant, as opposed to a vowel, and the way in which the cluster is formed. With reference to the following environment, we find that a following word that begins with a consonant will greatly increase the likelihood that the reduction process will operate. Thus, for example, we find reduction more frequent in a context such as *west coast* or *cold cuts* than in a context such as "west end" or "cold apple." Reduction takes place in both linguistic contexts, but is consistently favored when the following word begins with a consonant.

As mentioned earlier, cluster reduction is also influenced by the way in which the cluster is formed. Clusters that are a part of an inherent word base, such as *wind* or *guest*, are more likely to undergo reduction than clusters that are formed through the addition of an -*ed* suffix, such as *guessed* (which ends in [*st*] phonetically) and or *wined* (which ends in [nd] phonetically). Again, we note that fluctuation can be observed in both kinds of clusters, but that it is favored quantitatively in one type of cluster over the other type.

When we compare different linguistic effects on the relative frequency of a pattern such as cluster reduction, we find that some linguistic variables will have a greater effect on the pattern than others. Thus, in some dialects of English, the influence of the following segment (consonant versus vowel) is more influential than the cluster formation type (-*ed* versus non-*ed*). In a sense, this is comparable to the effect of different social variables, such as social status, region, gender, and so forth, which may all affect the incidence of reduction, but not in equal proportions.

In many cases, the linguistic constraints on variation can be found to operate across different varieties of English. Table 4–3 presents an inventory of representative dialects in their incidence of cluster reduction, based on a compilation of sociolinguistic studies conducted in these varieties during the past two decades. As we see in Table 4–3, all the varieties of English represented here are systematically influenced in the same way by the following linguistic environment and the formation of the cluster, although the proportional differences and the relationship between the linguistic variables is not always the same.

Table 4–3.   Comparison of Consonant Cluster Simplification in Representative Vernacular Dialects

	Linguistic Context			
	Followed by Consonant		*Followed by Vowel*	
Language Variety	*Not -ed % Reduction*	*-ed % Reduction*	*Not -ed % Reduction*	*-ed % Reduction*
Standard English	66	36	12	3
Northern White Working Class	67	23	19	3
Southern White Working Class	56	16	25	10
Appalachian Working Class	74	67	17	5
Northern Black Working Class	97	76	72	34
Southern Black Working Class	88	50	72	36
Chicano Working Working Class	91	61	66	22
Puerto Rican Working Class	93	78	63	23
Italian-American Working Class	67	39	14	10
American Indian Puebloan English	98	92	88	81
Vietnamese English	98	93	75	60

To understand the nature of differentiation among different varieties of English, it is necessary to appreciate the quantitative dimensions of some of these differences, as indicated earlier, and the systematic social and linguistic effects on variability. We see that the actual relationships of the forms are not nearly as simple as the categorical judgments people are prone to make, but instead they are highly structured in some rather subtle ways. The systematic nature of social and linguistic influences on fluctuating forms indicates one aspect of this detailed patterning.

Implicational Relationships

Systematic aspects of the quantitative dimension of language differences is not the only way in which the orderly relationships of dialects can be viewed. Another way of looking at the relationship between varieties is through the combinations of language structures. The forms that differentiate one variety from another are not distributed randomly throughout the system; instead, there are often *implicational relations* that hold between various forms in particular varieties.

An implicational relation in language variation holds when the presence of a particular characteristic in any variety of language implies the presence of another characteristic in that same variety. When form *B* is always present whenever form *A* is present, we say that "*A* implies *B*." However, the converse is not true, so that *B* may exist with or without the presence of *A*.

As an example of an implicational relation, we can consider the case of copula deletion, as it is called (i.e., the absence of the verb *be* in the present tense of forms such as *You ugly* (*You're ugly*) or *He reading the book* (*He's reading the book*). Varieties of American English differ in the amount of copula deletion they show, and there is a systematic implicational relationship between copula deletion involving *is* and *are*. Copula deletion of *is* necessarily implies the absence of *are*, but the converse is not true. In other words, if a variety of English shows the absence of *is* in sentences such as *He ugly*, it will also show absence in sentences with *are*, such as *You ugly*. However, a variety may have sentences such as *You ugly* without having sentences such as *He ugly*. An implicational array for this relationship, which is found in vernacular Black English and vernacular white Southern speech is found in Table 4–4, where "1" stands for the presence of the characteristic (in this case, the operation of the copula deletion rule), and "O" the absence of the characteristic. Also included in the array is standard English, which has neither *is* nor *are* deletion. In the array, the column to the left implies the column to the right.

Table 4–4. **Implicational Relationship Between** *Is* **and** *Are* **Deletion**

Language Variety	*is* Deletion	*are* Deletion
Standard English	0	0
Vernacular Southern White English	0	1
Vernacular Black English	1	1

As we might expect, the implicational relationships that hold between structures in the varieties of American English can sometimes be much more complex than the simple illustrative case, and sociolinguistic analyses have provided some fairly involved cases. More importantly, we find that implicational relationships demonstrate two important dimensions with respect to language relationships. First of all, this model provides a systematic basis for looking at the orderly relationships that exist among dialects. Our illustrative case shows several steps in the orderly differentiation of standard English, vernacular Southern white speech, and vernacular Black English. Given various steps in an implicational array, it is possible to determine the relative distance between dialects. For example, we see in Table 4–4 that vernacular Black English is closer to vernacular Southern white English than it is to standard English in its use of copula deletion. Vernacular Southern white English, however, is closer to standard English than vernacular Black English.

The second dimension added by implicational analysis relates to language change. As stated at the outset of our discussion, language change is an ongoing, dynamic process that takes place in a systematic way. Generally, this change will proceed through the orderly steps that are reflected in the implicational array. For example, suppose that a dialect is moving toward the standard variety by eliminating the rule of copula deletion. We would expect the progressive steps in the change to first eliminate the copula deletion rule for *is*, and then for *are*. In fact, there is evidence that some Black English varieties are moving toward standard white English in exactly this way, as *are* copula deletion is still operative but *is* deletion has been eliminated. Although this is a simplified picture, given other social and linguistic complexities, it provides an important ideal profile of the progressive steps that so typically characterize language change.

Our survey of sociolinguistic variation has been brief and relatively nontechnical, but it should be sufficient to demonstrate that variation within and across varieties of English is ultimately very systematic in its structure. It does not always conform to our preconceived ways of viewing language patterns, but the patterning of forms and relationships once again provides testimony to the intricate capabilities of the human mind in its adaptation to its social context. Our understanding of its patterning is, no doubt, limited only by our finite powers of investigation and our reticence in yielding our procrustean notions of how language variation operates. We have made considerable strides in understanding sociolinguistic variation in the past couple of decades, but we have probably just scratched the surface of ultimate comprehension and understanding.

A SELECTIVE INVENTORY OF VERNACULAR STRUCTURES

In the following section, we shall briefly inventory some of the major phonological and grammatical structures of vernacular English dialects. For the most part, this description is derived from more extensive sociolinguistic studies such as those of Labov, Cohen, Robins, and Lewis (1968), Wolfram and Fasold (1974), Baugh (1983), Wolfram and Christian (1976), and Christian and colleagues (1984), and these works should be consulted for more elaborate analyses. Our intent is simply to give a cursory overview that updates inventories such as those of Wolfram and Fasold (1974), Williams and Wolfram (1977), and Christian and Wolfram (1979). Many of these structures demonstrate the principles of linguistic change and differentiation we presented earlier. Our focus is on those dialects that are fairly stable and not on those that are transitory or the result of second language learning processes. For each of the structures, we shall make a brief general comment about the nature of the rule governing the structure, cite several illustrations, and then comment on its dialectal distribution. We concentrate upon those items that are socially significant in terms of the standard-vernacular continuum, so that we do not typically include items that are exclusively regional in their distribution. To the extent possible, we have attempted to use traditional orthography in representing items, but this is not possible in all cases.

PHONOLOGICAL STRUCTURES

Consonants

Final Cluster Reduction. Word-final consonant clusters ending in a stop can be reduced when both members of the cluster are either voiced (e.g., *find, cold*) or voiceless (*act, test*). This rule affects both clusters that are a part of the base word (e.g., *find, act*) and those clusters formed through the addition of an *-ed* suffix (e.g., *guessed, liked*). In standard English, this rule may operate when the following word begins in a consonant (e.g., *best kind*), but in vernacular dialects, it is extended to include following words beginning in a vowel as well (e.g., *best apple*).

This rule is quite prominent in vernacular Black English and in dialects of English that retain influence from another language, such as Chicano English and Vietnamese English. It is not particularly obtrusive in most Anglo-based dialects, such as vernacular Southern and Northern white varieties.

Plurals Following Clusters. Words ending in -*sp* (e.g., *wasp*), -*sk* (e.g., *desk*), and -*st* (e.g., *test*) may take the -*es* (i.e., [Iz] plural (e.g., *tesses, desses*) in many of these vernacular varieties. In such cases, the regular English plural simply operates after the application of the cluster reduction rule, since -*es* is the form that regularly occurs following *s* like sounds (i.e., sibilants).

In vernacular Appalachian English, an intrusive stop may be retained, thus resulting in items such as *postes* and *testes*. Such forms are considerably more rare in vernacular Black English, and seem to be a function of "overlearning" standard English plural forms.

Intrusive *t*. A small set of items, typically ending in *s* (and sometimes (*f*) may retain an earlier English version with *t*. This results in a final consonant cluster. Typical items affected by this process are *oncet, twicet, clifft,* and *acrosst.* This is found typically in Appalachian varieties and those other rural varieties retaining more relic forms.

***th* Sounds.** A number of different processes affect the *th* sounds. The phonetic realization is typically sensitive to the position of *th* in the word and the sounds adjacent to the *th*. At the beginning of the word, *th* is typically realized as a corresponding stop, such as *dey* for *they* (the voiced interdental fricative) and *ting* for *thing* (the voiceless interdental fricative). These productions are fairly typical of a wide range of vernaculars, although there are some differences in the distribution of the voiceless and voiced *th*. The *t* for *thing* tends to be most characteristic of selected Anglo-based and second language influenced varieties, whereas the *d* for *they* is spread across the full spectrum of vernacular varieties.

Before nasals, *th* participates in a rule in which a range of fricatives, including *z*, ð, and *v*, may also become stops. This results in forms such as *aritmetic* for *arithmetic* or *headn* for *heathen*, as well as *wadn't* for *wasn't*, *idn't* for *isn't*, and *sebm* for *seven*. This rule is typically found in Southern-based vernacular varieties, including Southern white and Black English.

In word-final and word-medial intervocalic position, *th* may be *f* or *v*, as in *efer* for *ether, toof* for *tooth, brover* for *brother,* and *smoov* for *smooth.* This production is typical of vernacular Black English, with the *v* for voiced *th* production more typical of Eastern varieties of the vernacular. Scattered Anglo-based and certain other varieties influenced by other languages in the recent past, such as Chicano English, also show limited evidence of the *f* production in *tooth*.

Some restricted Anglo-based varieties use a stop *d* for intervocalic voiced *th*, as in *oder* for *other* or *broder* for *brother*.

r and l. A number of different linguistic contexts occur in which *r* and *l* may be lost or reduced to a vowel-like vestige. After a vowel, as in *sister* or *steal*, the *r* and *l* may be reduced or lost. This feature intersects strongly with a regional dimension and is quite typical of Southern-based and New England varieties

Intervocalically, an *r* also may be lost, as in *Ca'ol* for *Carol* or *sto'y* for *story*. This intervocalic *r* loss is more socially stigmatized than the simple postvocalic version of the rule cited previously and is found in rural, Southern-based vernaculars.

Following a consonant, the *r* may be lost if it precedes a round vowel, such as *u* or *o*. This results in pronunciations of *through* as *thu* and *throw* as *tho*. Postconsonantal *r* loss may also be noted if it occurs in an unstressed syllable, such as *p'ofessor* for *professor* or *sec'etary* for *secretary*. This *r*-lessness also has a strong intersection with a regional Southern variable.

Before a labial sounds, *l* may be lost completely, giving *woof* for *wolf* or *hep* for *help*. Again, this is only characteristic of Southern-based Black and white varieties.

Some vocabulary items also have been affected by *r*-lessness, so that *they* for *their* as in *theyself* or *they book* apparently have been derived from the process of *r*-lessness historically.

Initial *w* Reduction. In unstressed positions within the sentence, an initial *w* may be lost in items such as *was* and *one*. This results in items such as *he's* for *he was* and *young 'uns* for *young ones*. This appears to be a generalization of the restricted process affecting the modals *will* and *would* in standard varieties of English (e.g., *he will* → *he'll; he would* → *he'd*). This process is found in Southern-based vernaculars.

Unstressed Initial Syllable Loss. The general process of deleting unstressed initial syllables in informal speech styles of standard English (e.g., *because* → *'cause; around* → *'round*) is extended in vernacular varieties so that a wider range of word classes (e.g., verbs such as *'member* for *remember* or nouns such as *'taters* for *potatoes*) and word-initial forms (e.g., *re-, po-, to-, sus-*) are affected in this rule.

***Initial h* Retention.**The retention of *h* on the pronoun *it* (*hit*) and the auxiliary *ain't* (*hain't*) is still found in vernacular varieties retaining some older English forms, such as Appalachian. This form is more prominent in stressed positions within a sentence. The pronunciation seems to be dying out among some younger speakers.

Nasals. A number of processes affect nasal sounds or items influenced by the presence of nasals in the surrounding linguistic environment.

One process that is very general in most vernacular varieties is the so-called "*g*-dropping," in which the back nasal represented as *ng* in spelling (phonetically [ŋ]) is pronounced as [n]. This process takes place when the *ng* occurs in an unstressed syllable, as in *swimmin'* for *swimming* or *buyin'* for *buying*.

Another widespread characteristic affecting nasals is the generalization of the form of the indefinite article *a* before both vowels and consonants (e.g., *a apple, a pear*).

A less widespread phenomenon affecting nasals is the use of a nasalized vowel (as in the production of the French nasalized vowel) when a nasal segment is in word-final position, particularly when the item is in relatively unstressed position within the sentence. Thus *man, bum,* or *ring* may be pronounced as *ma', bu',* or *ri',* respectively, with the vowel carrying a nasal quality. Most frequently, this process affects the segment *n*, although all final nasal segments may be affected to some extent. This process is typical of vernacular Black English.

There are other nasal processes (e.g., the collapsing of the contrast between [I] and [ɛ] before nasals as in *pin* and *pen*), but these tend to be much more regionally than socially sensitive.

Other Consonants. A number of other consonantal patterns affect limited sets of items or single items. For example, the retention of the older form *aks* for *ask* is observed in several vernacular varieties, including vernacular Black English. The form *chimley* or *chimbley* for *chimney* is also found in a number of Southern-based vernaculars. The use of *k* in initial *(s)tr* clusters as in *skreet* for *street* or *skring* for *string* is found in vernacular Black English, particularly rural Southern varieties. Such items are quite socially obtrusive, but they occur with such limited sets of items that they are best considered on an item-by-item basis.

Vowels

There are many vowel patterns that differentiate the dialects of English, but the majority of these are more regionally than socially significant. The back vowel [ɔ] of *bought* or *coffee* and front vowel [æ] in *cat* and *ran* are particularly sensitive to regional variation, as are vowels before *r* (e.g., compare pronunciations of *merry, marry, Mary, Murray*) and *l* (compare *wheel, will, well, whale,* etc.). Despite the primacy of the regional variable, some vowel differences have become associated with representative vernaculars.

Vowel Ungliding. The vowel glides, as in *ay* (e.g., *side, time*) and *oy* (e.g., *boy, toy*) may be unglided in items such as [tam] for *time* and [bɔ] for *boy*. Absence of the glide is more frequent when the following segment is voiced (e.g., *side, time*) than when it is voiceless (e.g., *sight, rice*). This variable is characteristic of practically all Southern-based vernaculars, and it is not particularly socially significant in the South.

Final Unstressed *ow*. In word-final position, standard English *ow*, as in *hollow* or *yellow*, may take an *r*, giving *holler* or *yeller*, respectively. This "intrusive" *r* also occurs when suffixes are attached, as in *fellers* for *fellows* or *narrers* for *narrows*. This production is characteristic of highland varieties, such as those found in Appalachia or the Ozarks, although it is found to some extent in other rural varieties as well.

Final Unstressed *a* Raising. A final unstressed *a* (phonetically a schwa [ə]), as in *soda* or *extra*, may be raised to a high front vowel [i], giving productions such as *sody* (phonetically [sodi]) and *extry* [ɛk-stri]). Again, this is a production found in highland and rural vernaculars of the South.

-*ire* Collapse. The sequence *ire*, which is usually produced as a two-syllable sequence in standard English, including a diphthong [ay] (e.g., [taɚ] "tire"; [faɚ] "fire," can be collapsed into a one syllable sequence, without the glide, as in *fa'r* [far] and *ta'r* [far]. This process also affects those sequences formed by the addition of an -*er* suffix, such as *buyer* [bar] and *retired* [ritard].

GRAMMATICAL STRUCTURES

The Verb Phrase

Many of the socially significant grammatical structures concern the construction of the verb phrase. Some of the variations involve readjustments following the linguistic principles set forth earlier, but there are also a few items that are unique to some vernacular varieties because of historical contact situations.

Irregular Verbs. Five categories of irregular verb patterns differentiate the usage of these forms in vernacular varieties. For the most part, the shifts in subclasses of irregular forms have resulted from the process of analogy, including both regularization and minority pattern shifts. These differences are (1) past as participle form, (2) participle as past form, (3) bare root as past form, (4) regularization, and (5) different irregular form. Examples for each follow.

Category	Example
1	I had *went* down there.
	He may have *took* the wagon.
2	He *seen* something out there.
	She *done* her homework.
3	She *come* to my house yesterday.
	She give him a nice present last year.
4	Everybody *knowed* he was late.
	They *throwed* out the old food.
5	I *hearn* something shut the church house door.
	She just *retch* up on the fireplace.

Various vernaculars of English participate in these patterns in slightly different ways, with the majority of vernaculars in the North and South having categories 1, 2, and 3. Southern-based vernaculars are more likely to have category 5. Varieties subject to the influence of second language learning strategies (e.g., Vietnamese English) will often reveal a higher incidence of regularization (category 4).

Verb Subclass Shifts. There are a number of different types of verb patterns that include analogical shifts among subclasses of verbs. Patterns found in vernacular varieties include the following: (1) shifts in the transitive status of verbs (i.e., whether or not the verb is required to take an object), (2) verbs derived from other parts of speech (e.g., verbs derived from nouns), (3) the formation of verb complement structures (i.e., the structures of items that co-occur with the verb), (4) verb plus verb particle formations, and (5) the semantic domain covered by the meaning of the verb form. Illustrations of each of these follow:

Category	Example
1	If we *beat*, we will be champs.
	She *learned* the students how to do math.
2	Our dog *treed* a coon.
	We *doctored* the sickness ourselves.

3   The kitchen *needs remodeled.*
       The students *started to messing* around.
4   He *happened in* on the party.
       The coach *blessed out* his players.
5   He *carried* her to the movies.
       My kids *took* the chicken pox when they were young.
       I was *fixin'* to go there.
       I been *aimin'* to go there.

For the most part, the shifts in verb subclasses and the semantic reference of various verbs have to be dealt with on an item-by-item basis. Although all vernaculars participate in these patterns to varying degrees, some researchers contend that Southern-based vernaculars show a more representative range of shifts. More extensive shifts of different word classes into verbs (category 2) seem to be found in vernacular Appalachian English.

Completive *done*. The form *done* may function to mark a completed action or event in a way somewhat different from simple past, as in a sentence such as "There was one in there that done rotted away" or "I done forgot what you wanted." In this use, the emphasis is upon the "completive" aspect. It may also add intensification to the activity, as in "I done told you not to mess around." This form is typically found in Southern white and Black vernaculars.

Habitual *be*. The form *be* in sentences such as "Sometimes my ears be itching" or "She usually be home in the evening" may signify "an event or activity distributed intermittently over time or space." This unique aspectual meaning of *be* is typically associated with vernacular Black English.

Remote Time *been*. The form *been* can also serve to mark a special aspectual function, indicating that the event or activity took place in the "distant past." In structures such as *I been had it there for about three years* or *I been known her*, the reference is to the event taking place, literally or figuratively, in some distant time frame. Its use, which is associated with vernacular Black English, is dying out in some varieties of the vernacular, but still prominent in those varieties more closely aligned with the creole predecessor, which used the form much more extensively.

***a*-Prefixing.** An *a-* prefix may occur on *-ing* participles functioning as progressives (e.g., *He was a-comin' home*) or adverbial complements to the verb, as in *He kept a-wantin' to go out, She makes money a-sewin'* or *He starts a-laughin' at you*. This form cannot occur on *-ing* forms that function as nouns or adjectives (i.e., sentences such as *He likes a-sailin'* or *The movie was a-charmin'* do *not* occur). The form is also restricted phonologically, in that it occurs only on forms beginning with a consonant (i.e., sentences such as *He was a-drinkin'* but not *He was a-eatin'*) and forms in which the first syllable of the form is relatively stressed (e.g., sentences such as *She was a-following the trail* but *not* sentences such as *she was a-discoverin' the cave*). This structure may be used to indicate intensity by some speakers, but it does not appear to have any unique aspectual marking analogous to habitual *be* or completive *done*. It is quite characteristic of vernacular Appalachian English.

Double Modals. Double modals involve constructions of two modal forms such as *might could, useta could, might should,* or *might oughta*. Sentences such as *I might could go there* or *You might oughta take it* are typically Southern vernacular structures; only modal clustering with *useta*, as in *He useta couldn't do it* or *He didn't useta go there* is found in Northern varieties.

Special Modals. The forms *liketa* and *(su)poseta* may be used as a special verb modifier to mark special speaker perceptions relating to significant events that were on the verge of happening. *Liketa* is a "counterfactual," in that it is used to indicate that an event about to take place actually did not happen, as in the sentence *She liketa scared me to death* or *I liketa froze it was so cold in there*. It usually carries with it an exaggerated connotation. *(Sup)poseta*, in sentences such as *You (su)poseta went there*, is used in a sense parallel to the standard English construction *supposed to have*.

Absence of *be* Forms. Where contracted forms of *is* or *are* may occur in standard English, these same forms may be deleted in some vernacular varieties. Thus, we get structures such as *You ugly* or *She taking the dog out* corresponding to the standard English structures *You're ugly* and *She's taking the dog out*, respectively. It is important to note that this absence only takes place on "contractable" forms (e.g., It does not affect forms such as *are* in *That's where they are*), and does not typically affect forms of *am* (e.g., Sentences such as *I ugly* do not typically occur). The deletion of *are* is typical of both white Southern and Black English vernaculars, and is often found in varieties developing from second language learning processes as well (e.g., Vietnamese English, Chicano English).

Subject-Verb Agreement. A number of different subject-verb agreement patterns enter into the social differentiation of dialects. These include (1) agreement with the expletive *there*, (2) agreement patterns with the general present and past tense forms of *be*, (3) agreement with the form *don't*, (4) agreement with *have*, (5) agreement with special kinds of plural subjects, and (6) agreement with regular third person singular. These are illustrated in the following examples.

Category	*Example*
1	*There was* five people there.
	There's two women in the lobby.
2	The cars *was* out on the street.
	Most of the kids *is* younger up there.
3	She *don't* like the cat in the house.
	It *don't* seem like a holiday.
4	My nerves *has* been on edge.
	My children *hasn't* been there much.
5	*Some people likes* to talk a lot.
	Me and my brother gets in a fight.
6	The dog *stay* outside in the afternoon.
	He usually *like* the evening news.

Different vernacular varieties participate in different ways in those various of subject-verb agreement patterns. Virtually all vernacular varieties participate to some extent in categories 1, 2, and 3 (In fact, standard varieties are moving toward the pattern found in category 1), but in different degrees. The patterns illustrated in categories 4 and 5 are most characteristic of highland Southern and rural varieties in the South, and those found in category 6 are most typical of vernacular Black English.

Past Tense Absence. Much of the past tense absence in regular verb forms such as *Yesterday he mess up* or *she like the book that she got for a present* can be accounted for by phonological processes discussed earlier (e.g., consonant cluster reduction). However, there are some instances in which past tense is unmarked as a function of a grammatical difference. This is particularly true of varieties influenced by other languages in the subject's recent past. Thus, structures such as *He bring the food yesterday* or *He play a new song last night* may be the result of a grammatical process rather than a phonological one. In some cases, both phonological and grammatical processes operate in a convergent way. Grammatically based tense unmarking tends to be more frequent on regular verb forms than irregular forms, so that a structure such as *Yesterday he play a new song* is more likely than *Yesterday he is in a new store*, although both may occur.

Tense unmarking has been found to be prominent in varieties such as Vietnamese English and American Indian English. In the latter case, unmarking is favored in habitual contexts (e.g., *In those days, we play a different kind of game*) as opposed to simple past time (e.g., *Yesterday, we play at a friend's house*).

Adverbs

There are several different patterns that distinguish adverb usage among vernacular varieties. These involve, for the most part, differences in the placement of adverbs within the sentence, differences in the formation of adverbs, and differences in the use or meaning of particular vocabulary items.

Adverb Placement. Several differences occur in terms of the position of the adverb within the sentence, including the placement of certain time adverbs within the verb phrase, as in *We were all the time talking* or *We watched all the time "Little House on the Prairie."* These cases do not hold great social significance, and are not particularly socially stigmatized. More obtrusive is the change in order with various forms of *ever*, as in *everwhat, everwho,* or *everwhich* (e.g., *Everwho wanted to go could go*). These retentions of older English forms are generally found only in vernaculars retaining relic forms of English, such as Appalachian, but even in these contexts they are currently dying out.

Comparatives and Superlatives. Most vernacular varieties of English participate in adaptations of irregular comparative and superlative forms. One natural extension is the regularization of irregular forms, giving *badder* or *mostest*. Another extension involves the use of *-er* and *-est* on two or more syllable words where the standard English rule uses *more* and *most* (e.g., *beautifulest, awfulest*). In some instances, the extension may result in double marking as in *most awfulest* or *more nicer*. Such natural regularization and generalization processes cut across the different kinds of vernacular varieties of English.

***-ly* Absence.** In present-day American English, some of the adverbs formed at an earlier period through the addition of the *-ly* suffix are losing the *-ly* (e.g., in informal standard English, most speakers say *He answered wrong* instead of *He answered wrongly*). The range of items affected by this absence can be extended to various degrees in different vernacular dialects, ranging from a relatively inobtrusive item such as *awful* in *He enjoyed life awful well* to a quite obtrusive form such as *original* in *I come from Virginia original*. Northern vernaculars tend to be less expansive in their extension of the items affected by this *-ly* absence than their southern counterparts, particularly the Southern highland varieties.

Intensifying Adverbs. A set of adverbs occurs in Southern-based vernaculars that can intensify particular attributes or activities. *Right* (which is currently limited to location or time in standard English as in *He is right around the corner*) intensifies the degree of an attribute (e.g., *She is right pretty*) whereas *plumb* intensifies the attribute in totality (e.g., *He fell plumb asleep*). Other adverbial intensifiers found in these varieties include items such as *big old, little old, right smart*, and *right much*, among others.

Other Adverbial Forms. In a number of other cases the adverbial forms of vernacular varieties differ from their standard counterparts. Some of these involve word class changes, as in the use of *but* as an adverb meaning "only" as in *He ain't but 13 years old*. In other cases, there are simply differences in the kinds of lexical items in the adverbial word class, such as *yonder* (e.g., *It's up yonder*) or *yet* (e.g., *I yet eat a lot of honey*). Another difference comes from the phonological fusion of items, such as *t'all* from *at all* (e.g., *It's not coming up t'all*), *pert' near* (e.g., She's pert' near seventy), or *druther* (e.g., *Druther than lose the farm, he fought*). Again, such differences must be considered on an item-by-item basis.

Negation

The two major differences in negation involve the formation of the so-called "double negatives," which involve the marking of negative elements at more than one point in the sentence, and the use of the lexical item *ain't*. Other forms, resulting directly from the acquisition of English as a second language (e.g., *He no like the man*) are found in the interlanguage of some developing varieties, but do not seem to be perpetuated as a continuing part of the English-based variety apart from this transitional process. (An exception may be the negative tag *no* as found in some Hispanic English varieties as in *He's going to the store, no?*).

Multiple Negation. There are four different kinds of negative marking patterns found in the vernacular varieties of English: (1) marking of the negative in the verb phrase and the indefinite(s) following the verb, (2) negative marking of an indefinite before the verb phrase and the verb phrase, (3) inversion of the negative element from the verb phrase and the pre-verbal indefinite, and (4) multiple negative marking across different clauses. These are illustrated in the following sentences.

Category	Example
1	The man *wasn't* saying *nothing.* He *didn't* say *nothing* about *no* people bothering him or *nothing* like that.
2	*Nobody didn't* like the mess. *Nothing can't* stop him from failing the course.
3	*Didn't nobody* like the mess! *Can't nothing* stop him from failing the course!
4	There *wasn't* much that I *couldn't* do (meaning "There wasn't much I could do") I *wasn't* sure that *nothing wasn't* going to come up. (meaning "I wasn't sure that anything was going to come up")

Virtually all vernacular varieties of English participate in the multiple negation, such as in category 1 in the foregoing inventory: restricted Northern and most Southern vernaculars participate in category 2, most Southern vernaculars participate in category 3, and restricted Southern and Black English varieties participate in category 4.

The Auxiliary *ain't*. The item *ain't* may be used as a correspondence for various forms of standard English auxiliaries, including forms of *be + not* (e.g., *She ain't here now, I ain't gonna do it*), forms of *have + not* (e.g., *I ain't seen her in a long time, She ain't gone to the movies in a long time*), and *do + not* (e.g., *He ain't tell him he was sorry, I ain't go to school yesterday*). The first two types are found in most vernacular varieties to one degree or another, but the third type, as the correspondence of standard *didn't*, has only been found in vernacular Black English varieties.

Nominals

The major word class of nominals, including various aspects of pronouns, is another that is affected by socially significant dialect variation. The major types of differences involve the attachment of various suffixes and the various case markings of forms.

Plurals. Plurals may be differentiated in several different ways from the patterns found in standard varieties of English. These include (1) general absence of plural suffix, (2) absence of plural suffix with restricted subclasses of nouns, and (3) regularization of various irregular plural noun forms. These are illustrated in the following sentences:

Category	Example
1	Lots of boy_ go to the school.
	All the girl_ liked the movie.
2	The station is four mile_ down the road.
	They hauled in a lotta bushel_ of corn.
3	They saw the *deers* running across the field.
	The *firemans* liked the convention.

Category 1 is found only among varieties in which another language was spoken in the recent past and, to a limited degree, in vernacular Black English. In category 2, plural suffix absence is limited to nouns of weights (e.g., *four pound, three ton*) and measures (*two foot, many mile, lotta acre*), including some temporal nouns (e.g., *two year, five month*); this pattern is found in many Southern-based vernaculars. Category 3 includes regularization of plurals that are not marked overtly in standard English (e.g., *deers, sheep*), forms marked with irregular suffixes in the standard (e.g., *oxes*), and forms marked by nonsuffixial plurals (e.g., *firemans, snowmans*). In the last case, plurals may be marked with both plural forms, as in *mens* or *childrens*. Some kinds of plurals in category 3 are quite widespread among the vernacular varieties of English (e.g., regularizing the nonmarked plurals such as *deers*), whereas others (e.g., the double marking in *mens*) are more limited.

Possessives. There are several patterns involving the possessive nouns and pronouns, including the absence of the possessive suffix, as in *The man hat is on the chair* or *John coat is here*, regularization of the possessive pronoun (*mines*) on the basis of analogy with *yours, his, hers*, and so forth, and the use of the special possessive form *his'n* or *your'n* (this form can only be found in "absolute" sentence position, as in *It is his'n*; it is *not* found in structures such as *It is his'n book*). The first two types of possessives are typical of vernacular Black English, and the third type is found in vernacular Appalachian English, although it is restricted to older speakers.

Pronouns. Pronoun differences typically originate in changes to the "case" forms or regularization by analogy. The categories of differences include (1) regularization of reflexive forms by analogy with possessive pronouns, (2) extension of object forms to coordinate subjects, (3) adoption of a second person plural form to "fill out" the number-person paradigm, (4) extension of object forms to demonstratives, and (5) a special "benefactive" use of the object pronoun form.

Category	Example
1	He hit *hisself* on the head.
	They shaved *theirselves* with the new razor.
2	*Me and him* will do it.
	John and them will be home soon.
3a	*Y'all* won the game.
	I'm going to leave *y'all* now.
b	*Youse* won the game.
	I'm going to leave *youse* now.
c	*You'uns* won the game.
	I'm going to leave *you'uns* now.
4	*Them* books are on the shelf.
	He didn't like *them there* boys.
5	*I* got *me* a new car.
	We had *us* a little old dog.

The first four types of pronominal differences are well represented in most vernacular dialects of English, with the particular kind of second person plural pronoun sensitive to the regional locale; category 3a is, of course, the Southern form and category 3b the Northern form, with some specific regions (e.g., western Pennsylvania) using category 3c. The so-called "personal dative" illustrated in category 5 is a Southern feature, but it is not particularly stigmatized in that context.

Other pronoun forms, such as the use of an object form with a simple subject (e.g., *Her in the house*) and the use of subject or object forms in possessive structures (e.g., *It is she book; It is he book*) are quite rare in most current vernaculars, except for those still closely related to a prior Creole state.

Relative Pronouns. Differences affecting relative pronouns include the extension of relative pronoun forms and the generalized absence of relative pronouns under certain conditions. Form differences may range from the socially insignificant use of *that* for human subjects (e.g., *The man that I was telling you about is here*) to the quite stigmatized use of *what*, as in *The man what I was telling you about is here*). One form that is becoming more common, and spreading into informal varieties of standard English, is the "conjunctive" use of *which*, as in the sentence *He gave me this cigar, which he knows I don't smoke cigars*.

In standard English, relative pronouns may be deleted if they are the object in the relative clause, so that *That's the dog that I bought* could alternately be rendered as *That's the dog I bought*. In most cases in which it is the subject, however, the relative pronoun must be retained, as in *That's the dog that bit me*. A number of Southern-based varieties may delete the relative pronoun in varying degrees, whether object or subject, so that these varieties use *That's the dog bit me* or *The man come in here is my father*.

Expletive *it* or *they*. The standard English form *there*, in sentences such as *There are four people in school* or *There's a picture on TV* functions as an expletive, or "existential" rather than a locational adverb. In these cases, vernacular variations may use *it* (*It's a picture on TV*) or *they* (*They's a picture on TV*) as the corresponding expletive form. *They* for *there* seems to be found only in Southern-based vernaculars.

Other Grammatical Structures. There are a number of structures that might be considered here, but we will not treat them in detail. In some cases, empirical sociolinguistic investigation indicates that the presumed vernacular forms are more common in informal standard varieties than had been thought originally, so they are not discussed in detail here. For example, pronominal apposition, as in *My mother, she made my breakfast*, is such a case, as it is found in the spoken language of practically all social groups of American English speakers. Furthermore, it is not particularly obtrusive in spoken language. It has also been found that indirect questions such as *He asked could he go to the movies* (as compared with *He asked if he could go to the movies*) are becoming a part of informal spoken English standard varieties and are not socially stigmatized. Other differences, such as those affecting prepositions, have to be treated item by item, and these really qualify as lexical rather than grammatical differences. Thus, forms such as *of the evening* ("in the evening"), *upside the head* ("on the side of the head"), *leave out of there* ("leave there"), *the matter of him* ("the matter with him"), and so forth, have to be treated individually. In most cases, their social significance is also secondary to their regional variation, so that we have not discussed them fully in this account. Standard linguistic atlas studies give much more adequate detail about these forms than could be given in this overview.

SUMMARY

Our overview of language variation in the United States has shown that there are a number of social and linguistic parameters that have to be considered in a realistic account of this variation. On a social level, we must consider variables such as region, status, ethnicity, gender, age, and style as they intersect with one another in defining the social dimensions of language variation. On a linguistic level, we have seen that a number of cognitive processes are at work to effect variation, including the principles of linguistic generalization, regularization, redundancy reduction, and analogy. The end result is intricate, systematically patterned language behavior.

One of the ironies of our understanding of linguistic variation is the fact that this complex behavior has so often been reduced to simplistic and uninformed explanation, being attributed to ignorance and simplicity. Nothing could be farther from the truth; instead, linguistic variation deserves our utmost respect as a representation of the complex workings of the human mind and human social adaptive mechanism. There are few behaviors that demonstrate as well the intricate and complex nature of the unique systematic human character as it functions in society.

REFERENCES

Bailey, G. (1985). Invariant *be* in Eastern Louisiana. In M. Montgomery and G. Bailey (eds.), *Proceedings of Conference on Black and White Speech in the South.* University, AL: University of Alabama Press.

Bell, A. (1984). Language style as audience design. *Language in Society, 13,* 145–205.

Baugh, J. (1983). *Black street speech.* Austin: The University of Texas Press.

Christian, D., and Wolfram, W. (1979). *Exploring dialects.* Washington, DC: Center for Applied Linguistics.

Christian, D., Wolfram, W., and Dube, N. (1984). *Variation and change in geographically isolated communities: Appalachian and Ozark English.* Final Report, NSF Grant BNS 8208916.

Dillard, J.L. (1972). *Black English: Its history and usage in the United States.* New York: Random House.

Fasold, R.W. (1981). The relation between black and white speech in the south. *American Speech, 56,* 163–90.

Feagin, C. (1979). *Variation and change in Alabama English: A sociolinguistic study of the white community.* Washington, DC: Georgetown University Press.

Frank, F., and Anshen, F. (1984). *Language and the sexes.* Albany: State University of New York Press.

Giles, H., and Powesland, P. *Speech style and social evaluation.* London: Academic Press.

Gold, D.L. (1981). The speech and writing of Jews. In C. Ferguson and S.B. Heath (eds.), *Language in the USA.* New York: Cambridge University Press.

Kramarae, C. (1981). *Women and men speaking.* Rowley, MA: Newbury House.

Labov, W. (1972). Some principles of linguistic methodology. *Language in Society, 1*, 97–120.

Labov, W., Cohen, P., Robins, C., and Lewis, J. (1968). *A study of nonstandard English of Negro and Puerto Rican speakers in New York City.* USOE Final Report Project No. 3288.

Labov, W., Yaeger, M., and Steiner, R. (1972). *A quantitative study of sound change in progress.* Final Report, NSF Grant GS-3287.

Leap, W.L. (ed.). 1977. *Studies in Southwestern Indian English.* San Antonio, TX: Trinity University Press.

Ornstein-Galicia, J. (ed.). (1984). *Form and function in Chicano English.* Rowley, MA: Newbury House.

Penalosa, J. (ed.). (1980). Chicano sociolinguistics. Rowley, MA: Newbury House.

Romaine, S. (1980). Stylistic variation and evaluative reactions to speech. *Language and Speech, 23*, 213–232.

Smith, P.M. (1985). *Language, the sexes, and society.* New York: Basil Blackwell.

Stewart, W.A. (1970). Continuity and change in American Negro dialects. In F. Williams (ed.), *Language and poverty: Perspectives on a theme.* Chicago: Markham.

Trudgill, P. (1972). Sex, covert prestige, and linguistic change in the urban British English of Norwich. *Language in Society, 1*, 179–95.

Williams, R., and Wolfram, W. (1977). *Social dialects: Difference versus disorder.* Rockville, MD: American Speech-Hearing-Language Association.

Wolfram, W. (1969). *A sociolinguistic description of Detroit Negro speech.* Washington, DC: Center for Applied Linguistics.

Wolfram, W. (1981). Varieties of American English. In C. Ferguson and S.B. Heath (Eds.), *Language in the USA.* New York: Cambridge University Press.

Wolfram, W. (1984). Unmarked tense in American Indian English. *American Speech, 59*, 31–50.

Wolfram, W., and Christian, D. (1976). *Appalachian speech.* Washington, DC: Center for Applied Linguistics.

Wolfram, W., and Fasold, R.W. (1974). *The study of social dialects in American English.* Englewood Cliffs, NJ: Prentice-Hall.

Chapter 5

Language Acquisition in Culturally Diverse Populations: The Black Child as a Case Study

Ida J. Stockman

This chapter reviews language acquisition research in the context of assessment issues that are relevant to children who acquire a nonmainstream variety of English. The problem of assessing the language of nonmainstream speakers has been recognized, particularly in the case of Black children (see Vaughn-Cooke, 1983, for a review of assessment issues). In this chapter, the lack of adequate empirical definition of normal language behavior is viewed as the single most critical barrier to the appropriate language assessment of such speakers.

The goals of this chapter are twofold. First, it aims to highlight the contribution of language acquisition research to the development of a normative language data base in Black children. Second, it aims to provide a synthesis and critique of the normative data that acquisitional research has yielded so far.

The chapter is organized into four subdivisions. The first highlights language acquisition research as a foundation for language assessment and calls attention to assessment problems that result from the absence of developmental data on Black children. The second subdivision offers four guidelines as a framework for evaluating language research that can serve a normative purpose. The third summarizes and critiques representative acquisitional studies on Black children within the framework of these guidelines. The fourth section synthesizes findings from acquisitional studies in the form of state-of-the-art conclusions about Black children's language development and addresses the implications of these conclusions for language norming and assessment.

LANGUAGE ACQUISITION RESEARCH AS A FOUNDATION FOR LANGUAGE ASSESSMENT

Language Acquisition Research and Normative Data

Notions of normalcy influence every clinical decision made about speakers who exhibit language impairment. Clinical judgments about atypical language behavior must be guided by some explicit or implicit definition of what constitutes normal behavior. Likewise, the formulation of therapy goals and the evaluation of treatment progress are guided by assumptions about the requirements for normal language performance. It might be said figuratively that yardsticks of normalcy serve as the barometers for clinical judgment.

What is normal language? The normalcy of any phenomenon refers to its usual or typical state under a given set of natural conditions. Normal language is framed in terms of the kind of linguistic behavior that is typically exhibited by the majority of speakers in a given linguistic community.

Normalcy exists as a relative rather than absolute standard. With respect to language, the speaker's age is among the variables that contribute to the relative nature of normalcy. The age factor should not be a surprising one given that children acquire language over a period of time. What constitutes normal language, therefore, will necessarily vary across age levels due to expected differences in the amount of linguistic experience before the target language is acquired. It follows, then, that judgments about normalcy of children's language must be based on variable norms that take into account what the children know about language at different age-related stages of development. Such a knowlege base is provided by language acquisition research. Its general goal is to describe children's linguistic knowledge at different ages and reveal language specific and universal processes that can explain how language is learned. Language acquisition research, therefore, provides important input to empirical definitions of children's normalcy.

Language acquisition research has impacted dramatically on clinical assessment trends in the past decade. This impact is partly due to the explosive gains in knowledge about children's language that were stimulated by the emergence of developmental psycholinguistics as an academic discipline. Developmental psycholinguists has placed a priority on the analysis of primary linguistic data derived from intensive longitudinal observations of children's spontaneous language, beginning at an early age. Using this approach, ground-breaking acquisitional studies were conducted on linguistic form (syntax, morphology, and phonology) in the 1960s, on linguistic meaning and use in the 1970s, and on interactions among linguistic form, meaning, and use in the 1980s.

The impact of an expanding developmental knowledge base on language assessment has been reflected in the growing disenchantment with formal standardized tests as the sole data source for evaluating linguistic status (Butler, 1981; Seymour and Miller-Jones, 1981). The trend reflects recognition that many current standardized tests do not incorporate recent developmental findings, and their restricted language sampling format limits the adequacy with which they could ever sample certain dimensions of language (e.g., pragmatics).

The validity of spontaneous language sample analysis, which is advocated as a complement to formal tests, also rests on the adequacy of normative data at various ages. The analytical procedures attempt to place the child at some criterion referenced stage of behavior based on expectations about normal behavior. Miller's Assignment of Structural Stages (ASS) (1981) is a good example of a procedure of this type. The outcomes yielded by such procedures are expected to aid the formulation of intervention goals by identifying the language skills that have not been acquired.

Absence of Acquisitional Data as a Barrier to Language Assessment of Nonmainstream English Speakers

The bulk of the acquisitional research that has motivated changing language assessment trends is not based on children who acquire nonmainstream features of English. For such children who acquire vernacular Black English, fewer than a dozen studies have focused systematically on language acquisition.

Black English (BE, in contradistinction to SE or standard English) is used here to refer to that dialect variety spoken in the United States, which (1) is argued to be a decreolized derivative of an English vernacular having African based linguistic features (Alleyne, 1980), and (2) is most prominently represented among rural and urban working class Black speakers with little formal education (Labov, 1972; Dillard, 1972). Hence, BE does not refer to the spoken language of all Black speakers in the United States. It is recognized that not all Black speakers acquire a BE dialect, and that among those who do, the number and type of features vary along a continuum from most to least socially acceptable or standard (Taylor, 1971).

Linguistic features that are commonly attested to among such BE speakers include, for example, the use of invariant be, stress been, copula absence, go copula, multiple negation, /f/ for /ə/ substitution in word medial and final positions, and so forth. The works of Labov (1972), Vaughn-Cooke (1976), Wolfram (1969), and, more recently, Baugh (1983) are among those that have described various BE features. Cole (1980) gives a lucid summary of BE's origin and features.

Children who acquire BE provide a good example of the kind of assessment problems that arise when language research has not yielded normative data. In the absence of such data, Black children are likely to be at greater risk for inappropriate clinical diagnosis than their adult counterparts. This situation is due to the fact that the variable nature of a child's developing system can yield language behavior that is actually normal, but which may be judged as abnormal when it differs from standard English (SE) as well as adult BE. It is not surprising, therefore, that BE speaking children have been either over- or underrepresented in clinical service programs (Bartel, Grill and Bryen, 1973; Mercer and Brown, 1973; see also Williams and Wolfram, 1976, for a discussion of language differences versus disorders). Overrepresentation means that therapy is inappropriately recommended for some children whose language behavior can be accounted for by differences due to the acquisition of a nonmainstream language variety. Underrepresentation reflects a pendulum swing toward judging too many children as presenting language differences when, in fact, their language is pathological. Both types of judgment error result from unclear definition of what constitutes normal versus pathological behavior for BE speaking children.

Resolving the assessment problem either by adapting existing procedures or by constructing new ones cannot be guided by much empirical documentation of what Black children know about language at different ages. The inadequacy of normative data is not due to the lack of language research on the population. Black children's language has been the subject of more research and controversy than any other minority group in the United States. But, most of the studies have been oriented toward investigative frameworks that were not compatible with the goal of building a normative knowledge base. According to Stockman and Vaughn-Cooke (1982b), most language research has reflected one of three orientations: (1) the deficit, (2) the dialect proficiency, and (3) the language use orientations.

With respect to the deficit orientation, the goal of the studies was to determine if and how Black children's language differed from that of white children (Bereiter and Engelmann, 1966; Entwisle, 1968; Loban, 1966; Osser, Wang, and Zaid, 1969; Raph, 1967). The studies typically involved the comparison of white and Black children's verbal responses to structured elicitation tasks that were oriented toward SE. Observed group differences were explained in terms of Black children's acquisition of an undeveloped and incorrect form of English (i.e., a deficient form of English).

The dialect proficiency studies were designed to counter the claims of the deficit theory. They were based on the premise that BE is rule governed and conforms to the same constraints as all natural languages. Given the assumption that Black children acquire a legitimate language system that differs in systematic ways from SE, the goal of the dialect proficiency studies was to show that their language proficiencies varied with whether the verbal task was oriented toward SE or toward BE. This goal was achieved in some studies by intragroup comparison—that is, by comparing dialect proficiency on SE and BE tasks as exhibited by the same Black speakers (DeStefano, 1972; Henrie, 1969; Levy and Cook, 1973; Lewnau, 1973; Quay, 1971; Ramer and Rees, 1973). Other studies continued the intergroup comparison of Black and white children to determine if the verbal proficiency of both racial groups was equally affected when performance was required in an unfamiliar dialect (Baratz, 1969; Frazure and Entwisle, 1973; Marwit, 1977; Seymour and Seymour, 1981; Weener, 1969). Observed performance differences within and across racial groups were attributed to language differences as opposed to deficits.

Language use studies were stimulated by expanding linguistic theory, which viewed competency on specific linguistic forms or structures as subordinate to the more general notion of communicative competency. Communicative competency, broadly speaking, focuses on a speaker's ability to achieve purposeful communicative goals in real world sociocultural contexts. Linguistic forms function as one of the means by which communicative ends or goals can be achieved, and social interactions are assumed to impose critical constraints on how communicative goals are achieved.

This relatively new view of competency permitted investigative goals to shift from a focus on Black children's isolated use of specific linguistic forms or structures to a focus on how they use language to manage communicative interactions and the sociocultural context for these interactions. To accommodate the expanded focus on language use and socialization, the language use studies employed methods for sampling and analyzing language spoken in naturalistic contexts (Horner and Gussow, 1972; Mitchell-Kernan and Kernan, 1977; Ward, 1971) and in structured spontaneous contexts (Peters, 1983).

The study of Black children's spoken language in the sociocultural contexts in which language is used naturally represented a significant departure from the more commonly used structured elicitation procedures. Language use studies, therefore, differed from deficit and dialect proficiency studies in their essential focus and method. They, like the deficit and dialect proficiency studies, however, did not yield normative data. This outcome was due to the fact that some studies focused on aspects of the language socialization experience and not on the actual language behavior exhibited by children (e.g., Horner and Gussow, 1972). Studies that provided usable descriptions of children's pragmatic behaviors (e.g., Peters, 1983), did not focus on performance in relation to age.

The goals and methods of language research that can serve normative goals require an orientation that differs from that which characterizes the three categories of studies cited earlier. The kind of research that is required to address the practical problem posed by inadequate normative data on Black nonmainstream English speaking children should conform with the following four basic guidelines:

1. The investigative goal should have a developmental focus.
2. The mother tongue principle should guide the choice of language studied.
3. The investigative focus should be guided by a theoretical framework that permits the examination of linguistic forms in relation to their meaning and use.
4. The methodological orientation must reflect sensitivity to the sociocultural context in which children's language is learned and spoken.

The following section elaborates on each guideline. The reader should note that the guidelines do not apply uniquely to Black children. They conform with expectations for language acquisition research in any group of children. Yet, such guidelines have not been reflected in the language research on Black children given the social and political context in which their language, historically, has been learned and studied. It is instructive, therefore, to review the guidelines here as a framework for evaluating the adequacy of existing language acquisition research on this population.

GUIDELINES FOR CONSTRUCTING AND EVALUATING LANGUAGE ACQUISITION RESEARCH THAT CAN SERVE A NORMATIVE PURPOSE

The Investigative Goal Should Have a Developmental Focus

Language, like many other complex human skills, is learned over a period of time. Consequently, children's language is characterized by change and variability as it evolves toward a target language. Given the inherently temporal nature of the subject matter for study, a fundamental goal of language research must be one of describing the stages in the emergence and evolution of a language system.

Achieving the goal of a developmental study requires comparison of children's behavior at different points in time. This can be done cross-sectionally by observing independent groups of children who are at different ages, or longitudinally, by making repeated observations of the same children across time. Cross-sectional data, however, provide a static developmental perspective in that they reveal the linguistic knowledge already achieved at the age of observation.

Longitudinal data, on the other hand, provide a more dynamic developmental perspective; they reveal not only what the child has achieved by a certain age but also how elaboration of the same knowledge gives rise to new knowledge at various stages of language growth. Hence, longitudinal data permit the researcher to reveal the steps involved in achieving a particular knowledge stage.

The number of comparative time points chosen for observation is often determined by practical constraints. The more time points on which information is available, however, the more comprehensive will be the developmental description, irrespective of a cross-sectional or longitudinal sampling strategy.

Although the features of a developmental study are well known, they are reviewed here for contrast with the type of age comparison studies that are *not* developmentally focused. Results from these latter studies, nevertheless, have been used to make inferences about Black children's language. Reference is made here to studies in which disparate groups, differing on such status variables as race or social class, have been studied at different ages. Groups A and B, for instance, are compared at ages 1, 2, and 3 years. The comparative goal, however, is not to examine developmental continuity or discontinuity across time for either group, except in an incidental way. Rather, the goal is to determine the equivalence or lack of equivalence between groups that represent different linguistic or cultural backgrounds. (Refer to the brief review of deficit and dialect proficiency studies earlier in this chapter.) The motivation for including different age groups is to determine whether racial group differences or similarities are generalizable across ages.

A study by Anastasiow and Hanes (1974) illustrates this point. Given its title *(Cognitive Development and the Acquisition of Language in Three Subcultural Groups)*, the reader is led to expect a comparison of data trends across different ages. In fact, the 67 Black children selected for study were represented at different ages as correlated with their respective kindergarten and first and second grade school levels. Their performances on a sentence repetition task were compared to those of 60 middle class white children and 57 rural white children at the same age and grade levels. The task was tailored to a wide range of syntactic structures and Piagetian cognitive tasks. The authors explicitly stated that the grade-age factor was not of major significance to the hypotheses tested in the study. What emerges clearly is the primary goal of comparing three groups of children on the language and cognitive measures under study. A major conclusion, for example, was that Black children and middle class white children were at similar stages of development when allowances were made for dialect variation.

The comparative focus of the study of Anastasio and Hanes, though misleadingly labeled as developmental in focus, does not provide data on children's normative linguistic knowledge or on its acquisitional processes, except perhaps in an incidental way. Consequently, such data do not help to solve the practical problems of language assessment that are posed by the absence of developmental data.

The Mother Tongue Principle Should Guide the Choice of Language Studied

The choice of language to be studied is an issue for acquisitional research on all children who acquire nonmainstream dialects as the first language or *mother tongue.* This issue is due to the fact that the dialect used in the home and community for routine social interaction and group identity differs from that which is required for school, government, and commerce. Hence, the bidialectal experience is likely to be the norm rather than the exception for such children since they must achieve proficiency in more than one dialect to fully participate in the cultural and national institutions that govern their lives. It seems appropriate, therefore, to pose the question of whether SE or BE should be given priority in language acquisition studies on Black children.

Any recommendation should follow from knowledge about the medium for learning the two dialects and the purposes they serve. Unfortunately, we do not have the benefit of ethnographic studies of language function as they pertain to bidialecticism and the maintenance of cultural institutions among persons of Afro-American descent in the United States. Consequently, a recommendation can be forwarded only by making general assumptions about the way the BE and SE varieties appear to function for BE speaking children.

The argument here is that BE, as the mother tongue, should be given priority in language acquisition studies, particularly when they focus on Black children in the formative years (i.e., before the age of 6 years and the onset of formal schooling).

Although some SE proficiency is probably acquired without formal instruction, SE is assumed to be learned primarily as a second language, which serves more restricted purposes than those served by the native BE vernacular. In fact, before the onset of formal schooling, there is likely to be little demand to know SE forms except to comprehend television and radio programs.

BE, on the other hand, is assumed to be the principal dialect for establishing and maintaining social relationships in the home and community, cultural patterning, and self-identity for all Black children who learn it, including those who may rely on SE for school and work. Inasmuch as BE is not taught by formal instruction, it provides the most natural evidence for the types of strategies and hypotheses that guide children's learning of language. As a first language, it is expected to form the foundation for all subsequent language learning, both written and oral.

The acquisitional study of BE, therefore, should benefit language assessment in at least two ways. First, it should provide the normative data that are needed to detect language impairment at early ages, when BE is likely to be the main dialect spoken by the child. The benefits of early clinical diagnosis of language impairment are well recognized. Information about early linguistic performance also is relevant to decisions about school readiness and placement.

Second, the normative data yielded from acquisitional study of BE also should aid the diagnosis of language impairment among older children, particularly those for whom spoken language continues to be confined to the nonmainstream vernacular after schooling is begun. Even for older children who acquire SE as a second language, the researcher needs to refer to normative BE data when attempting to determine if language difficulty in the second dialect is due to language pathology or to native dialect interference. For example, a differential diagnosis, which draws on the expectation that problems due to clinical pathology affect both first and second language learning, requires knowledge of what constitutes normalcy in the native dialect.

The acquisitional focus on BE should not detract from the importance of obtaining more empirical data on Black children's acquisition of SE. Second language data are required for a comprehensive description of the linguistic competencies exhibited by children who acquire a nonstandard English vernacular because most are forced to achieve some proficiency in a mainstream dialect. As pointed out earlier, such data, used in concert with native dialect norms, can be useful for judging the presence or absence of language pathology for some children.

Second language data also can contribute to the exploration of such theoretical issues as language change, for which observations of language contact situations are relevant. For example, it is reasonable to expect language change to occur for one or both dialect systems that are spoken by the same speakers. However, the investigator should consider the importance of having normative knowledge about BE even for adequate exploration of theoretical issues pertaining to language change, as well as issues in other areas (e.g., interference phenomena).

The Investigative Focus Should be Guided by a Theoretical Framework that Permits Examination of Linguistic Forms in Relation to Meaning or Use, or Both

The characterization of the child's linguistic knowledge, as it develops over time, will undoubtedly mirror the strengths and weaknesses of the theoretical framework that guides the investigative process. For this reason, researchers must carefully evaluate available framework before selecting one to direct the focus and plan of data analysis. A central concern of the evaluation should be the framework's capacity to describe and explain the complex multidimensional nature of language and its learning. Although no single analytical approach is capable of achieving the ideal goal of providing a complete characterization of the vast set of knowledge required to speak a language, some come closer to attaining this goal than others. It is instructive to review the major frameworks that have been employed in language acquisition research.

The earliest approaches focused exclusively on linguistic forms (i.e., the grammatical rules that govern the juxtaposition of words in syntactic constructions). See for example, the works of Bellugi and Brown (1964), Braine (1963), Brown (1968), Brown and Bellugi (1964), Cazden (1968), Chomsky (1969), Menyuk (1963); and Miller and Ervin (1964). The focus on form, which dominated the research during the 1960s, was expanded in the 1970s to include analytical approaches that focused either on language meaning (Bloom, 1970; Bloom, Lightbown, and Hood, 1975; Bowerman, 1973; Brown, 1973) or on language use (Bates, 1976; Dore, 1973; Halliday, 1975; Limber, 1976; Ochs and Schieffelin, 1979; Sachs and Devin, 1976). These expanded approaches evolved partly from the creation of methods for examining the situational context surrounding the linguistic forms used. That is, from examining "what the child said in relation to what he talked about and the situation and behavior that co-occurred with what he said" (Bloom, 1970, p. 2).

The recognition that a comprehensive linguistic description requires an analysis of form, content, and use was followed in the 1980s by a shift toward frameworks that could capture the interaction among these dimensions. This focus is illustrated for the following hypothetical example of a child's utterance.

Context   *Child's Utterance*
(Mother and child playing with race track
and cars)

Mother: "Let me have a car; I want one too."

(Child takes one of two cars and holds it close
to his chest)   "This car mines."
Mother: "Okay then, I'll take the other one."

For the foregoing example, the form analysis would require classification of the utterance in terms of its syntactic and morphological features. For example, it could be noted that the elaborated noun phrase is represented by the demonstrative adjective *(this)* plus noun *(car)*. In addition, the analysis can specify what the utterance means and how it is used. This can be done by focusing on both the linguistic structure of the utterance and the context in which it occurs. With respect to utterance meaning in the foregoing example, the occurrence of the possessive pronoun, *mine,* and the nonlinguistic act of taking one of the two cars and holding it close to the chest provide evidence that the utterance refers to a possessive state. With respect to language use, the mother's preceding verbal request for a car could be seen as an appropriate context for the *informative* function of a child's response, which has the general effect of denying a request.

An interactional analysis would require that the distributions of features for one dimension be examined in relation to others so as to determine if and how performance in one area (e.g., form) is constrained or influenced by performance in another area (e.g., meaning or use). Such an analysis could reveal, for example, whether or not noun phrase elaboration occurs more or less often in semantic contexts that code states as opposed to actions. Furthermore, the investigator could explore whether or not elaborated noun phrases in utterances referring to states are differentially linked to the types of pragmatic goals (e.g., informatives versus requestives). This multidimensional approach is superior to unidimensional ones, not only because of the comprehensive description that it can yield but also because of its greater explanatory power. A study conducted by Bloom, Lahey, Hood, Lifter, and Fiess (1980) illustrates the explanatory feature of the framework.

The study by Bloom and colleagues demonstrated that the acquisition of syntactic connectives (e.g., conjunctions) in complex sentences was influenced by meaning and use. It was observed that the conjunctive form *and* is learned before the conjunctive form *then*. The earlier occurrence of *and* before *then* was explained in terms of conceptual differences underlying their meaning. The conjunction *and* codes an additive semantic notion (e.g., you do one and I do one) whereas the conjunction *then* codes a temporal semantic notion (e.g., you do one, then I do one). The investigators appealed to research that has shown that additive reactions are conceptually less complex than temporal ones in that "children learn to form collections of things (e.g., Sinclair, 1970) before they learn to form series of things that are ordered relative to one another (e.g., Inhelder and Piaget, 1964)."

The study by Bloom and colleagues revealed that the use of connective forms also was influenced by the types of discourse cohesion contexts in which complex sentences were used. Regardless of the conjunctive meaning expressed, complex sentences occurred most often in intraspeaker or child-child cohesion contexts (i.e., contexts in which the two clauses occurred within the same utterance or across two consecutive utterances produced by the child (e.g., *there's my eye, and there's my feet;* or *there's my eye and my feet*). Whenever complex utterances occurred in interspeaker cohesion contexts that involved adult-child or child-adult-child turn-taking events, they most often expressed causality and adversative meaning. The interspeaker cohesion pattern increased developmentally, and "appeared to reflect the children's ability to participate in discourse using newly or already learned linguistic forms" (Bloom, et al., 1980, p. 258).

Only a multidimensional interaction analysis could have revealed the kind of findings described earlier. Other studies that provide sharp illustrations of the explanatory power of multidimensional frameworks include those of Limber (1976), Antinucci and Miller (1976), and Johnston and Slobin (1979).

The Methodological Orientation Must be Sensitive to the Sociocultural Context in Which Children's Language is Learned and Spoken

The study of children's language within the dynamic framework of form-content-use interactions requires the use of data collection strategies that are sensitive to the context in which language is spoken. Context, in its narrowest sense, refers to the particular situations in which spoken language may be observed. It includes the physical setting for verbal exchange, the nonverbal and verbal behaviors of the participants, topics, role relations, and so forth. In its broadest sense, context refers to the culturally shared beliefs and values of a speech community that dictate the conditions under which verbal communication occurs and their respective social codes of interaction.

The research methodology can reflect sensitivity to sociocultural context by employing language data that characterize routine social interactions. This requirement can be met most easily by using naturalistic data — that is, data consisting of spontaneous spoken language as it may occur in its typical or untampered state during everyday talk. Such naturalistic sampling provides the kind of data that serve normative goals. Furthermore, because the resulting data require the investigator to make few asusmptions about their form prior to the study, they are particularly appropriate for initiating research on the language of speakers about which little is known.

On the other hand, structured elicitation tasks such as those modeled after Berko (1958) often do not require observation of spoken language in social interactive contexts. In fact, elicitation tasks usually are structured to elicit very specific linguistic features with known properties. Hence, the use of elicitation tasks requires prior knowledge about which linguistic features are relevant to study. For example, the investigator already has to know that past tense can be marked with the -ed form for such verb stems as "walk" and "laugh" before designing a task to elicit such markers in a research study.

Since structured elicitation tasks must be guided by prior knowledge of the relevant features for observation, they do not provide the most effective data gathering strategy for initiating research in an area about which little is known.

Let us now consider four requirements of using a naturalistic data sampling strategy. First, naturalistic data sampling requires more than a spontaneous speech sample. It also requires that the sample be collected in social contexts in which language is used routinely. Language is not used routinely to talk to investigators in small rooms or laboratories. It is used in the home, at school, or on the community playground to talk with family members and playmates about shared experiences in a speaker's culture. Language is used to request food, report ailments, ask questions, tease, play games, and so forth. Such communication acts cannot be studied unless language is observed in naturalistic settings.

Second, naturalistic data sampling requires the investigator to record the most relevant verbal and nonverbal details of the context in which language is spoken. Records of contextual data meet the demand of an expanded theoretical framework which relies on them to infer utterance meaning and use. The data record may include what is said before and after each of the child's linguistic responses, what the child and others are doing at the time of a language response, who the participants are and their relation to the child, and similar information. Although descriptive contextual detail may be recorded using on-site handwritten notes, audiovisual records obviously provide more complete and dynamic representation of speech events.

Third, a naturalistic data sampling strategy ideally requires data collection without informant knowledge because such knowledge could alter typical language behavior. It is impossible, however, to eliminate the effect of investigator presence altogether if firsthand observations are to be made, especially when audiovisual recording is used (see Labov, 1972, for a discussion of the observer paradox). The barrier created by investigator's presence can be minimized to some extent if the investigator assumes the role of participant-observer, a strategy used effectively by some ethnographers. An ethnographic approach permits the investigator to become a natural extention of the child's communicative environment and thereby experience directly the social interactive effects of the informant's language behavior. Naturally, this means that the investigator does not always structure the interaction. The success of a participant-observer approach depends partly on the type of informant-investigator relationship that is established prior to and during data collection.

Fourth, the investigator must have prior knowledge of the range and types of situations in which children typically talk as well as the general kind of social factors that impact on the frequency and quality of talking. In the absence of such information, an adequate language sample may not be obtained. For example, an earlier claim that Black children are nonverbal was made erroneously because investigators lacked knowledge about the way these children behave verbally when interacting with white interviewers, particularly in atypical, formal communicative situations (Labov, Cohen, and Robbins, 1968). The limited language samples obtained by Blount (1969) from Luo speaking children in Kenya showed that even in the familiar homestead, children in some cultures will reduce their verbal output when talking to strangers. Blount elicited about 200 utterances overall from more than six children across an 8 month period.

It is now well known that cultural groups are not homogeneous with respect to the types of social factors that impact on language behavior. The implication is that the investigator cannot impose his or her cultural orientation on the subjects under study without the danger of misrepresenting them.

REVIEW OF LANGUAGE ACQUISITION STUDIES ON THE BLACK CHILD

In the preceding section, four guidelines for conducting language development research were proposed. In this section, these guidelines provide a framework for describing and evaluating language acquisition research on Black children who acquire a nonstandard English vernacular.

Although language research on BE speaking Black children spans at least three decades, only a small subset of these studies has focused specifically on language development. Representative studies include those of Blake (1984), Bridgeforth (1984), Cole (1980), Kovac (1980), Reveron (1978), Steffensen (1974), Stockman (1984), Stockman and Vaughn-Cooke (1982a, 1982b, 1984), Stockman, Vaughn-Cooke, and Wolfram, 1982; and Stokes (1976).

The developmental focus on Black children's language is recent relative to the research on other groups of children. The studies just cited were among the earliest ones conducted on Black children. Note that they were not initiated until the mid- to late 1970s, whereas acquisitional research on other groups predated this period by several decades. For example, there was the work on white children's phonological and grammatical development in the 1940s and

1950s (Irwin, 1947; McCarthy, 1954; Templin, 1957), followed by the virtual explosion of child language research in the 1960s and 1970s.

The initiation of acquisitional research on Black children coincided with the peaking of a decade or more of sociolinguistic research that had defended BE's legitimacy as a language system. Evidence that Black children acquire a legitimately different variety of English sharply focused the practical need for developmental normative data, because in principle such data on other English varieties could no longer be applied unconditionally to them.

Although acquisitional research represented an important shift in the type of language research that historically had been conducted on Black children, it did not consistently conform to all four guidelines described in the previous section. All acquisitional studies of Black children's language met the requirement of the first guideline because they shared the common goal of describing what Black children know about language at different ages. All conformed to the second guideline by focusing on the acquisition of BE as the first language acquired. The studies differed primarily in theoretical and methodological orientation, the foci of the third and fourth guidelines.

Two groups of studies can be distinguished on the basis of research orientation. The earliest group of studies focused predominantly on linguistic form whereas a more recent group of studies has focused on form in relation to meaning or use. The two different investigative foci naturally reflected diverging notions about what was important to study and how to study it.

The form-focused studies reflected the influence of sociolinguistic frameworks that have revolved around the general goal of describing and explaining language differences in various social and cultural contexts. This orientation to language differences is reflected in the goal of form-focused developmental studies, which has been to determine the ages at which Black children acquire just those features that distinguish BE and SE. This research goal typically has been met by using quasi-experimental research methods that require the elicitation of specific linguistic features during a structured spoken language task. The linguistic features investigated are restricted to those that have been documented to occur in the spoken language of mature BE speakers. The task may be administered to relatively large groups of children of various ages. A group performance criterion is then used to determine the ages at which various features conform to the adult BE forms.

The theoretical and methodological orientation of the form-focused studies conforms less aptly to the third and fourth guidelines than the later initiated acquisitional studies that focused on form in relation to meaning or use. The latter studies reflect the research frameworks of developmental psycholinguistics. Consequently they are guided by the general goal of describing and accounting for the full range of linguistic knowledge acquired by children and the acquisitional order of such knowledge within and across languages. The methodology accommodates the expectation that the linguistic features used by children need not mirror those used by the mature speaker of a language at all developmental stages. Rather than construct tasks to elicit specific responses based on expected adult features, investigative methods typically have involved the collection and analysis of spoken language data gathered in naturalistic settings. The intensive analysis of longitudinal data on small numbers of children has been favored over the cross-sectional analysis of structured responses from large groups of children. This approach permits the discovery of childrens' typical language behavior. Discovery is aided by the use of investigative methods that exploit interpretive analysis to derive children's linguistic knowledge, particularly in the areas of meaning and use.

The following sections present descriptive summaries and critiques of studies that focused exclusively on linguistic form and studies that focused on form in relation to meaning and use.

Studies of Linguistic Form

The major findings from the form-focused studies are summarized in Table 5–1.

Steffensen (1974) observed the language of two boys, one covering the period of 20 to 26 months and the other covering the period of 17 to 26 months. The spoken language of each subject was sampled for about 1 hour every other week in the home setting. The goal of the study was to determine the age of emergence for BE forms associated with plural, possessive, third person singular, and past tense inflections, pronominals, copula, and auxiliary verbs. Steffenson reported that inflectional markers generally were not used to denote such features as plurality, possession, and so forth. However, the children's conceptual knowledge of these categories of knowledge was indicated by the semantic context of their utterances and the use of other linguistic forms that were not under study. Copula use stabilized in the final position of utterances having ostensive mean-

Table 5-1.   Summary of Major Findings from Form-Focused Studies

Age	Steffensen (1974) (No criterion for acquisition) (2 subjects per age)	Stokes (1976) (No criterion for mastery) (12 subjects per age)	Cole (1979) (90% group criterion for mastery) (20 subjects per age)	Reveron (1978) (80% group criterion for mastery) (20 subjects per age)	Kovak (1980) (No criterion for mastery) (8 subjects per age)
1½–2½ years	Uninflected -z for plural, possessive, and third person singular Uninflected past tense -ed Inflected -ing for visible action verbs (e.g., go) Full form copula final position of sentences having ostensive meaning (e.g., There Mary is) Full and contracted copula in medial position of sentences having ostensive meaning (e.g., There is Mary)				
3 years		Negativized constructions that include: modals invariant be progressive past participle copula tag questions indefinite problems	Copula absence Uninflected -z for third person singular Uninflected -ed for past tense Remote past tense *been*	Uninflected -z for plural possessive, third person singular Uninflected -ed for past tense (38% to 58%)	Contracted copula Deleted copula

4 years	All the above plus Emergence of negativized relative clauses embedded questions	All the above plus Regularization of indefinite article (a apple) Regularization of reflexive pronouns (hisself) Multiple negation (he don't like nobody)	Consistently uninflected -ed for past tense Consistently uninflected -z for third person singular	
5 years	All the above	All the above plus Regularization of demonstrative pronoun	Same as above	All the above
6 years			Same as above plus Uninflected -z for possessive (approaches criterion for low socioeconomic class children)	
7 years				All the above

ing (e.g., There the boy *is*), and it variably occurred as a contracted or full form in the medial position of sentences having the same meaning (e.g., There's the boy). Steffenson concluded that the forms exhibited by the subjects did not differ from those exhibited by white children of the same age who learn SE.

Stokes (1976) used a cued elicitation task and a one-half hour spontaneous speech sample to elicit negation constructions from 36 Black boys and girls, who were evenly distributed at 3, 4, and 5 years of age. The children were required to negativize affirmative statements that were presented in both BE and SE during individualized testing. The stimuli represented two to five aspects of four categories of constructions: (1) auxiliary verbs, (2) main verbs plus copula, regular and irregular verbs, (3) indefinites, and (4) multipropositions. The findings did not support a systematic sex differences on any feature category. Of the four categories, multipropositions, which included relative clauses and embedded questions, were the least often negated by 3 year old children and remained difficult even at 5 years. Some constructions in each of the remaining three categories could be negated as early as 3 years of age, but differences existed among age groups in the frequency with which various constructions were negated. Increments with age, however, were not linear in that the increase in negating some constructions at 4 years was followed by a decrease at 5 years. Overall, the children presented both differences from and similarities to SE speaking children as described in the literature.

Reveron (1978) examined the use of BE morphological rules for plural, possessive, past tense, and third person singular by 80 Black children who represented low and middle socioeconomic groups and four ages: 3, 4, 5, and 6 years. A Berko type elicitation task, which consisted of 24 nonsense monosyllables, was presented. The stimuli were represented visually by black and white drawings. They were audio recorded and presented in both SE and BE. Whereas each category of morphological markers was used by some children in every subject group, their frequencies varied with social class, age, and presentation mode. Middle and lower class Black children produced significantly more BE than SE morphological rules. The frequency of BE rule usage increased with age, reaching the 80 percent acquisitional criterion at 4 years only for past tense and third person singular in either social groups. The acquisition criterion was not met for SE morphological rules by either group at any age. Middle class children, however, produced fewer BE rules than did lower class children. Social class differences were significant above 4 years.

Cole (1979) observed the spontaneous speech of 60 Black girls who were distributed evenly at 3, 4, and 5 years of age. Using a structured picture elicitation task, the goal was to determine the ages at which the children exhibited 19 BE features, which included, for example, plural, possessive, and past tense inflections, and go copula. Whereas each feature was exhibited in varying frequency at every age, the 90 percent acquisitional criterion was reached on just eight features. At 3 years, these included the uninflected verbs for regular -ed past tense, third person singular, absence of present tense copula, and use of the remote past *been*. At older ages, the acquisitional criterion was reached for all four features observed at 3 years, plus the BE features of indefinite article regularization and multiple negation at 4 years, and the BE features of reflexive and pronominal regularization at 5 years. The failure of 11 features to reach the acquisitional criterion suggested that some BE features (e.g., go copula, hypercorrection, regularized demonstrative pronouns) are mastered after 5 years.

Kovac (1980) elicited spontaneous speech from 26 middle and working-class Black and white children, 3, 5, and 7 years old, to investigate the acquisition of auxillary and copula features within the framework of variation theory. Data were collected in day care and elementary school settings in three contexts involving (1) role playing dyads, (2) question and answer interviews and free conversation, and (3) picture book description. For both social classes of white subjects, contracted copula was highest in frequency of occurrence, followed in order by deleted and full forms. Middle class Black children exhibited a distribution that was similar to that of white children. The pattern for lower class children was similar to that of the other two groups only at the youngest ages. At 5 years, deleted forms were more frequent than contracted forms among lower class Black children. At 7 years, contracted forms were again more frequent than deleted or full forms. Kovac (1980) concluded that Black children's variable copula deletion at older ages conforms to expected BE variable constraints, but that at the youngest ages, it was impossible to separate developmental absence from dialect specific deletion patterns.

Critique of Form-Focused Studies

The form-focused studies have pioneering status as the earliest attempts to describe Black children's normal language development. They were, nevertheless, limited in their capacity to provide a comprehensive picture of developing language. The major limitation considered here is their collective focus on linguistic form in isolation from meaning and use. The isolated investigative focus on linguistic form does not reflect the theoretical and analytical framework offered by the third guideline. (see description earlier in this chapter.) Consequently, the resulting developmental data were restricted as considered here.

First, the exclusive focus on linguistic form does not take into account the fact that learning a language involves more than learning its sounds, words, and grammatical rules; it also requires learning about the meaning of underlying words and sentences, and how language is used pragmatically to accomplish communicative goals. It has been argued that linguistic forms exist to serve semantic and pragmatic goals, and as such are less primary than meaning and use. Thus, the isolated focus on form leaves important dimensions of a Black child's developing language undescribed, except in an incidental way.

Second, the preoccupation with just those forms that are characteristically BE limits the completeness with which linguistic forms even can be described. Dialect specific forms make up just a small subset of the complex grammatical system that is likely to be acquired by BE speaking children. Stockman (1984) noted that with respect to syntactic constitutent patterns for talking about locative events, characteristic BE patterns accounted for less than 25 percent of all the utterances used in language samples of children at 1 year 6 months, 3 years, and 4 years 6 months.

Furthermore, a number of the most salient BE markers include morphological features (e.g., the absence of inflectional word endings) that do not represent the most basic grammatical features acquired by the child. For example, the child probably learns rules for concatenating words to express basic semantic relations like action and state before he or she learns to inflect specific lexical forms to signal the time, aspect, or person connected with action or state. Morphological inflections are likely to represent the later learned modulations (in the sense of Brown, 1973) of basic syntactic structures. The restriction of acquisitional research just to the dialect specific forms, therefore, prevents researchers from answering fundamental questions about language learning, such as "When do Black children acquire two and three word utterances?", "When do they acquire complex sentences?", and so forth.

The methodological orientation of most form-focused studies did not conform to the fourth guideline. Consequently, the data yielded even on dialect specific forms may be less definitive than is optimal. The use of structured elicitation tasks raises at least two questions

about the BE features that have been observed in children's repertoires. First, do the BE features observed on structured tasks reflect
their distribution in spontaneous spoken language? Second, does the
use of noncontextualized responses prevent the investigators from
revealing rule-governed variability that influences the distribution
of observed features?

The notion of variable rule usage governing morphological and
phonological forms has been documented as an important BE feature (Labov, 1969). See also Kovac (1980) for an overview of the variability paradigm. As an example, reference can be made here to the
variable occurrence of the *-ed* marker depending on phonological factors such as the presence or absence of a succeeding consonant
(Fasold, 1972).

Failure to consider the variable through systematic occurrence of
-ed under certain conditions could lead to a normative description
that encourages erroneous judgments to be made about BE speaking
children. For example, the variable absence of this marker could be
interpreted erroneously as a pathological rather than normal language difference.

Acquisitional Studies of Form, Content, and Use

Since 1980, acquisitional studies on Black children were broad-
ened to include investigative focus on the meaning and use of language in addition to its form. Representative studies include the research of Stockman and Vaughn-Cooke (1982a, 1982b, 1984),
Stockman (1984), Blake (1984), and Bridgeforth (1984). These studies, unlike the form-focused studies, did not restrict observation only
to dialect specific features. Rather, their goals were to provide a comprehensive description of the linguistic feature selected for study.
The major findings from this set of studies are summarized
in Table 5–2.

Stockman and Vaughn-Cooke's research was initiated in 1980.
Their long-term investigation, which involves a coordinated series of
studies, is still in progress. Its goals are to document the age and acquisitional order in which working class Black children acquire major categories of meaning and the grammatical and phonological
forms for expressing meaning. A cross-sectional, longitudinal data
collection strategy was used to track the language development of 12
working class Black children across 18 months. Two boys and two
girls were represented at each of three ages that were separated by
an 18 month interval. At the onset of data collection, the children
were 1 year 6 months, 3 years, and 4 years 6 months.

Table 5-2. Summary of Major Findings from Form, Content, and Use Studies

Age	Stockman & Vaughn-Cooke (1982a) (Criterion of 5 responses) (4 subjects per age)	Stockman & Vaughn-Cooke (1984) (Criterion of 5 responses) (4 subjects per age)	Stockman (1985) (Criterion of 5 responses) (4 subjects per age)	Stockman, Vaughn-Cooke, & Wolfram (1982) (No criterion) (4 subjects per age)	Blake (1984) (Criterion of 3 responses) (3 subjects per age)			Bridgeforth (1984) (No criterion) (4 subjects per age)
1½–2 years	Action Existence	Dynamic directional locative meaning	Single words predominate multiword utterances (verb + locative implement)	/m/ initial word position /n/ initial word position	MLU = 1.3–2.0 Type Token Ratio = .32–.71	Major Semantic Relations: Action/Locative Action State/Locative State Existence Attribution Intention Minor Semantic Relations: Wh-Questions Place Other: Social Expressions	Inter-personal[R,P] Expressive Effective[R,P] Objective[R,P] Directive[R,P] Social and nonsocial self expressive[R,P] Participative[R]	
2–2½ years					MLU = 1.6–2.6+ Type Token Ratio .62–.78	All the above plus notice negation recurrence possession dative	All the above plus self-expressive[P] participative[P] attentive[P]	

	Action/Loca-tive action State/Locative state negation recurrence possession dative time	Dynamic directional meaning Dynamic positional destinative meaning Dynamic combinative meaning Dynamic original meaning Static positional meaning Static combinative meaning	Predominant use of multiword utterances (verb + locative complement) (verb + object + locative complement) (Subject + verb + locative complement) (Subject + verb + object = locative complement) (Subject + loctive complement here + go + object)	/m/ final word position preceding vowels /n/ final word preceding vowels			Informatives Reporting personal facts Reporting general facts Responding to questions Requestive/ Regulator direct requests Recycles Repeating Imitating Giving
3 years							
4½ years	All the above plus coordination causality epistemic[1Ss] antithesis[3Ss]	All the above plus Static directional meaning	All the above plus (there/here + go + object) (there/here + object + go)	/m/ same as above /n/ same as above			All the above plus Imaginatives Role playing

R = Real context
P = Pretend context

MLU = Mean length of utterance
Ss = Subjects

During monthly visits to the children's homes, 1 to 2 hour spontaneous language samples were obtained. Audiovisual recordings were made during these samples while the children engaged in routine conversations and loosely structured play activities with the investigators and familiar others. The utterances were extracted from the tapes and orthographically recorded along with relevant verbal and nonverbal contextual detail that could be used to infer utterance meaning.

The data analysis plan requires the reliable categorization of the utterances according to one or more broad semantic categories adapted from the taxonomy presented by Bloom and Lahey (1978). The taxonomy included semantic categories, such as action, state, possession, causality, location, and so forth.

Once the semantic categories are assigned to children's utterances, all grammatical features for coding the semantic categories are identified and compared across ages. So far, results have been reported for the cross-sectional analysis of the baseline or initial sampling period of the 18 month longitudinal data base. The preliminary findings have focused on four areas as described later in this chapter, and they are summarized in Table 5–2.

One set of findings pertained to the number and types of semantic categories represented at each age cross-section in the first sampling period (see Stockman and Vaughn-Cooke, 1982a, and 1982b). Of the 17 categories studied, 88 percent, 76 percent, and 41 percent were represented at the ages of 4 years 6 months, 3 years, and 1 year six months, respectively. The multipropositional categories of causality, antithesis, coordination, and epistemic distinguished children at 4 years 6 months and 3 years, whereas the categories of quantity, possession, and mood, which are coordinated with the major categories of action, state, and location, differentiated children at 1 year 6 months and 3 years.

A second set of findings pertained to the type of developmental changes that take place once a major semantic category emerges (Stockman and Vaughn-Cooke, 1984). To illustrate, it was observed that children who productively coded the major semantic category of location differed in the type of locative meaning expressed (see Stockman and Vaughn-Cooke, 1984). In the baseline sampling period, children at 1 year 6 months talked about location in terms of the movement that displaced an object from one position to another (dynamic locative events or locative action). For example, the utterances referred to objects *going up, coming down, going away, moving back,* and the like. In addition to object displacement, children at 3 years and 4 years 6 months talked about the fixed spatial position of objects (i.e., static locative events or locative state). For example, utterances referred to objects' locative positions as being *in, on, under,* or *between* other objects.

Within the dynamic and static locative categories, the meanings of the utterances were differentiated further. Depending on the child's age, dynamic locative utterances referred to the object's locative displacement in terms of one of four referent subcategories. The subcategories included (1) the *origin* of the locative displacement (e.g., ball fell from the tree); (2) the *direction* of locative displacement (e.g., ball fell down); (3) the *destinative position* of locative displacement (e.g., ball fell to the ground); or (4) some combination of the three subcategories (e.g., the ball fell down to the ground). Analogous subcategories of locative reference were observed for static locative events.

At 1 year 6 months, the criterion of productive usage (i.e., at least five different utterances in the same sampling session) was met only for the directional subcategory of dynamic locative events. This was the most frequently coded aspect of dynamic locative utterances at 3 years, although the children at this age also productively coded object displacement in terms of its origin, destination, or some combination of the subcategories. The children at 4 years 6 months had productive usage of the four dynamic locative subcategories in the first sampling period. However, they exhibited noticeably higher utterance frequencies than 3 year old children for the subcategories of destinative position and combinative reference.

With respect to static locative meaning, the criterion of productive usage was not met by the 1 year 6 month old children for any subcategory in the first sampling period. At 3 years and 4 years 6 months, productive usage was observed consistently and most frequently across all subjects for the positional and combinative subcategories.

A third set of findings pertained to the kind of grammatical forms that were used to talk about locative events (Stockman, 1984), Syntactic constructions were characterized by the type and order of major grammatical constituents (e.g., subject, verb, object, verb complement). Seven patterns accounted for at least 90 percent of the multiword utterances. Dynamic locative meaning, irrespective of the referent subcategory, was encoded by four types of constructions. These constructions included the following:

1. verb + locative complement (e.g., fell down)
2. verb + object + locative complement (e.g., put the ball down)
3. subject + verb + locative complement (e.g., ball fell down)
4. subject + verb + object + locative complement (e.g., boy put ball down)

Category 1 constructions were used exclusively by children at 1 year 6 months, whereas all four types of constructions were observed among 3 year and 4 year 6 month old children, albeit with different frequencies.

Static locative events were coded by the same types of constructions in categories 1 through 4, in addition to the following three types:

5. subject + locative complement (e.g., the ball in)
6. here/there + go + object (e.g., here go the ball, there go the ball)
7. here/there + object + go (e.g., here the ball go, there the ball go)

None of the 1 year 6 month old children used static locative constructions whereas children at 3 years and 4 years 6 months used all three constructions with varying frequencies. Significantly more static locative utterances were observed at 4 years 6 months than at 3 years.

Children's ability to use a pattern to encode both dynamic and static locative events increased with age and constituted one differnce between the 3 year old and 4 year 6 month old children.

Stockman's results showed that by 3 years, a multiword grammatical system was well in place for talking about locative events. None of the utterances used at 1 year 6 months could be accounted for by dialect specific features, and fewer than 25 percent of utterances made at older ages conformed with dialect specific features.

A fourth set of findings pertained to the phonological patterns used in the baseline sampling period. Analysis of nasal consonants (Stockman et al., 1982) among 3 year and 4 year 6 month old children revealed that the /m/ and /n/ segments were used as early as 1 year 6 months, but not in word final position. At 3 years, final nasal consonants were observed under certain conditions. They were present most often when followed by words beginning with a vowel and deleted most often when followed by a consonant or no segment at all. The /n/ segment was more subject to deletion than /m/. When deleted, nasal segments were marked by vowel nazalization. The data suggest that by 3 years, nasal segments had already begun to conform to a BE rule governed variable pattern of usage.

Blake studied three Black children (two boys and one girl) who were between 18 and 27 months of age. Longitudinal samples (8 to 20 per child) of their language, taken in mother-child dyads in a low structure playroom setting, were videotaped for 1 hour every four weeks.

The analysis of linguistic form revealed that MLU increments with age were comparable to that reported for white children.

Changes in type or token ratios also indicated increments in the diversity of forms used as age increased. Five BE features were observed, but rarely was the same BE form used by every subject, and none reached a criterion of productive usage in any child's speech.

With respect to meaning, major semantic categories (e.g., action, state, location, negation) reached the criterion of productive usage at earlier ages than did minor semantic categories (e.g., recurrence, coordination, and causality).

With respect to language use, at least eight major functions were required to describe the language of all three subjects. The functions that accounted for most of the utterances included interpersonal expressive, affective, objective, and directive. The number of functions increased with age for both real and pretend contexts.

To examine the interaction among form, content, and use, a quantitative measure of mean length of utterance (MLU) shifts was compared with performance shifts in semantic-syntactic relations and pragmatic functions within the same time period. It was observed that smaller shifts in MLU were associated with greater shifts in language content and use. This finding suggested that learning something new in one area of language has a certain cost that is reflected in less comparable gains in other areas.

Bridgeforth (1984) examined the language functions of eight working class Black children at two age cross-sections, 3 years and 4 years 6 months. The subject data were the same as those used in the Stockman and Vaughn-Cooke studies cited earlier. The analysis was restricted to spontaneous utterances in the first of the 18 sampling periods. The analytical scheme involved conceptualization of functions on two levels. *Microfunctions,* such as reporting personal facts or requesting clarification, were subsumed under five *macrofunctions:* informatives, requests and regulators, recycles, imaginatives, and social conventions. Bridgeforth's pragmatic categories were broadly analogous to those derived by Blake (1984). Blake's objective, directive, and self-expressive categories, corresponded respectively to the microfunctions of reporting general facts, reporting personal facts, and reporting personal feelings that were subsumed under the macrofunction of informatives. Blake's affective, participative, and attentive categories correspond to microfunctions subsumed under the macrofunction of requests and regulators. Bridgeforth's macrofunction of social conventions appears to be most analogous to Blake's interpersonal expressive category.

Among macrofunctions studied by Bridgeforth, the informative and imaginative functions were used most frequently by the older group, whereas the request or regulator and recycling functions were used most frequently at 3 years. The informative function at both ages was used to report general facts more frequently than it was used to serve any other microfunction. Direct directives was the most frequently used microfunction in the request or regulator macrofunction.

Bridgeforth's results for 4 year 6 month old children were similar to those obtained by Peters (1983). Peters studied the pragmatic functions of 4 year old Black children from low and middle class backgrounds. She showed that for both social classes, the informative function ranked higher in frequency of use than did the regulative, social, imaginative, requestive, and emotional functions.

Critique of Form-Content-Use Studies

The form-content-use studies undoubtedly come closest to meeting the requirements of all the guidelines posed in the preceding section. By extending the analysis beyond linguistic form, particularly those that are dialect specific, they overcome certain limitations of earlier developmental studies. Given that form-content-use studies are still few in number and represent a small sample of children, it is not surprising that they do not provide a complete picture of Black children's developing language. In fact, no one or two studies can examine all the features that are relevant to a developmental description.

It appears that specific aspects of grammatical and phonological forms have been less well investigated in those studies that have focused on form, meaning, and use than in those that have focused solely on form. Blake (1984), for example, used global measures of form (i.e., MLU and Type Token Ratio (TTR) while the specific morphosyntactic features examined were restricted to BE. Stockman (1984), on the other hand, described some syntactic constituent patterns used by BE speaking children, but these analyses were restricted to just the subset of utterances that coded locative meaning. Although it is expected that the same patterns will be reflected in other utterances (i.e., those that code action, states, and so forth), this expectation needs to be documented. Bridgeforth's study ignored linguistic forms altogether.

Therefore, there is still limited information about the normative characteristics of Black children's general syntactic features as they relate, for example, to noun and verb phrase elaboration and the coding of complex propositions. Such features should be examined in utterances that exhibit BE features and in those that do not. Although BE features seem to account for just a subset of the utterances used by the Black children, their impact, if any, on the acquisitional time and order of non-BE features remains an important research issue to be explored as well.

SUMMARY AND CONCLUSIONS

This chapter has called attention to the role that language acquisition research can and does play in building the normative data base that is so critical to the language assessment process. It has also attempted to make obvious the need to expand the number and types of developmental studies on Black children who acquire a nonstandard English vernacular.

The four guidelines offered as a framework for evaluating language acquisition research on Black children that can serve a normative purpose included the following: (1) the investigative goal should have a developmental focus, (2) the mother tongue principle should guide the choice of language studied, (3) the investigative focus should be guided by a theoretical framework that permits examination of linguistic forms in relation to their meaning and use, and (4) the methodological orientation of the research should be sensitive to the sociocultural context in which language is learned and spoken.

Eight acquisitional studies on Black children were summarized and critiqued within the framework of these four guidelines. These studies included those that have focused solely on linguistic forms and those that have focused on linguistic form in the context of meaning or use. Collectively, they provide converging evidence for several generalizations about the language development of BE speaking children.

1. Black children, not surprisingly, develop language over a time period. Language learning for some children is well under way by 18 months in the sense that one and two word utterances can be found (Blake, 1984; Steffensen, 1974; Stockman, 1984; Stockman and Vaughn-Cooke, 1982a).

2. Black children acquire language for coding the same early domains of meaning as those acquired by SE speaking children (Blake, 1984; Stockman and Vaughn-Cooke, 1982a; also see Steffensen's 1974 examination of ostensive, locative, and state categories [1974]). The number of semantic categories represented increases with age. The semantic categories of action and existence are among the earliest ones acquired, whereas categories

underlying multipropositions such as coordination or causality
are among the latest acquired (Blake, 1984, Stockman and
Vaughn-Cooke, 1982a).

3. Before 3 years of age, BE speaking children use language to accomplish a broad range of pragmatic functions that provide for
(1) commenting on the environment (informatives), (2) getting
others to do something (directives and requestives), and (3) maintaining or regulating social interactions (Blake, 1984; Bridgeforth, 1984). (Also see the selected study of questions by Steffensen [1974] and corroborating evidence from Peters [1984].)

4. BE speaking children appear to acquire a diverse system of
grammatical forms for expressing semantic and pragmatic goals.
The MLU increases with age and up to at least 2 years 6 months,
the increments are similar to that reported for white SE speaking children (Blake, 1984). By the time Black children are 3
years, well-formed multiwork constructions having subject, verb,
and object complement are well in place (Stockman, 1984). The
bulk of the utterances at 3 years are expected to be single verb or
simple constructions, although a few complex utterances can be
observed as well.

5. Before 3 years, BE features are not prominent and, in fact, the
data suggest that the earliest patterns exhibited do not differ
from those that have been observed for children who acquire SE
(Blake, 1984; Steffensen, 1974; Stockman, 1984). However, BE
features increase with age (Cole, 1979; Kovac, 1980; Stokes,
1976). Between 3 and 7 years, children acquire some of the dialect specific rules for plural, possessive, tense, third person singular, indefinite article, and pronominalization in addition to variable rules for copula deletion and final consonant segment
deletion (Cole, 1979; Kovac, 1980; Reveron, 1978; Stockman,
Vaughn-Cooke, and Wolfram, 1982). They also acquire dialect
specific rules for negating affirmative utterances (Stokes, 1976).

6. There is variation among Black children in the types of developmental patterns presented. Although no sex differences have
been reported (e.g., see Stokes, 1976), differences related to social
class have been reported (Kovac, 1980; Reveron, 1978; see also
corroborating data on 4 year old children from Peters [1984]). Social class differences appear more pronounced after 4 years when
low SES children begin to show more marked used of BE features
than those from middle SES groups. Children present individual
differences in the frequency and type of specific linguistic features exhibited even within the same SES group (Blake, 1984;
Steffensen, 1974; Stockman, 1984; Stockman and Vaughn-Cooke,

1982a). This observation is due presumably to differences in language environment, learning, and data sampling conditions.

Implications for Assessment

The language acquisition data just summarized have obvious implications for assessing Black children's language. They provide at least a rudimentary empirical basis for shaping expectations about what they ought to know about language at an early age, at least in very broad terms. Such expectations should be taken into account when constructing new language assessment tests and when using informal, criterion referenced procedures to make judgments about language status. For example, consider what is known about the language of 3 year old children who acquire BE. Three years is the earliest age at which children typically are referred for speech and language services. Tables 5–1 and 5–2 indicate that by 3 years, an intact, functional, multiword language system would be expected that allows the child to code all major categories of meaning at some level. The linguistic system is also mature enough to allow the child to achieve the major pragmatic goals of commenting about the state of affairs at some level, getting others to do something (i.e., answer a question or follow a command), and maintaining routine social relations (e.g., greetings) in real and pretend situations. The older the child is, the more obligatory these features should be in the child's system in addition to dialect specific ones.

The data suggest, then, that a Black child's failure to exhibit the above-mentioned features by 3 years is more likely to reflect a pathological rather than a dialect difference. In fact, there is converging evidence to indicate that dialect specific features, except perhaps in the area of phonology, are either absent or lack prominence at the earliest stages of Black children's language development (i.e., before the age of about 4 years). The grammatical forms used, regardless of social class, seem to be indistinguishable from those used by children who acquire an SE vernacular. This should not be surprising given the assumption that all children probably first acquire the most basic and universal features of a language system before they acquire those features that mark the dialect specific characteristics.

Evidence that children who acquire BE and those who acquire SE exhibit the same types of linguistic features at the early stages of development naturally raises the question of whether Black children's language at early developmental stages can be appropriately assessed using the standardized tests that are already in place and normed on SE speakers.

There are at least two reasons to be extremely cautious about using existing tests that were designed initially for SE speakers, even
within an early restricted age range. First, conclusions about the
similarity of early BE and SE development have been based mainly
on spoken language in situations that optimized the occurrence of
natural responses. Standardized tests employ highly structured for-
mats that place constraints on the kind of responses offered by children and, in addition, involve child-examiner interactions that contrast sharply with the interactional requirements of naturalistic
language sampling. In clinical testing situations, it is not always
possible to isolate the child's linguistic knowledge from the contexts
for displaying such knowledge. Consequently, a child could still be
judged erroneously to have a clinical pathology even if he or she has
a certain knowledge but does not display it in the situation offered.
Thus, the appropriate application of existing tests to BE speakers at
an early age requires careful prior documentation that the conditions for eliciting responses are normative for them, just as their linguistic knowledge is expected to be.

A second reason for caution about the indiscriminate use of existing tests with Black children at early developmental stages recognizes how little is still known about their early normal development.
In the absence of an adequate data base, we cannot be sure that development is similar enough to justify appropriate use of existing
tests. Inspection of Table 5–1 shows that only one study of two boys
has focused on Black children's development of linguistic forms before the age of 3 years. Table 5–2 shows that two studies have focused
on development of meaning and use prior to 3 years.

The studies summarized in Tables 5–1 and 5–2 are particularly
limited in that they do not provide a comprehensive description of
the wide range of grammatical structures that undoubtedly characterize the developing language of children who acquire BE, particularly those structures that are not characteristically BE. What little
is known focuses more on morphological than on syntactic and phonological features. To date there has been no major normative study
of phonological development in any age range.

Much is yet to be learned even about those features that have
been described. Many details remain to be disclosed about the order
in which various form, meaning, and use features emerge. For example, little is known about the rule governed variable occurrence of
forms that are known to be conditioned by linguistic variables and to
be differentially distributed in SE and BE. With respect to the latter
point, for example, it is documented that BE and SE adult systems
both include the voiceless *th* sound. Whereas /ə/ occurs in word initial, medial, and final positions in SE, it occurs in just word initial

positions in BE. The study by Stockman, and colleagues (1982) showed further that children's productions of nasal consonants as early as 3 years exhibited variable features that coincided with the adult system. It was observed that nasal consonant deletion in final word position varied with whether the succeeding sound was a consonant or a vowel. Thus, in addition to the issue of social interactional context, linguistic context presents yet another factor that is likely to influence the conditions under which specific linguistic performances will occur on standardized tests.

Data such as those cited earlier suggest that certain linguistic contexts may favor the elicitation of a particular linguistic feature more readily than others at certain developmental stages. For example, a final nasal such as /m/ is more likely to be elicited when it is followed by a vowel than when it is followed by consonant or no other sound. The implication is that a given test will not be able to tap speakers' linguistic knowledge unless it provides the proper linguistic context for its elicitation.

Rule governed contextual constraints are likely to be equally relevant to SE speaking children. The type, frequency, and the developmental impact of such constraints may not be the same across dialect groups. Consequently, the investigator must be careful about applying the same test to different groups because most current tests are unlikely to be sensitive to variable constraints that operate differentially across speaker groups. In the absence of such sensitivity, a standardized test may inadvertently favor the occurrence of a given feature in one group and not the other. As a result, the one group whose contextual conditions are met will exhibit the feature and be credited with knowledge of the feature. The group whose contextual conditions are not met will not exhibit the expected feature and, as a result, will not be credited with knowledge of a feature even when, in fact, it has knowledge of the feature. The negative consequence of this result for clinical decisions should be obvious.

Linguistic contextual constraints on language acquisition are expected to receive more emphasis as child language research moves toward dynamic models of description and analysis that require observations of form, meaning, and use interactions.

REFERENCES

Alleyne, M.C. (1980). Linguistic issues in black communication. In B. Williams and O.L. Taylor (Eds.), *International Conference on Black Communication. The Rockefeller Foundation,* Bellagio, Italy, pp. 23–51.

Anastasiow, N.J., and Hanes, M.L. (1974). Cognitive development and the acquisition of language in three subcultural groups. *Developmental Psychology, 10*(5), 703–709.

Antinucci, F., and Miller, R. (1976). How children learned to talk about what happened. *Journal of Child Language, 3,* 167–189.

Baratz, J.C. (1969). A bi-dialectal task for determining language proficiency in economically disadvantaged Negro children. *Child Development, 40*(3), 889–901.

Bartel, N., Grill, J., and Bryen, D.N. (1973). Language characteristics of Black children: Implications for assessment. *Journal of School Psychology, 11,* 351–364.

Bates, E. (1976). *Language in context.* New York: Academic Press.

Baugh, J. (1983). *Black street speech: Its history, structure, and survival.* Austin: University of Texas Press.

Bellugi, U., and Brown, R. (Eds.) (1964). The acquisition of language. *Monographs of the Society for Research in Child Development, 29*(1), 5–191.

Bereiter, C., and Engelmann, S. (1966). *Teaching disadvantaged children in the preschool.* Englewood Cliffs, NJ: Prentice-Hall.

Berko, J. (1958). The child's learning of English morphology. *Word, 14,* 150–177.

Blake, I.K. (1984). *Language development in working-class Black children: An examination of form, content, and use.* Unpublished doctoral dissertation, Columbia University, New York.

Bloom, L. (1970). *Language development: Form and function in emerging grammars.* Cambridge, MA: MIT Press.

Bloom, L., Lightbown, P., and Hood, L. (1975). Structure and variation in child language. *Monographs of the Society for Research in Child Development, 40.*

Bloom, L., and Lahey, M. (1978). *Language development and language disorders.* New York: John Wiley & Sons.

Bloom, L., Lahey, M., Hood, L., Lifter, K., and Fiess, K. (1980. Complex sentences: Acquisition of syntactic connectives and the semantic relations they encode. *Journal of Child Language, 7,* 235–262.

Blount, B.G. (1969). *Acquisition of language by Luo children.* Unpublished doctoral dissertation, University of California, Berkeley.

Bowerman, M.F. (1973). *Early syntactic development: A cross-linguistic study with special reference to Finnish.* London: Cambridge University Press.

Braine, M. (1963). The ontogeny of English phrase structure: the first phase. *Language, 39,* 1–13.

Bridgeforth, C. (1984). *The development of language functions among Black children from working class families.* Paper presented at the pre-session of the 35th Annual Georgetown University Round Table on Language and Linguistics, Georgetown University, Washington, DC.

Brown, R. (1968). The development of wh questions in child speech. *Journal of Verbal Learning and Verbal Behavior, 7,* 279–290.

Brown, R. (1973). *A first language: the early stages.* Cambridge, MA: Harvard University Press.

Brown, R., and Bellugi, U. (1964). Three processes in the child's acquisition of syntax. *Harvard Educational Review, 34,* 133–151.

Butler, K.G. (Ed.) (1981). Language assessment: Selected critical issues. *Topics in Language Disorders, 3,* 1–100.

Cazden, C. (1968). The acquisition of noun and verb inflections. *Child Development, 39*, 433–448.

Chomsky, C. (1969). *The acquisition of syntax in children from 5 to 10.* Cambridge, MA: MIT Press.

Cole, L. (1980). Developmental analysis of social dialect features in the spontaneous language of preschool Black children. Unpublished doctoral dissertation, Northwestern University, Evanston.

DeStefano, J.S. (1972). Productive language differences in fifth grade Black students' syntactic forms. *Elementary English, 49*(4), 552–58.

Dillard, J.L. (1972). *Black English: Its history and usage in the United States.* New York: Vintage Books.

Dore, J. (1973). *The development of speech acts.* Unpublished dissertation, City University of New York.

Entwisle, D.R. (1968). Subcultural differences in children's language development. *International Journal of Psychology, 3*, 13–22.

Fasold, R.W. (1972). *Tense marking in Black English: A linguistic and social analysis.* Arlington, VA: Center for Applied Linguistics.

Frasure, N., and Entwisle, D. (1973). Semantic and syntactic development in children. *Developmental Psychology, 9*,(2), 236–245.

Halliday, M.A.K. (1973). *Explorations in the functions of language.* London: Edward F. Arnold Publishers.

Henrie, S.N. (1969). *A study of verb phrases used by five-year-old non-standard Negro English speaking children.* Unpublished doctoral dissertation, University of California Berkeley.

Horner, V.M., and Gussow, J.D. (1972). John and Mary: A pilot study in linguistic ecology. In C. Cazden, V. John, and D. Hymes (Eds.), *Functions of language in the classroom.* New York: Teachers College Press.

Inhelder, B., Piaget, J. (1964). *The early growth of logic in the child.* New York: Harper and Row.

Irwin, O.C. (1947). Development of speech during infancy: Curve of phonemic frequencies. *Journal of Experimental Psychology, 37*, 187–193.

Johnston, J.R., and Slobin, D. (1979). The development of locative expressions in English, Italian, Serbo-Croatian, and Turkish. *Journal of Child Language, 6*, 529–545.

Kovac, C. (1980). *Children's acquisition of variable features.* Unpublished doctoral dissertation, Georgetown University, Washington, DC.

Labov, W. (1969). Contraction, deletion, and inherent variability of the English copula. *Language, 45*, 715–762.

Labov, W. (1972). *Language in the inner city: Studies in the Black English vernacular.* Philadelphia: University of Pennsylvania Press.

Labov, W., Cohen, P., and Robbins, C. (1968). *A Study of the non-standard English of Negro and Puerto Rican speakers in New York City.* Cooperative Project No. 3288, Vols. 1 and 2. New York: Columbia University Press.

Levy, B., and Cook, H. (1973). Dialect proficiency and auditory comprehension in standard and Black nonstandard English. *Journal of Speech and Hearing Research, 16*, 642–49.

Lewnau, L. (1973). *Bidialectal skills of Black children.* Unpublished doctoral dissertation, Columbia University, New York.

Limber, J. (1976). Unravelling competence, performance, and pragmatics in the speech of young children. *Journal of Child Language, 3*, 309–18.

Loban, W.D. (1966). *Problems in oral English*. Champaign, IL: National Council of Teachers of English.

Marwit, S.T. (1977). Black and white children's use of standard English at 7, 9, and 12 years of age. *Developmental Psychology, 13*,(1), 81–82.

McCarthy, D. (1954). Language development in children. In P. Mussen (Ed.), *Carmichael's Manual of Child Psychology*. New York: John Wiley & Sons.

Menyuk, P. (1963). Syntactic structures in the language of children. *Child Development, 34*,(1), 407–422.

Mercer, J.R., and Brown, W.C. (1973). Racial differences in I.Q.: Fact or artifact? In C. Senna (Ed.), *The fallacy of I.Q.* New York: Third Press.

Miller, J. (1981). *Assessing language production in children*. Baltimore: University Park Press.

Miller, W., and Ervin, S. (1964). The development of grammar in child language. In U. Bellugi and R. Brown (Eds.), The acquisition of language. *Monographs of the Society for Research in Child Development, 29*, 9–34.

Mitchell-Kernan, C., and Kernan, K.T. (1977). Pragmatics of directive choice among children. In S. Ervin-Tripp and C. Mitchell-Kernan (Eds.), *Child discourse*. New York: Academic Press.

Ochs, E., and Schieffelin, B. (1979). *Developmental pragmatics*. New York: Academic Press.

Osser, H., Wang, M., and Zaid, F. (1969). The young child's ability to imitate and comprehend speech: A comparison of two sub-cultural groups. *Child Development, 40*, 1063–1976.

Peters, C. (1983). *A pragmatic investigation of the speech of selected Black children*. Unpublished dissertation, Howard University, Washington, DC.

Quay, L. (1971). Language dialect, reinforcement and the intelligence test performance of Negro children. *Child Development, 42*, 5–15.

Ramer, A., and Rees, N. (1973). Selected aspects of the development of English morphology in black American children of low socioeconomic status background. *Journal of Speech and Hearing Research, 16*, 569–577.

Raph, J. (1967). Language and speech deficits in culturally disadvantaged children: Implications for the speech clinician. *Journal of Speech and Hearing Disorders, 32*, 203–214.

Reveron, W.W. (1978). *The acquisition of four Black English morphological rules by Black preschool children*. Unpublished doctoral dissertation, Ohio State University, Columbus.

Sachs, J., and Devin, J. (1976). Young children's use of age appropriate speech styles in social interaction and role playing. *Journal of Child Language, 3*, 81–98.

Seymour, H.N., and Miller-Jones, D. (1981). Language and cognitive assessment of Black children. In N.J. Lass (Ed.), *Speech and language: Advances in basic research and practice, 6*, 203–263.

Seymour, H., and Seymour, C. (1981). Black English and standard American English contrasts in consonantal development of four and five year old children. *Journal of Speech and Hearing Disorders, 46*, 274–280.

Sinclair, H. (1970). The transition from sensori-motor behavior to symbolic activity. *Interchange, 1*, 119–126.

Steffensen, M. (1974). *The acquisition of Black English*. Unpublished doctoral dissertation, University of Illinois, Evanston.

Stockman, I. (1984, September). *The development of linguistic norms for nonmainstream populations.* Paper presented at the National Conference on Concerns for Minority Groups in Communication Disorders, Vanderbilt University.

Stockman, I., and Vaughn-Cooke,F. (1982a). Semantic categories in the language of working class Black children. In C.E. Johnson, and Thew, C. L., *Proceedings of the Second International Child Language Conference,* Vol. 1, pp. 312–327.

Stockman, I., and Vaughn-Coke, F. (1982b). A re-examination of research on the language of Black children: The need for a new framework. *Journal of Education, 164,* 157–172.

Stockman, I. and Vaughn-Cooke, F. (1984, July). *A closer look at the dynamic and static locative distinctions.* Paper presented at the Third International Child Language Congress, Austin, Texas.

Stockman, I., Vaughn-Cooke, F., and Wolfram, W. (1982). *Development of Black English: The first phase.* Final Research Report, National Institute of Education — NIE-G-80-0135. (ERIC Clearinghouse on Language and Linguistics — microfiche No. 2455556)

Stokes, N.H. (1976). *A cross sectional study of the acquisition of negation structures in Black children.* Unpublished doctoral dissertation, Georgetown University, Washington, DC.

Taylor, O.L. (1971). A response to social dialects and the field of speech. In *Sociolinguistics: A cross-disciplinary perspective.* Washington, DC, Center for Applied Linguistics.

Templin, M. (1957). *Certain language skills in children.* Minneapolis, University of Minnesota Press.

Vaughn-Cooke, F. (1976). *The implementation of a phonological change: The case of resyllabification in Black English.* Unpublished doctoral dissertation, Georgetown University, Washington, DC.

Vaughn-Cooke, F. (1983). Improving language assessment in minority children. *ASHA, 25,* 29–34.

Ward, M.C. (1971). *Them children.* New York: Holt, Rinehart & Winston.

Weener, P.D. (1969). Social dialect differences and the recall of verbal messages. *Journal of Educational Psychology, 60,* 194–199.

Williams, R., and Wolfram, W. (1976). *Social dialect: Differences versus disorders.* Rockville, MD: The American Speech and Hearing Association.

Wolfram, W. (1969). *A sociolinguistic description of Detroit Negro speech.* Washington, DC: Center for Applied Linguistics.

PART III
PREVALENCE AND NATURE

Chapter 6

Speech, Language, and Hearing Disorders in Black* Populations

Cassandra A. Peters-Johnson
and Orlando L. Taylor

Scholars from a variety of disciplines attempt to describe communication and generate models of communication that portend to show how people communicate, how they learn to interact verbally and nonverbally with one another, and what happens when communication breaks down. Some of these researchers and practitioners have begun to focus on pathologies of speech and language that interfere with an individual's ability to communicate with others in the environment. In recent years, particular attention has been given to issues pertaining to communication dysfunction as a function of a number of cultural and social variables, and, where appropriate, as a function of race linked variables. For example, there has been a marked increase of interest since the 1960s in communication disorders in nonwhite, non-English speaking populations, especially Black populations.

The purpose of this chapter is to review the state of the art of speech, language, and hearing disorders in Black populations around the world. The chapter will focus specifically on (1) the definition of communication disorders in Black populations; (2) the identification, description, and characteristics of communication disorders in Black populations; (3) types of communication disorders found in Black populations; (4) approaches to testing and remedia-

---

*As used throughout this chapter, the word "Black" is used to refer to indigenous African peoples who live in sub-Saharan Africa and to their descendants who reside throughout the world (the African diaspora).

tion of communication disorders in Black populations; and (5) suggestions for future research.

Speech and language functions are uniquely human phenomena. Researchers from disciplines such as psychology, education, linguistics, anthropology, and sociology have greatly increased our understanding of language structure and use. In addition, they have provided insights into the nature of speech and language disorders and have attempted to develop approaches for diagnosis and management of these disorders in children and adults. In the United States, as in other parts of the world, it is difficult to get an accurate picture of the nature of speech and language disorders in Blacks. Research and clinical procedures have been so influenced by the majority white culture that any claims regarding these disorders in Blacks have to be weighed carefully against what are thought to be culturally valid norms of Black communication. In fact, many researchers (Peters, 1979; Reveron, 1984; Seymour and Miller-Jones, 1981; Vaughn-Cooke, 1980) have demonstrated that most assessment procedures in speech-language pathology are culturally and linguistically biased toward middle class white Americans and biased against an overwhelming number of Black Americans.

Speech-language disorders may be defined generally as deviations from the linguistic and communicative norms of a given society. Societies may differ, however, in their definition of what they consider abnormal communicative behavior and how it should be treated. For this reason, it is unreasonable to impose the communicative standards of one society to determine "normalcy" in another society. This notion is particularly relevant to a discussion of "pathologies" in Black American populations for which there is strong reason to believe that there are significant linguistic and communicative differences from the dominant white population. Therefore, it is difficult to accept reports of communication disorders in Blacks at face value. To judge the validity of such reports, we must look carefully at the criteria used to determine pathology, the assessment instruments, and the standards within the particular Black community for determining normal speech and language behavior.

CULTURAL BASIS OF COMMUNICATION DISORDERS IN BLACK POPULATIONS

This chapter is presented from a sociocultural perspective suggesting that communication and communication disorders must be defined, studied, and discussed from a cultural orientation. Since pathological communication is defined as a deviation from the norm, that norm has to be culturally based. In a largely Black community, the standards against which individual communicative behaviors are evaluated must obviously include rules of Black communication for such evaluations to be valid. Of course, some Black persons communicate according to the rules of some other community, usually the economically, politically, or socially dominant white community. For example, a Black person — especially an educated Black person — in a colonized state, such as the French colony of Martinique, might choose to communicate in a manner deemed appropriate by the white power structure, in this case the French colonizers, rather than by the indigenous Black population. Instead of limiting an individual Black person to using only communicative behaviors characteristic of the local Black community to be judged normal, our definitions of communication disorders must be sufficiently broad to permit the use of an appropriate set of Black communication norms according to the rules of a specific speech community to determine the presence or absence of pathology. It would be ethnocentric to exclude such norms.

RACE-LINKED DISEASES IN BLACKS

In addition to the cultural argument discussed earlier, race-linked disease tendencies represent a second, and equally impelling, reason for advancing the concept of Black communication disorders. It is a well-documented fact that racial groups, probably because of different environmental conditions, are subject to different incidences, prevalences, and, in some cases, severities of physical, social, and psychological disorders. For example, Williams (1975) reports that Blacks suffer from hypertension at higher rates than whites at all age levels. This condition frequently results in strokes, a major cause of aphasia (a disorder of language encoding or decoding), agnosia (a disorder of sensory perception), apraxia (a disorder of motor programing for speech), and dysarthria (a disorder of motor speech movements).

Holland (1983) suggests that the incidence and prevalence of cerebrovascular disease for Blacks in the United States are considerably higher than for whites. The odds suggest, therefore, that a disproportionately large percentage of Blacks have aphasia and related disorders in relation to national averages. On the other hand, Holland notes that with the exception of Parkinson's disease and possibly multiple sclerosis, the incidences of neurological diseases that produce language problems do not vary with race in the United States. Holland notes finally that there is practically no sociolinguistic literature associated with aging, a predisposing factor in cerebrovascular accidents.

Sickle cell disease is another disease that has a much larger incidence among Blacks than other populations. Williams (1975) reports that 1 in every 10 to 12 Blacks in the United States carries the sickle cell trait, and approximately 1 in every 600 has sickle cell disease. He reports further that more than 28 million Africans carry the sickle cell trait of a total population of more than 250 million. Speech and hearing disorders may result from neurological damage associated with a sickle cell crisis. Payne and Stockman (1979) report that the sickling of red blood cells impedes or halts blood supply to vital body organs and tissues, including those related to normal speech and hearing functioning. Of course, race-related disease tendencies are not limited to Blacks. For example, otosclerosis, a hardening of the bones of the middle ear leading to a conductive-type hearing loss, and other pathological disorders of the middle and inner ear appear to be much more prevalent among whites than among American Blacks (Weddington and Meyerson, 1984).

Johnson and Griffiths (1981) note that the inability of many physicians to accurately diagnose certain pathological conditions in Black infants can contribute to the development of handicapping conditions that could otherwise have been prevented. In other cases, the effects of an already adverse situation are compounded by inaccurate diagnoses. Jaundice, for example, which is caused by elevated blood levels of bilirubin (bilirubinemia), is often not recognized in a dark-complexioned newborn child because the standard diagnostic sign in Western medicine is the presence of yellow skin. An accurate diagnosis of jaundice can be made by inspecting the color of the lip and cheek tissue *inside* the oral cavity or the sclerae (white fibrous membrane covering the eyeball). High levels of bilirubin in the brain can lead to varying degrees of brain damage, which can cause mental retardation, cerebral palsy, deafness, and, in less severe cases, minimal brain dysfunction (Marlon, 1965, cited in Johnson and Griffiths, 1981). Other diseases that may be overlooked or misdiagnosed in Black children are cyanosis (presence of blue skin) and scarlet fever (presence of pinkish-red skin) (Johnson and Griffiths, 1981).

Inappropriate Diagnostic Procedures and Misdiagnoses

Because of varying communication rules among different cultural groups, approaches to the examination and treatment of communication disorders are much more likely to be effective if the instruments, interpersonal interactions, and testing and treatment models of clinical practice are consistent with the communication rules of the group from which the communicatively impaired individual comes. For this reason, effective clinical practice in Black populations is correlated with sensitivity to and use of culturally relevant materials and orientations.

In 1969, a group of Black professionals in speech pathology and audiology recognized the need for increased sensitivity to Black communicatively impaired persons and formed the Black Caucus of the American Speech and Hearing Association. Using data and theory from the field of sociolinguistics, the Black Caucus argued as follows:

> Unfortunately, far too many speech pathologists view legitimate language differences among Afro-Americans from a pathology model. The result is that a number of Black children are receiving speech and language therapy, particularly in urban areas, when they, in fact, have no pathology. Negative psychological effects on the Black child are obvious. In order to develop a more intelligent approach to recognizing legitimate linguistic differences and satisfactory methods for second language instruction as a skill, clinicians need training in sociolinguistics and the historical and cultural roots of Black children. All too often clinicians fail to understand the Black child's language, as well as the child himself.
>
> (Taylor, Stroud, Hurst, Moore, and Williams, 1969)

Reveron (1984) points out that the factor of linguistic differences has a pervasive effect on language assessment and that most tests have been normed on populations of children who speak standard English. Few valid tests have been designed specifically for children who speak nonmainstream English dialects. Notable exceptions include the *Screening Kit of Language Development (SKOLD)* by Bliss and Allen (1983) and the *Black English Sentence Scoring (BESS)* procedure by Nelson (1983) (see Reveron, 1984, for a critique of these instruments). As a result, Black children are often misevaluated owing to the inability of these measures to differentiate between language differences and language disorders. Several researchers have analyzed the validity of using tests standardized on standard English speakers for the assessment of children who speak other English dialects (e.g., Reveron, 1984; Vaughn-Cooke, 1983; Wolfram, 1983).

Bartel and Grill (1973) observe that there exists a paradoxical situation in which errors of overdiagnosis (Type I errors) and underdiagnosis (Type II errors) occur with undesirable frequency, particularly in children from nonwhite, non–middle class populations.

There are two possibilities that may lead to errors of overdiagnosis. First, the child is identified as having a speech or language disorder through the use of a test standardized on a population other than his or her own. Second, the child is diagnosed as having a speech or language disorder from a test of standard English (SE) in which a subgroup of the normative sample consists of speakers of Black English vernacular. In this latter instance, the presence of Black English vernacular speaking children in the normative sample is obscured by the averaging of their responses into the remainder of the sample (Reveron, 1984).

The second type of error is one of underdiagnosis, in which the child has a speech or language disorder, but the assessment procedures are insufficiently sensitive to detect it. That is, the procedures fail to provide a standard within the child's own linguistic system against which normalcy or abnormalcy can be determined. An error of underdiagnosis may also occur if the speech-language pathologist is unaware of the specific way the child's dialect differs systematically from standard English and attributes any variance in the child's linguistic system to the dialect that he or she speaks. There are two serious ramifications of either type of diagnostic error. In the first, the child may be labeled as speech or language disordered and inappropriately placed into a speech-language therapy program. In the second, the child may suffer educationally by not receiving the therapeutic intervention needed (Reveron, 1984).

Another problem of misdiagnosis is that Black children are obviously part of the speech-language disabled population, yet descriptions of the specific problems encountered by them from the vantage point of their indigenous linguistic systems are practically nonexistent. It is apparent that Black children have been diagnosed and placed in speech-language services based on norms collected from other populations (Cole, 1984). Assessment biases preclude accurate determinations of prevalence, incidence, and service delivery figures for minority speech and language disordered populations.

In an effort to differentiate between Black children with communicative disorders and those with normal communication, Seymour and Miller-Jones (1981) introduced a bidialectal model of communication in which children's utterances that do not vary from either Black English or standard English references would be acceptable. Their model is based on the premise that Black children's language is determined by their larger speech community. They note that as with adult Black English (BE), the child's language is characterized by both Black English and standard English (SE) features. Seymour and Miller-Jones introduce the concept of variance into their model to establish differences between a communicatively disordered and a normal child. The model shows that there are forms that are variant from BE and SE and other forms that are invariant from either BE or SE. BE and SE variant forms would be produced by the communicatively disordered bidialectal child. The model depicts pathology and development as sources of variance.

OTHER FACTORS ASSOCIATED WITH IDENTIFICATION AND TREATMENT

Besides the issue of assessment bias, there are several other factors that may interface in the assessment and treatment of communication disorders in Black populations. These possible factors include (1) culturally inappropriate settings and communicative interactions within the diagnostic-therapy process; (2) cultural misinterpretations of communicative behaviors; and (3) negative linguistic attitudes or expectancies on the part of the clinicians. Some of these problems have been discussed by Murphy (1978) and Taylor (in press).

Among Blacks in the United States and in many other parts of the world, especially the Caribbean and the African continent itself, there are sociocultural, geographical, and value constraints that impede identification and treatment of communication disorders. Services by trained professionals are often unavailable. Clients may be embarrassed by certain disorders or have superstitions or religious beliefs about them. Some anomalies lead to natural or induced mortality (e.g., children may die owing to inadequate feeding and aspiration). Folk medicines may be considered the "cure-all" for certain diseases. Taylor and Samara (1985) have identified several possible barriers to the delivery of clinical services to communicatively disordered Black persons in developing nations. Many barriers they cite with Black majority populations fall within cultural, political, health-educational, and professional domains.

Cultural barriers include fatalism, low priorities placed on communication disorders, intermarriage, and colonial mentality. Two major political barriers cited are lack of trained personnel in policy and decision making positions and lack of adequate national infrastructures for service delivery, such as telephones, postal services, transportation, and health care systems. In the health-education area, there are barriers such as inadequate public education on communication disorders, insufficient research on communication disorders associated with high-frequency indigenous diseases, and an overabundance of foreign professionals in the health-educational work force. Finally, possible professional barriers include a lack of normative communication data on indigenous populations, lack of locally normed and culturally valid assessment procedures, and absence of incidence and prevalence data.

TOWARD A DEFINITION OF COMMUNICATION DISORDERS IN BLACKS

Clinical observations of Black children and adults around the world have revealed the presence of a universal set of communicative disorders. These disorders usually involve speech, language, or hearing and typically result from psychological, sociological, or biological causes. Although disorders of communication are apparently worldwide in distribution, this universality is more easily observed for those disorders associated with physical factors than for those associated with psychological or sociological causes. For example, hearing loss and aphasia — communication disorders that have distinct physical bases — probably exist throughout the world. However, stuttering, as we know it in the United States, is a disorder believed to have a strong cultural base and may not be of universal occurrence. Although the physical-psychological-sociological dichotomy is a valid point of departure, it is perhaps too simplistic to provide an accurate view of communication disorders in different ethnic or social groups.

With respect to the physical dimension, it was established earlier in this chapter that there are different incidences of diseases and disease histories for different cultural groups: sickle-cell disease in Blacks, for instance, and otosclerosis in whites. Furthermore, there is some evidence to suggest that societies have different values for determining minimally proficient (or normal) communication and, more importantly, what to do about conditions of abnormal communication. In some societies, for example, mild deviations in communicative behavior may hardly be considered cause for alarm in the context of other cultural priorities.

The point here is that societies may have different criteria for determining when a difference makes a difference and what to do if one exists. Some societies may believe that little or nothing should be done about a communication disorder except to keep it hidden from the public, since such disorders are perceived as acts of God. Unfortunately, there has been little research reported on what different societies, especially Black societies, consider pathological communication and what to do about it. Therefore, virtually all present-day concepts pertaining to these topics have a Eurocentric orientation from the United States, Canada, Western Europe, Australia, and South Africa. Interestingly, speech pathology and audiology exist as disciplines in few places outside the Eurocentric world, and the overwhelming bulk of the literature on the subject of communication disorders is oriented toward white and middle-class populations. Research on other populations, especially Black populations, is clearly needed. Also, culturally appropriate clinical services need to be developed for these other populations.

The American Speech-Language-Hearing Association's (ASHA) 1983 position paper on social dialects makes it clear that the speech-language pathologist must distinguish between those aspects of linguistic variation that represent the diversity of the standard language from those that represent speech, language, and hearing disorders. The Minority Concerns Office of the American Speech-Language-Hearing Association is currently developing a project to focus on the full range of communication disorders and service delivery issues in Black as well as in American Indian, Asian, and Hispanic populations. The project will provide information on such topics as the epidemiology of hearing loss related to sickle cell anemia; the effect of anthropomorphic differences and wound healing on the manifestation of orofacial anomalies cross-racially; folklore and superstition associated with communicative disorders; and the professional policies and governmental legislation needs relative to multicultural populations.

RESEARCH ON COMMUNICATION DISORDERS IN BLACK POPULATIONS

To date, a small but significant body of literature on the subject of communication disorders in Blacks throughout the world has emerged in English language journals and monographs. Most of the publications come primarily from the United States, although there are some publications on communication disorders from Jamaica, Trinidad, Kenya, Uganda, Zambia, Nigeria, and Egypt. Some of this research will be discussed on the next several pages.

TYPES OF COMMUNICATION DISORDERS AMONG BLACKS

In terms of types of communication disorders among Blacks, it was reported earlier in this chapter that Blacks suffer from the same types of communication disorders as any other human population, although incidence and prevalence figures, causes, and clinical findings may vary as a function of race or culture. Keeping in mind the culture and test-bias problems associated with assessing communicative behavior in Blacks discussed earlier, scattered statistical data have been reported in the literature.

Fajemisin (1980) reports, for example, that even such disorders as stuttering, otosclerosis, and Meniere's disease, which have been previously reported by some to be virtually nonexistent in Black populations, do in fact exist in African populations, at least in Nigeria, where he conducts his otolaryngology research and clinical practice. However, both Fajemisin and Okeowo and Nwanze (1978) have observed that many persons in Nigeria who stutter, or even those who have an articulatory problem, do not typically find it necessary to seek professional help for such disorders because of a general societal acceptance of them. Although this impression needs to be confirmed by formal research rather than by anecdotal clinical reports, cultural definitions and priorities for normal speech and language function, especially when disorders are the result of nonorganic causes, may differ greatly from population to population. These differences may be a contributing factor to the tendency by many minority persons, including many in the United States to not find it necessary to take advantage of clinical services, even when they are made available free of charge and provided at convenient times and in accessible places.

Hearing Disorders

In a number of studies, the prevalence and incidence of hearing disorders in African and Caribbean populations are reported to be similar to that for white populations in Europe and the United States. In some cases, however, hearing disorders are reported to occur less often.

For example, Rosen's research (1966) on the Mabaan people in Southeast Sudan suggests lower incidence rates. Rosen reports that the Mabaan, a dramatically quiet people who eat a low-cholesterol diet with almost no red meat, have a very low incidence of hearing loss. They also seem to age more slowly than Western people, have longer life spans, and a low incidence of arteriosclerosis. There is virtually no difference in their diastolic blood pressures between the ages of 15 and 75 years, and coronary heart disease is unknown. Rosen's data show that at all age levels (10 to 70 years), Mabaans' hearing acuity is significantly more acute than that of people of corresponding ages living in urban areas in the United States, in Dusseldorf, Germany, and in Cairo, Egypt. Furthermore, Mabaans reportedly have a 50 percent smaller air-bone gap at 4,000 cps at age 55 years than do whites. Indeed, the 4,000 cps air-bone gap of 12 db (long considered to be normal by age 55) does not occur in Mabaans until age 75!

Refusing to attribute all of the Mabaans' extraordinary hearing to a quiet environment, Rosen explored the diet variable by studying changes in Finnish persons after changing their diets to correspond with that of the Mabaans. Finland was chosen for the study because the Finns are known to have diets containing large quantities of saturated fat, mainly from whole milk and butter. The dietary alterations resulted in many positive physical changes in the experimental group, such as lower serum cholesterol levels, lengthened blood coagulation time, slightly lowered myocardial ischemia levels, and significantly lower levels of new coronary heart disease. For our purposes, however, the most remarkable finding was that 5 years after the dietary changes, the hearing of individuals in the experimental group, for all age groups under study (40 to 49 years and 50 to 59 years), was superior at all frequencies. Indeed, experimental subjects demonstrated hearing levels comparable to whites 10 years younger. Further, the aforementioned air-bone gap at 4,000 cps was much smaller for the experimental group.

Rosen's research is important not only because it documents the extraordinary hearing of a group of African people but also because it supports an apparent link between diet, arteriosclerosis, and coronary heart disease. Since these problems can be improved with diet, a strong case can be made for making serious attempts to alter dietary habits among Black people around the world who are known to have high-cholesterol diets.

The relationship between diet and sensorineural hearing loss has also been highlighted by the reports of Monekosso (1963), Monekosso and Wilson (1966), Osuntokun and colleagues (1969), and Hinchcliffe (1972). In oto-neuro-ophthalmological syndrome in Nigerians and neuropathy in Jamaicans, a cyanide-containing fruit, cassava, is thought to be an etiological factor. In both countries cassava is consumed liberally.

In addition to the aforementioned articles, there are several scattered reports of major etiological factors associated with hearing loss in Africa. These reports have been summarized as follows by Hinchcliffe (1972) of the University of London:

Kenya: meningococcal meningitis (Ormerod, unpublished data)
Tanzania: pneumococcal meningitis (Ormerod, unpublished

data) and ataxic neurological syndrome (Haddock et al., 1962)

Malawi: arbovirus encephalitis and chronic suppurative otitis media (Drummond, 1968)

Uganda: chronic suppurative otitis media (Roland, 1960; Martin, 1967)

Nigeria: oto-neuro-ophthalmological syndrome (Monekosso, 1963; Osuntokun, 1968)

Seychelles and Mauritius: neuro-otological patterns

In addition, Sellars, Beighton, Horan, and Beighton (1977) have provided some data on hearing disorders in Black children in Southern Africa associated with a number of etiological factors: Waardenburg syndrome, vitiligo, Hunter's syndrome, Crouzon's disease, Pendred's syndrome, and trichorhinophalangeal syndrome. Other causes of deafness were listed as cryptogenic, meningoencephalitis, bilateral mastoid surgery, and familial deafness.

Hinchcliffe (1972) has also reported that African people generally show a different pattern of neuro-otological hearing disorders than Europeans, probably for genetic reasons, and that their incidence of hearing loss is generally lower. Among Jamaicans, he reports that poor hearing levels of many persons in that country, especially women, are associated with neurological and ophthalmological defects that characterize the ataxic type of Jamaican neuropathy, which is possibly identical to the ataxic neuromyelopathy reported by Osuntokun, Monekosso, and Wilson (1969) in Nigeria. There may be dietary factors related to this phenomenon. In any case, both samples are too small to generate definitive conclusions on the generalizability of this trait in the genetic pool of African people. Obviously, more research data are needed to evaluate this idea.

The issue of the relationship between sickle-cell disease and hearing loss has also been documented by some research conducted on African and Caribbean populations. In 1969, Morgenstein and Manance, working in the United States, observed many pathological temporal bone findings in patients with sickle cell disease, including absence and abnormality of many inner and outer hair cells, sickle cell engorgement of striate vessels, and venous and capillary blockage by clumped sickle cells throughout the temporal bone. Morgenstein and Manance speculated that their findings probably represented progressive or degenerative changes associated with sickle cell crisis. They were believed to be cumulative following several sickle cell attacks during the life of the child.

Todd, Sergeant, and Larson (1973) have published some of the most extensive data on hearing loss associated with sickle cell disease. Reporting on the hearing of 83 Jamaicans between 10 and 39 years of age, Todd and colleagues found that 22 percent of the persons with sickle cell disease demonstrated a sensorineural hearing loss of 25 db or greater in one or more frequencies in at least one ear, compared with a prevalence figure of only 4 percent for normal controls. Both sexes were affected, and the higher frequencies were most vulnerable. Interestingly, the losses seemed to be slow in onset, probably increasing with each sickle cell crisis. These researchers argued that anemia and thromboses (clots) are probably the two most important causative factors for hearing loss following sickle cell crisis.

Most recently, Sharp and Orchik (1978), who compared nine Black subjects with sickle cell anemia with a control population, found no differences in measures of hearing acuity and undistorted speech discrimination. However, some evidence suggested reduced eighth nerve and central auditory function in the sickle cell group. Sharp and Orchik recommend further investigation into the correlations between the number, duration, and severity of crisis episodes and the audiologic manifestations observed in sickle cell anemia. They also suggest that future research examine the influence of other hemolytic disorders on auditory function.

Although more research is needed on the relationship between sickle cell disease and hearing loss, this disease provides an excellent example of how data from international sources in Africa and the Caribbean can shed light on important issues in communication disorders in the United States.

Maxillofacial Anomalies (Cleft Lip and Palate)

Clefts of the lip and palate, together with other structural anomalies of the head and face, are major causes of articulation and voice problems. For the most part, these anomalies are caused by genetic factors or by intrauterine teratogenic factors. Study and treatment of communication disorders associated with maxillofacial anomalies represents a major subspecialty within the disciplines of speech pathology and audiology.

There are conflicting data on the incidence of cleft lip and cleft palate in Blacks. Some clinicians have reported that such conditions rarely occur in Blacks and when they do are more likely to occur in those Blacks with some type of Caucasian genetic history. Several writers (e.g., Cole, 1980) have called this impression into serious question. Weddington and Meyerson (1984) reported an incidence of 1 in 700 for cleft lip or palate in Blacks in the United States.

Reports of maxillofacial anomalies in Africa also are not rare. For example, David, Edoo, Mustaffah, and Hinchcliffe (1971) reported a high incidence of maxillofacial anomalies associated with profound congenital deafness among the Adamarobe villagers in Southern Ghana. Gupta (1969) found a prevalence of facial clefts of 1 in 1,055 among newborns in a large general hospital in a western region of Nigeria (an unselected population of neonates). Oluwasanmi and Adekunle (1970) and Oluwasanmi and Kogbe (1975) have also reported cases of congenital facial clefts in Nigerians. Fajemisin (1980) has reported that teratogenic infections and drugs seem to affect pregnant Black women in the same way as white women. He observes further that many cases of maxillofacial anomalies might be overlooked in Nigeria because babies with severe cases aspirate and die during forced feeding, the traditional way of artificially feeding babies in certain parts of the country. Robinson and Shepherd (1970) estimated a minimum prevalence for cleft lip or palate to be 0.8 per 1,000 births in Uganda.

There are two major studies on maxillofacial anomalies in the Caribbean. Robertson (1963) reports a 1 in 1,888 prevalence rate in Trinidad for Blacks and, interestingly, an astoundingly high rate of 1 in 500 for the East Indian population of that country. Millard and McNeill (1965) conducted a rather thorough analysis of 56,000 births at the Victoria Jubilee Hospital in Jamaica from 1960 to 1963 to project the following prevalence figures for maxillofacial anomalies among Jamaicans: cleft lip, 1 in 6,250; cleft palate, 1 in 9,091; cleft lip and palate, 1 in 3,704; all types of maxillofacial anomalies, 1 in 1,887. Millard and McNeill suggest three interesting, although unsubstantiated, reasons for the relatively low prevalence of maxillofacial anomalies among Blacks, especially in the Americas. First, the authors suggest that infanticide was practiced on deformed infants in some African cultures. Second, they argue that only the strongest persons were selected by Europeans to be brought to the Americas as slaves. Third, Millard and McNeill advance the notion that the institution of slavery itself resulted in a weeding out of the physically weak from the Black population.

The Waardenburg syndrome is occasionally mentioned in the literature as one that occurs from time to time in African populations. Hagerman (1980) reports that this autosomal dominant hereditary condition may cause maxillofacial anomalies; pigment disorders of the eyes, hair, and skin; and congenital deafness. One type of patient (Type I) seems to have maxillofacial anomalies, specifically a lateral displacement of the medial corners of the eye, a broad nasal root, and confluent eyebrows. Type II patients reportedly do not have maxillo-facial anomalies.

Hagerman asserts that congenital bilateral deafness is the most serious characteristic of the Waardenburg syndrome, occurring in 25 percent of the Type I patients and in 50 percent of the Type II patients. Reporting on his research on 16 of 19 schools for the deaf in Kenya, Hagerman reports that of 724 subjects, 11 cases (1.5 percent of the population) were found. Although the Waardenburg syndrome is not limited to persons of African ancestry, it appears to occur in sufficient numbers to warrant more research on the subject, particularly on the speech, language, and hearing disorders that accompany the disease.

Articulation Disorders

Excluding studies that inaccurately label nonstandard Black phonological features as pathological and those which are associated with such physical anomalies as cleft lip and palate, there are virtually no studies of so-called functional articulation disorders among Blacks. In the 1950s, however, one such study (Everhart, 1953) reported that Black children with articulatory defects showed no significant differences from white children in terms of the characteristics or developmental patterns of the disorder. It is not known, however, what various Black communities perceive as the appropriate standard for determining whether articulatory behavior is normal, nor is it known what priority Black communities place on eradicating mild to moderate articulation abnormalities. The whole area of community-based standards for various Black communities and cultures around the world emerges as requiring major research relating to the examination, diagnosis, and management of communication disorders in Blacks.

Stuttering

Although the incidence of stuttering is not particularly great among the various types of communication disorders, the disorder continues to be the one that many people find the most intriguing and speech pathologists consider the most complex. Although there are many theories on the pathogenesis of stuttering, the most popular theories claim that the disorder is a learned phenomenon associated with stress. As pointed out earlier, claims have been made that stuttering does not exist in some countries, including some African societies. These claims are beginning to receive less credulity as more research and clinical reports emerge, particularly from indigenous people. More research is needed to determine the tenability of these claims, especially as they relate to Blacks who live outside major metropolitan areas and outside the United States.

There is one major discussion of cultural influences on the development of stuttering in Blacks (Leith and Mims, 1975). In their treatise on Black stutterers in the United States, these writers note a sharp difference in stuttering patterns between Blacks and whites. Whites, they report, show a strong tendency for what they call Type I stuttering behavior, characterized by overt (audible) repetitions and prolongations with a moderate number of overt secondary characteristics, such as word phrase repetitions, accelerated speaking rates, and so on. Blacks, by contrast, show a strong tendency for Type II stuttering, a stuttering behavior characterized by more covert (nonaudible) prolongations and repetitions and a large number of relatively severe secondary characteristics, including total avoidance of speech. Black stutterers, like all Type II stutterers, often appear to have either a mild handicap or no handicap whatsoever, although they tend to appear tense and anxious. The major point is that the Type II stutterer works very hard to appear not to stutter.

Leith and Mims argue that Blacks engage in Type II stuttering behavior far more than whites because, as pointed out by several sociolinguists (e.g., Mitchell, 1969; Kochman, 1970, 1981; Labov and Robins, 1969; Labov, 1983), the Black culture in the United States places a high premium on oral proficiency and "being cool." Indeed, a substantial part of the Black male self-concept is built around proficiency in such oral skills as ritual insults, rapping, and verbal routines with women, including the ability to perform these skills in such a "cool" way as to always appear to be in control and never ruffled. Obviously, stuttering behavior runs counter to these social values, and, therefore, the Black stutterer would naturally try to mask stuttering behavior and the resultant emotional reactions.

Aphasia

Aphasia is a disorder of language expression or comprehension caused by damage to the central nervous system. Strokes, many of which are caused by hypertension and arteriosclerosis, are a major cause of aphasia, particularly among the aged. Given the high incidence of hypertension among Blacks, at least in the United States, it is rather incredible to note the paucity of research on aphasia in Blacks. There are no definitive studies on the prevalence or incidence of aphasia among Blacks in the world, nor any studies of the patterns of language dissolution following brain damage among the myriad languages, dialects, and patois spoken by Blacks around the world.

There are, however, two studies that demonstrate the difficulty of determining the degree and type of aphasia following brain damage among Blacks when test instruments designed for whites are used (Anderson and Ulatowska, 1978; Warrick, 1975). In both studies, the investigators found that instruments commonly used to examine for aphasia are incapable of differentiating aphasic-like responses from responses that indicate normal language variation among many Black speakers. Indeed, many existing tests of aphasia are so insensitive to this problem that they would give the false impression that many perfectly normal Black people with no brain injury are aphasic! Obviously, test instruments and assessment procedures are needed for Black populations that would reflect greater cultural and sociolinguistic sophistication.

In the area of childhood aphasia, Payne and Stockman (1979) report data that suggest that the neurological damage that can accompany recurrent sickle cell crisis may result in language defects (perhaps aphasic-like) in Black children. Again, much more research is needed to evaluate this hypothesis. It is also possible that lead poisoning, resulting from ingestion of certain paints or crayons, inhalation of fumes from burning batteries or automobile exhausts, and so on, is another source of brain injury resulting in aphasia for many poor Blacks, especially in urban ghettos in the United States and England. Williams (1975) claims that many Black children are prone to ingestion of these toxins because of a high incidence of pica — an inordinate craving for unusual articles of food. Williams suggests that pica is somewhat prevalent among Blacks because of a relatively common practice of using a chewing stick in many parts of West Africa. However, formal support for this claim is unavailable.

DIAGNOSIS AND MANAGEMENT OF COMMUNICATION DISORDERS

The area of clinical management has received by far the least amount of attention by researchers and clinicians interested in communication disorders in Blacks. The few published papers that do exist are largely anecdotal in nature. Taylor (1978, in press) and Adler (1973) have argued that the interpersonal dimension is a vital component in any type of effective clinical management of communication disorders. For this reason, differences in the verbal and nonverbal rules between clinician and client can result in unintended episodes of insult, discomfort, or hypersensitivity, which could negatively affect the interpersonal dynamics needed for effective clinical work. Scholars in the fields of intercultural and interpersonal communication could be very helpful to speech pathologists and audiologists by providing them with the knowledge and skills needed to improve their ability to communicate with clients from various backgrounds.

As stated, there are a few anecdotal clinical reports in the literature. For example, Okeowo and Nwanze (1978) have described their encouraging results from speech and language therapy in Nigeria. Milstein (1976) has shown how a knowledge of the conversational and linguistic rules of "Coloured" children in South Africa can be used to improve the quality of speech and language testing and therapy for children of this racial designation.

Despite the dearth of scientific literature on speech and language therapy designed specifically for Blacks, there are several position papers in which it is argued that such therapy should be based on the appropriate sociolinguistic developmental norms for the clients' cultural group. Taylor (1973), for instance, writes that it is not enough to know the sociolinguistic behaviors of adult speakers in a population to conduct culturally appropriate speech or language therapy. Instead, he asserts that developmental patterns of that language must be known in order to determine (1) differences between developmental variants and pathological deviations, (2) the appropriate time to begin speech or language therapy for pathological features, and (3) the course of therapy once it has started.

Seymour and Seymour (1977) have developed one of the few models for providing therapy for Blacks who have speech or language disorders which take language variation into account. In their treatise, Seymour and Seymour argue that because many of the features of so-called standard English and Black English vernacular in the United States overlap, therapy goals for Black English speaking children should be congruent with educational goals and social expectations. Therefore, their model is constructed in such a way that the modification of particular linguistic features is sought for both Black English vernacular and standard English. The intriguing feature of the Seymour and Seymour model is its recognition of the possibility of pathological deviations from both vernacular and standard English and that true linguistic competency in the culture probably requires proficiency in both systems (see Seymour, 1986, for a bidialectal model for clinical intervention).

Leith and Mims (1975) have developed a culturally oriented therapeutic program for the Black stutterer based on the previously described differences in stuttering patterns between Blacks and whites. These authors argue that the more popular approaches to stuttering therapy in the United States may prove to be unpopular and ineffective with Black stutterers. These approaches typically encourage the stutterer to be overt in his stuttering behavior and discourage any avoidance of nonfluency, on the assumption that the stutterer can only develop a control of his or her stuttering behavior by recognizing its existence and allowing it to happen. Presumably, through such techniques as operant or classical conditioning, the client will become more fluent by learning to control the stuttering behavior.

Because of the arguments presented in an earlier section of this paper, it can be deduced that the Black stutterer may be unwilling to pay the price of permitting more overt stuttering, with possible loss of self-esteem, for the possible long-term reward of more fluent speech. Leith and Mims note from their clinical experiences that Black stutterers in the United States, especially during the teenage and young adult years, frequently reject stuttering therapy when it requires movement of overt stuttering behavior outside the clinic to peers in the community. They explain this withdrawal from therapy as a conflict between clinical and cultural needs.

Although Leith and Mims's notions need to be subjected to rigorous research, their hypotheses are interesting. If true, they offer many implications for the development of culture-based therapeutic programs for the Black stutterer. It may well be the case, of course, that therapy for all types of communicative disorders in Blacks, particularly those with psychological or sociological causes, might be enhanced by the introduction of culturally based regimens.

SUMMARY AND CONCLUSIONS

On the basis of literature reported to date on communicative disorders in the United States, Africa and the Caribbean, the following conclusions can be made:

1. Blacks suffer from most, if not all, of the speech, language, and hearing disorders suffered by members of other racial groups.
2. Contrary to popular belief, communication disorders previously thought not to exist at all, or to exist rarely, in African peoples (e.g., stuttering and maxillofacial anomalies) do indeed exist, although at different prevalence and incidence rates.

3. The prevalence and incidence of speech, language, and hearing disorders in African and Caribbean peoples is unknown, owing in part to biased instruments, lack of national surveys, and inadequate knowledge of various cultural definitions of communication pathology. Among Blacks in the United States, there is some evidence suggesting that previous figures on the prevalence and incidence of speech-language disorders in Blacks are too high, and that these figures can be brought closer to reality when culturally valid norms and assessment procedures are employed.

In addition to the foregoing conclusions, it can be also observed that although no specific therapy models have been advanced for African or Caribbean populations, considerable progress has been reported from these locations on second language instruction that uses indigenous language systems. These advancements may be of particular value to speech-language pathologists in the United States who are interested in becoming competent to teach standard English as a second dialect or who are interested in providing services to bilingual persons.

Finally, there is a strong need for research on Black populations in the United States, Africa, and the Caribbean on the following topics:

1. Definitions of and priorities placed on various types of communication disorders.
2. Developmental sociolinguistic norms.
3. Culturally and linguistically valid assessment procedures.
4. Incidence of various types of communication disorders.
5. Clinical descriptions of behavioral characteristics of communication disorders associated with disease entities, environmental conditions, and social phenomena that greatly impact on Black populations.
6. Culturally based therapeutic models for providing treatment services for persons with communication disorders.

Although this chapter has focused on communication disorders in Black populations around the world, the issues discussed provide good evidence for not allowing national political boundaries to limit where research on communication disorders is conducted for any population. It appears that comparative studies among populations in the United States with their "Old World" counterparts can be quite significant in determining etiological factors associated with communicative disorders that may be in the genetic pool of a particular racial or ethnic group. Of course, this research could result in important benefits to communicatively handicapped persons inside and outside the United States.

REFERENCES

Adler, S. (1973). Data Gathering: The reliability and validity of test data from culturally different children. *Journal of Learning Disabilities, 6*(7), 429–434.

Anderson, E., and Ulatowska, H. (1978). A problem of diagnosis: Black English or aphasia. In R. Brookshire (Ed.), *Clinical aphasiology — collected proceedings, 1972–1976* (pp. 125–138). Minneapolis: BRK Publishers.

Bartel, N., and Grill, J. (1973). Language characteristics of Black children: Implications for assessment. *Journal of School Psychology, 11*, 351–364.

Bliss, L., and Allen, D. (1983). *Screening kit of language development.* Baltimore: University Park Press.

Cole, L. (1980). Blacks with orofacial clefts: The state of the dilemma. *ASHA, 22*, 557–560.

Cole, P. (1984). Language/learning disabilities and the Black primary school age child: An investigation. Unpublished paper.

David, J., Edoo, B., Mustaffah, J., and Hinchcliffe, R. (1971). Adamarobe — a "deaf" village. Sound 5(5), 70–72.

Drummond, A., *Deafness in Malawi.* Report to the Commonwealth Foundation (unpublished).

Everhart, R. (1953). *The growth and development of Negro and white elementary children with articulatory defects.* Unpublished doctoral thesis. Ann Arbor: University of Michigan.

Fajemisin, B. (1980). Comments on communication disorders in Blacks. In O. Taylor and B. Williams (Eds.), *International issues in Black communication.* New York: Rockefeller Foundation.

Gupta, B. (1969). Incidence of congenital malformations in Nigerian children. *West African Medical Journal, 18*, 22–27.

Haddock, D.R., Ebrahim, G.J., and Kapur, B.B. (1962). Ataxic neurological syndrome found in Tanganyika. *British Medical Journal, 2*, 1442.

Hagerman, M. (1980). Heterogeneity of Waardenburg syndrome in Kenyan Africans. *Metabolic Pediatric Ophthalmology, 4*, 1983–1984.

Hinchcliffe, R. (1972). Some geographical aspects of neuro-otology with particular reference to the African. *African Journal of Medical Sciences, 3*, 137–148.

Holland, A. (1983). Nonbiased assessment and treatment of adults who have neurological speech and language problems. *Topics in Language Disorders, 3*, 67–75.

Johnson, R., and Griffiths, V. (1981). *Early intervention with handicapped Black infants from low socio-economic families: Issues and concerns.* Paper presented at the Council for Exceptional Children Conference on The Exceptional Black Child, New Orleans.

Kochman, T. (1970). Towards an ethnography of Black speech behavior. In N.E. Whitten and J. Szwed (Eds.), *Afro-American anthology.* Englewood Cliffs, NJ: Prentice-Hall.

Kochman, T. (1981). *Black and white: Styles and conflict.* Chicago: University of Chicago Press.

Labov, W. (1983). *De facto segregation of Black and white vernaculars.* Unpublished paper. Annual meetings of new ways to analyze variation in language, Montreal, October 27.

Labov, W., and Robins, C. (1969). A note on the relation of reading failure to peer-group status in urban ghettos. *The Teachers College Record, 70,* 396–405.

Leith, W., and Mims, H. (1975). Cultural influences in the development and treatment of stuttering: A preliminary report on the Black stutterer. *Journal of Speech and Hearing Research, 40*(4), 459–466.

Martin, J.A. (1967). Deaf children in East Africa. *Hearing, 22,* 68–87.

Millard, D., and McNeil, K. (1965). The incidence of cleft lip and palate in Jamaica. *Cleft Palate Journal, 2,* 384–388.

Milstein, R.)1976). Language of the English speaking coloured child. *Journal of South African Speech and Hearing Association, 23,* 13–28.

Mitchell, C. (1969). Language behavior and the Black urban community. Unpublished doctoral thesis. Berkeley: University of California.

Monekosso, G.L. (1963). An epidemiological relationship between stomatoglossitis and defective vision. *Journal of Tropical Medicine and Hygiene, 66,* 255.

Monekosso, G., and Wilson, J. (1966). Plasma thiocyanate and vitamin B_{12} in Nigerian patients with degenerative neurological disease. *Lancet, 1,* 1062.

Morgenstein, K., and Manance, P. (1969). Temporal bone histopathy in sickle cell disease. *Laryngoscope, ;79,* 2172–2180.

Murphy, R. (1978). Why minority individuals with developmental disabilities drop out of the service system. A report. Madison, WI: State Council on Developmental Disabilities.

Nelson, N. (1983). Black English sentence scoring: A tool for non-biased assessment. Paper presented at the Annual Convention of American Speech-Language-Hearing Association, Cincinnati.

Okeowo, P., and Nwanze, H. (1978). Therapy of speech disorders — the state of the art in Nigeria. *Nigerian Medical Journal, 8*(3), 259–262.

Oluwasanmi, J., and Adekunle, M. (1970). Congenital clefts of the face in Nigeria. *Plastic and Reconstructive Surgery, 46,* 245–251.

Oluwasanmi, J., and Kogbe, O. (1975). Rarer clefts of the face in Ibadan, Nigeria. *Medical Journal of Zambia, 1,* 25–28.

Osuntokun, B., Monekosso, G., and Wilson, J. (1969). An ataxic neuropathy in Nigeria: A clinical, biochemical, and electrophysiological study. *Brain, 91,* 215.

Payne, J., and Stockman, I. (1979). Sickle cell disease recommendations for research and clinical services in speech pathology and audiology. *Journal of Allied Health, 2*(3) 257–264.

Peters, C. (1979, December). Some communication problems related to testing minority populations with standardized instruments. *Resources in Education, 14* (12), 249. (ERIC Document No. ED 173 849)

Reveron, W. (1984). Language assessment of Black children: The state of the art. *Papers in the Social Sciences, 4,* 79–94.

Robertson, E. (1963). Racial incidence of cleft lip and palate in Trinidad. In *Transactions of the Third International Congress of Plastic Surgery.* Washington, DC: Exerpta Medica Foundation.

Robinson, D., and Shepherd, J. (1970). The prevalence and natural history of cleft lips and palate in Uganda. *Developmental Medicine and Child Neurology, 12*, 637–641.

Roland, P.E. (1960). Otological problem in Uganda. *Journal of Laryngology, 74*, 678.

Rosen, S. (1966). Hearing studies in selected urban and rural populations. *Transactions of the New York Academy of Sciences, 29*, 9–21.

Sellars, S., Beighton, G., Horan, F., and Beighton, P. (1977). Deafness in Black children in Southern Africa. *African Medical Journal, 55*(10) 309–312.

Seymour, H. (1986). Clinical intervention for language disorders among nonstandard English speaking children. In O. Taylor (Ed.), *Treatment of communication disorders in culturally and linguistically diverse populations.* San Diego: College-Hill Press.

Seymour, H., and Miller-Jones, D. (1981). Language and cognitive assessment of black children. In N. Lass (Ed.), *Speech and language: Advances in basic research and practice,* vol. 6. New York: Academic Press, 203–263.

Seymour, H., and Seymour, C. (1977). A therapeutic model for communicative disorders among children who speak Black vernacular. *Journal of Speech and Hearing Disorders, 42*(2), 247–256.

Sharp, M., and Orchik, D. (1978). Auditory function in sickle cell anemia. *Archives of Otolaryngology, 104*, 322–324.

Taylor, O. (1973). Sociolinguistics and the practice of speech pathology. *Rehabilitation Record, 14*(3), 14–17.

Taylor, O. (in press). Clinical practice as a social occasion: An ethnographic model. ASHA Reports.

Taylor, O. (1978). The sociolinguistic dimension in standardized testing. In M. Saville-Troike (Ed.), *Linguistics and Anthropology.* Washington, DC: Georgetown University Press.

Taylor, O., and Samara, R. (1985). Communication disorders in underserved populations: Developing nations. Unpublished paper.

Taylor, O., Stroud, R., Hurst, G., Moore, E., and Williams, R. (1969). Philosophies and goals of the ASHA Black caucus. *ASHA, 11*, 221–225.

Todd, G., Sergeant, G., and Larson, M. (1973). Sensori-neural hearing loss in Jamaicans with SS disease. *Acta Otolaryngologica, 76*, 268–272.

Vaughn-Cooke, E. (1980). Evaluating the language of Black English speakers: Implications of the Ann Arbor decision. In M.F. Whiteman (Ed.), *Reactions to Ann Arbor: Vernacular Black English and Education.* Washington, DC: Center for Applied Linguistics.

Vaughn-Cooke, F. (1983). Improving language assessment in minority children. *ASHA, 25*, 29–34.

Warrick, E. (1975). *The effects of scoring the language modalities for aphasia in accordance with sociolinguistic data on Black English.* Unpublished master's thesis. Washington, DC: Howard University.

Weddington, G., and Meyerson, M. (1984). Syndrome-related speech and hearing disorders in Black children. Paper presented at the 1984 ASHA Convention in San Francisco, November.

Williams, R. (1975). *Textbook of Black related diseases.* New York: McGraw-Hill.

Wolfram, W. (1983). Test interpretation and sociolinguistic differences. *Topics i ι Language Disorders, 3*, 21–34.

Chapter 7

Assessment of Communication Disorders in Non-English Proficient Children

Joan Good Erickson and Aquiles Iglesias

As specialists in communication we are challenged to evaluate the most elusive of behaviors, human verbal and nonverbal interactions. These phenomena communicate feelings, thoughts, and knowledge; modify and extend thinking; and facilitate social and intellectual intercourse. Verbal and nonverbal interactions intertwine with culture, provide solidarity for group identification, and offer or deny access to participation in the mainstream society of a particular country. Parents and researchers are fascinated by their development. Nations are understood and misunderstood through their use. Professionals in education are charged with their measurement and, when indicated, their remediation.

Our responsibility to children impels us to search for the most appropriate and fair assessment of an individual's communication skills. A common-sense approach, supported by research, suggests that language use varies depending on the interactors, topics, and situations; is related to culture; and is affected by the language learning environment to which a child is exposed during the language acquisition process. An awareness of these factors would dictate assessment procedures that go beyond the diagnostic room, beyond a few tests probing only a limited number of linguistic skills, and beyond a single testing interaction. As professionals we recognize that our diagnostic decisions affect the educational future of mainstream English speaking children. Certainly the assessment of children who speak a language other than English, or two languages at varying levels of proficiency, who come from families whose cultural beliefs and practices vary from those of the mainstream group within our society, offers an even greater challenge, if not a greater opportunity to err.

Analogous to Bloom's explanation (1970) of how context is crucial to the understanding of "mommy sock," knowledge of the context in which the assessment of LEP-NEP (Limited English Proficient or Non-English Proficient) children occurs is crucial to an understanding of the quagmire surrounding the communication assessment of language minority children. To help you understand current and proposed assessment procedures for this population, the first section of this chapter will place the assessment of LEP-NEP children within a cultural, linguistic, and historical context. This information will provide a rationale for why traditional approaches to language assessment should be evaluated and modified for the language minority child. The second section addresses assessment of LEP-NEP children from a decision-making paradigm. According to Tomblin and Liljegreen (1985), "a major component of any clinical activity consists of a decision making process" (p. 221). This process includes making decisions regarding the approaches used to collect information as well as how to interpret the information obtained.

We now explore the many questions regarding communication assessment of LEP-NEP children. Some questions have answers; others raise more questions. We hope that the reader will both experience soul-searching and find solutions regarding communication assessment of language minority children.

ASSESSMENT CONTEXT

Since children's communication abilities do not develop independently of their environments, communication assessments should not take place in a vacuum. Therefore, it is imperative that factors that impinge on the communication skills of LEP-NEP children be considered. Following is a brief discussion of the cultural, linguistic, and historical contexts in which the assessment of LEP-NEP children must be placed.

Cultural and Linguistic Context

Within any group of people, be it a nation, state, or community, there are subgroups of people whose behaviors or physical characteristics, or both, set them apart from other members of the group.

When the relative size of the group is small or the economic-political power of the group is weak, the group is referred to as a "minority." In the last few years, the term minority has been used primarily to refer to those individuals who have been denied the opportunity to fully participate within our society. Some linguistic and cultural groups — such as LEP-NEP — can be classified as minorities in the full sense of the definition; their relative size is small, their economic and political power is weak, and their access to full participation in our society has been limited. Let us begin by providing descriptions of the two major factors, culture and language, that make LEP-NEP children different from the majority group within our society.

Saville-Troike (1978) defines culture as "all of the rules for appropriate behavior which are learned by people as a result of being members of the same group or community, and also the values and beliefs which underlie overt behaviors and are themselves shared products of group membership" (p. 1). Using Watzlawic, Beavin, and Jackson's notion (1967) that all behavior in an interactional situation has a message value, it is impossible to talk about culture independently from communication. Birdwhistell (1970) explains the relationship between culture and communication as follows: "Culture and communication are terms which represent two different viewpoints or methods of representing patterned and structured human interconnectedness. As 'culture' the focus is upon structure; as 'communication' it is upon process" (p.318).

Thus, culture can be viewed as a grammar; it is a template generating and interpreting behavior. The verbal and nonverbal behaviors generated from this template vary across different cultural groups (Schieffelin and Eisenberg, 1984). Although differences are evident at all ages, they are most evident in the child socialization patterns used by the socialization agent of the child. Owing to the paucity of data on cross-cultural child socialization patterns, and in some cases plain ethnocentrism, there are certain behaviors that are assumed to be "universals." In reality, they are merely behaviors that are typical of the cultural groups that have been studied extensively, primarily behaviors exhibited by white, middle class Americans. As will be pointed out in the next section, our present assessment protocols assume that any child who does not exhibit these "universal" behaviors would be considered to have a disorder.

One illustration of a "universal" communication behavior is the use of verbal labels. The literature is replete with reference to the importance of the child's ability to label; all objects have labels, and the child is expected to know the specific label of a large number of objects. Somehow, this aspect of communication is considered significant enough that the majority of language tests directly or indirectly assess this ability. It is also considered to be an integral part of any verbal measure of intelligence. But what if the child comes from a culture in which responding to questions for which the adult knows the answer is thought of as purposeless; in which the socialization agent does not engage in "What is this?" routines; in which the use of nonspecific vocabulary supported by gestures is the rule rather than the exception; in which stating the function of the object is as acceptable as labeling the object? Obviously, in this type of culture the importance of labels, as presently defined in assessment protocols, is high irrelevant.

It is difficult, if not impossible, to find within our society a truly homogeneous cultural group that differs from the white, middle class American culture in totality. Even recent immigrants begin to adapt, consciously or unconsciously, to the behavior patterns of the dominant society. This does not mean, however, that all behaviors that existed in their native cultures cease to exist. Some behaviors, especially those related to child socialization, appear to be less adaptable and continue to be transmitted from generation to generation. It is these behaviors that, if not accounted for, will render an assessment culturally biased.

Perhaps the greatest adaptation made by many cultural groups, and the one viewed by many as the true measure of Americanization, is the acquisition of English. We must be aware, however, that, in general, cultural minority children and their parents are a linguistically heterogeneous group. Some members are monolingual speakers of the minority language, some are monolingual speakers of the majority language, and most fall between the two ends of the continuum. Present estimates of the size of the linguistic minority population vary as a function of the definition used, the data collection method, and the age range of the population investigated. As such, estimates of the size of the population should be viewed with extreme caution.

In 1980, the United States Census Bureau asked respondents to state whether they were native speakers of a language other than English. According to the United States Department of Commerce (1983) census data, 41.7 million or 18 percent of the population is composed of individuals who speak a language other than English at home. Forty-eight percent of this group self-reported speaking English "not well" or "not at all." Thus, it is estimated that the size of the "true" linguistic minority population is 20.4 million. Of this number, 733,290 are children between the ages of 5 and 17 years,

Table 7-1.   Language Other than English Spoken at Home and Reported Difficulty with English (Source: U.S. Department of Commerce, 1983)

Language	Persons 5–17 Years Old		Persons 18 Years Old and Over	
	Total (1,000)	Difficulty* (Percent)	Total (1,000)	Difficulty (Percent)
Spanish	4,568	14.0	18,492	19.4
Italian	147	5.4	8,164	27.6
French	223	6.8	1,328	7.2
German	192	6.2	1,395	4.7
Polish	41	5.7	780	10.6
Chinese	114	20.9	516	31.6
Greek	65	5.2	336	17.0
Philippine languages	63	8.9	411	9.4
Portuguese	68	10.3	284	31.6
Japanese	34	18.7	303	19.6
Korean	60	17.0	207	32.4
All others	608	14.8	3,298	12.3

*Persons reported as speaking English "not well" or "not at all."

and 19.6 million are individuals over the age of 18 years. No information is available on the linguistic skills of children under the age of 5 years. The lack of data for children under 5 is distressing considering that the "under 5" group accounts for 10 percent of the racial-ethnic minority of the United States (11.3 percent of Hispanics, 9.2 percent of Blacks, and 10.5% of American Indians, Eskimos, and Aleuts). The language background of the linguistic minority population of age 5 years and older is given in Table 7–1.

Besides the age-range limitations, there are two additional problems with these data. First, the data on linguistic proficiency in English are based on self-evaluations. As such, they must be viewed with caution since a self-judgment of proficiency in another language is largely based on what is considered to be adequate. Second, and perhaps more important, the definition focuses only on linguistic and not communicative proficiency in a language. This type of definition of what constitutes a linguistic minority population is based on a narrow view of communication. A definition based on "linguistic proficiency" rather than "communicative proficiency" also suggests that the problems encountered by this group are due solely to their lack of knowledge of specific linguistic skills, and that when these skills are mastered the "problem" is eliminated.

A perhaps more valid, although more limited, estimate of linguistic minorities was obtained by O'Malley (1976). These data, the

Table 7-2. Estimated Numbers of Limited English Proficient Children Ages 5 to 14, in 1976, and Projected Numbers to the Year 2000, by Language Background (Numbers in Thousands)

Language Background	1976	1985	2000
Total	2,520.4	2,439.9	3,400.0
Chinese	34.3	30.3	36.2
Philippine languages	36.4	32.1	38.3
French	97.6	86.0	102.9
German	97.4	86.0	102.6
Greek	29.0	25.6	30.6
Italian	104.1	91.9	109.6
Japanese	14.5	12.8	15.3
Korean	13.4	11.8	14.1
Navajo	26.6	23.5	28.1
Polish	26.3	23.2	27.7
Portuguese	26.1	23.1	27.5
Spanish	1,789.0	1,794.3	2,630.0
Vietnamese	27.3	24.1	28.7
Yiddish	24.6	21.8	26.0
Other languages	173.3	153.2	182.4

largest and most comprehensive to date, attempted to estimate the number of school-aged children with limited-English proficiency in the United States. According to these data, approximately 2.5 million school-aged children have sufficient difficulty speaking, reading, and understanding the English language to deny them the opportunity to learn successfully in classrooms in which the language of instruction is English. Table 7-2 illustrates the language background of these children and the projected increase of this population for the years 1985 and 2000.

Considerable differences exist between the 1980 census data and O'Malley's data. According to O'Malley's findings, the number of LEP children was 2.5 million, almost three times the estimate from the 1980 United States census. The difference is more significant when we consider that O'Malley's data were collected 4 years prior to the 1980 census and that he sampled 5 to 14 year old students, compared with the sample of 5 to 17 year olds reported in the 1980 United States census.

Table 7-3 illustrates the linguistic minority student population across states (O'Malley, 1976). As can be seen from this table, the 10 states with the largest minority populations are California, Texas, New York, Illinois, Florida, Arizona, New Mexico, Pennsylvania, and Massachusetts. The states of California, Texas and New York contain 62.4 percent of the LED population. An additional factor to con-

Table 7–3. Estimated Numbers of LEP Children Ages 5 to 14, in 1976, and Projected Numbers to the Year 2000, by State* (Numbers in Thousands)

State	1976	1985	2000
All states*	2,520.4	2,439.9	3,400.0
Alaska	5.4	6.0	7.8
Arizona	73.4	86.7	133.2
California	609.9	606.8	902.5
Colorado	33.7	37.2	57.5
Connecticut	31.3	25.1	34.0
Delaware	2.7	2.4	3.3
District of Columbia	2.9	2.3	2.2
Florida	84.1	99.9	160.6
Georgia	11.0	11.1	13.5
Hawaii	21.0	20.8	25.8
Idaho	5.5	6.0	8.6
Illinois	84.5	78.0	101.8
Indiana	25.1	22.7	28.1
Iowa	6.0	5.0	6.4
Kansas	8.2	7.4	9.3
Louisiana	41.0	37.5	42.9
Maine	7.7	6.9	8.7
Maryland	18.0	16.1	21.7
Massachusetts	44.8	36.9	50.8
Michigan	29.4	25.8	31.9
Minnesota	10.2	8.7	11.5
Missouri	8.1	6.9	8.3
Montana	3.4	3.2	3.9
Nebraska	5.8	5.6	8.0
Nevada	5.3	5.7	8.3
New Hampshire	5.6	4.9	6.4
New Jersey	83.3	77.0	109.1
New Mexico	69.2	73.9	106.4
New York	455.1	394.2	526.4
North Dakota	2.4	2.0	2.4
Ohio	41.4	34.6	40.5
Oklahoma	15.8	15.7	19.7
Oregon	10.5	10.0	13.5
Pennsylvania	65.9	55.5	69.5
Rhode Island	7.1	6.4	8.4
South Dakota	1.8	1.5	1.7
Texas	509.4	571.8	853.5
Utah	7.2	8.5	11.5
Vermont	2.2	2.0	2.5
Virginia	14.6	13.8	19.1
Washington	17.8	16.6	22.6
Wisconsin	8.2	7.0	9.4
Wyoming	2.1	2.2	3.0

*Data on eight states were not presented. From O'Malley, M. (1976).

sider is the relative size of the population. In some states (Arizona, California, Colorado, New Mexico, New York, and Texas) the linguistic minority population exceeds 15 percent of the student population. In contrast, in the majority of the states the linguistic minority never exceeds 5 percent.

The demographic characteristics of the linguistic minority population have had an effect on the assessment policies that have been developed in various states. In states in which the linguistic minority population is large, there appear to be established procedures for the identification and placement of the normal and handicapped school-age linguistic minority population. These state guidelines parallel federal legal mandates, and implementation is closely monitored at the state level. In contrast, in states in which the linguistic minority population is small in proportion, state policies do not exist. The lack of guidelines has resulted in numerous communities having policies that are contradictory to federal mandates. Since monitoring of these local policies is not done at the state level, and monitoring of local policies from the federal level is almost impossible, numerous communities in these states continue to have policies that violate the legal rights of handicapped LEP-NEP children.

No studies specifically designed to ascertain the national prevalence of communication disorders in the linguistic minority population are available. The closest we can get to those data are the child-count numbers obtained by each state. Unfortunately, these data tend to be reported in terms of racial or ethnic background of the child rather than linguistic background, and they are often based on inappropriate testing procedures.

Additional factors make these state child-count data even more difficult to interpret. Owing to the historical overrepresentation of certain ethnic groups in special education classes, some states have strongly encouraged school districts to limit the number of racial or ethnic minority students who are identified as handicapped. In some school districts, the number of students classified as Educable Mentally Retarded (EMR) cannot exceed the percentage of Hispanics in the school district. Thus, the incidence of EMR in the Hispanic population, rather than the true prevalence, determines the number of children served and thus counted. Another interesting trend occurs when there is a shift in the incidence of particular types of disorders among minorities. Tucker (1980), in a study of school-aged children, found an increase in the ethnic representation of minorities diagnosed as having learning disabilities. We can only speculate as to what changes more — tests, policies, or children.

There is also a tendency in some school districts not to classify a child as handicapped until the child is enrolled in English-only classes. This policy is the result of several factors: (1) the assumption that all difficulties encountered by linguistic minority children are due to their lack of English skills, (2) the inability of the school district to find qualified personnel to assess the child in his or her native language, and (3) the assumption that "double counting" (LEP and handicapped) is not allowed under local, state, and federal regulations. Most important, how language dominance and disorders are identified will affect prevalence data as well as the educational future of a child.

In 1981, the American Speech, Language, and Hearing Association (ASHA) Task Force on the Prevalence of Communicative Disorders (Healey, Ackerman, Chappell, Perrin, and Stormer, 1981) concluded that the prevalence and incidence data available on communication disorders were "inconsistent, at best, and conflicting, at worst" (p. 76). It is not surprising, therefore, that the same can be said about the data presently available for communication disorders in the linguistic minority population.

In addition to the problems discussed in the ASHA report and the state child-count data, other factors exist that make valid and reliable data on the prevalence of communication disorders in the heterogeneous cultural-linguistic minority population almost impossible to obtain. First, there is no clear agreement as to what constitutes a disorder within a particular population. For example, a voice that is judged disordered in one culture might be considered normal in another culture; reluctance to speak or maintain eye contact with adults may be appropriate in one culture and thought of as disordered in another. Second, developmental data on non-English speaking populations as well as children learning two languages simultaneously are increasing (McLaughlin, 1977) but remain limited compared with information on English. In addition, language systems may be so complicated (e.g., Navajo) or variant from English (e.g., Vietnamese), as well as lacking in specific normative or descriptive information, that comparable developmental levels and thus disorders are difficult to ascertain. Finally, the assessment procedures used to assess "normalcy" may be culturally and linguistically biased. Before discussing how to identify handicapped language minority children most appropriately, let us briefly explore another contextual factor, the history of bilingualism and bilingual education in the United States.

Historical Context

Many people have the mistaken belief that bilingualism and bilingual education are new and controversial issues in the United States. In reality, the issue has been the subject of spirited debate over many decades. Although the United States was founded on principles of religious and individual freedom, attitudes toward linguistic and cultural diversity have varied. A theme often heard within our society is that America is a "melting pot." This view is best exemplified in the words of Zangwill (1909):

> America is God's Crucible, the great Melting Pot where all races of Europe are melting and reforming! Here you stand, good folk, think I, when I see them at Ellis Island, here you stand in your fifty groups with your fifty languages and histories, and your fifty hatreds and rivalries, but you won't be long like that, brother, for these are the fires of God. (p. 37)

Zangwill's view of America as a melting pot has often been supported by government policy that stresses cultural conformity and linguistic assimilation. Diversity, especially in languages, has been seen as an insurmountable barrier to national unity. Speaking English has become a badge of Americanism. This attitude, sometimes amounting to xenophobia, is interesting considering that the rest of the world is characteristically bilingual or multilingual. Grosjean (1982) states that "it is practically impossible to locate a genuinely monolingual country, that is, one that does not contain one or several linguistic minorities whose members use, to some extent at least, both the majority and minority language" (p. 5).

Although bilingualism in the United States was tolerated until the middle of the nineteenth century, the acceptance of cultural and linguistic pluralism declined considerably after this period. Examples of governmental policy designed to eradicate anything that is not "American" include the following: The establishment of "off reservation boarding schools" in 1879 for the purpose of eradicating Indian languages and customs; the English-only rule established in Puerto Rico as soon as the United States occupied Puerto Rico during the Spanish-American War and again in 1905; the introduction of English into the legal and educational system of Hawaii as soon as it was annexed to the United States in 1898; the establishment of English as the official language of the Philippines in 1901; the restriction of bilingual schools from before World War I until after World War II; the 1940 Nationality Act requiring English literacy as a condition for naturalization (Castellanos, 1984).

Even the founding fathers of speech-language pathology (Travis, Johnson, and Shover, 1937) contributed to the belief that speaking another language might be detrimental to a child's normal speech development. Van Riper (1947) stated "some parents deliberately attempt to teach their children two languages at the same time, a procedure which is usually disastrous" (p. 108). In 1961, the American

Speech and Hearing Association listed bilingualism as a disorder when reporting "speech defects" in public school populations. Thus, politicians and professionals perpetuated the ideal of monolingualism in this country.

Despite attempts to eradicate the various cultural and linguistic subgroups, many of these subgroups survived. Their survival was due to people's unwillingness or inability to assimilate into the dominant subgroup within our society. Indeed, bilingualism was never eradicated, particularly in geographical areas with large ethnic populations or strong religious organizations (U.S. Commission on Civil Rights, 1975). In many families, a language other than English continued to be spoken. Ethnic customs were handed down from generation to generation. Even now it is not unusual for individuals to refer to their cultural heritage (e.g., "I'm Irish and German"), albeit lacking the linguistic ability of their forebears.

In the last three decades we have seen the acceptance of the view that our society is pluralistic; that it is not melting but is a society that is unique and rich because of its diversity. The acceptance, or more realistically the tolerance, of this view was not won without considerable sacrifice.

During the 1960s and 1970s a number of significant cases (e.g., *Lau v. Nichols,* 1974, and *Dianna v. State Board of Education,* 1973) defined the process by which LEP and handicapped students were to be identified, evaluated, and served by educational agencies. The judicial principles that emerged from these and other court proceedings are included in the two major pieces of legislation affecting the rights of the handicapped linguistic minority population: The Bilingual Education Act of 1984 (preceded by Title VII of the 1965 Elementary and Secondary Education Act, which became law in 1968 and was amended in 1974), and the Education of All Handicapped Children Act of 1975 (Public Law 94–142). For a full description of the laws and judicial mandates that apply to the linguistic minority population, see Leibowitz (1982) and Baca and Cervantes (1984).

In general, the Bilingual Education Act of 1968 was established as a way to assist children who were "educationally disadvantaged because of their inability to speak English." Although compensatory in nature, this federal law recognized the need for instruction in a language other than English and is credited with providing the impetus for bilingual education in the United States. Subsequent legislation — the Bilingual Education Act of 1974 — further expanded the population to be served to include migrant workers, the handicapped, and adults and indicated that instructional models include "maintenance" and "transitional" bilingual programs. The 1984

Act expanded the type of instruction to include "immersion" programs.

The Education of All Handicapped Children Act required, among other directives, that procedures used for evaluation and placement of handicapped children be selected and administered so as not to be racially or culturally discriminatory. This directive also indicated that the administration of these procedures be in the native language or mode of communication of the child. Native language, as defined by the Bilingual Education Act, means the language normally used by an individual, or, in the case of a young child, the language used by the parents of the child.

Legal and judicial mandates have resulted in numerous policies that have had both a positive and a negative effect on the education of the linguistic minority population, both handicapped and nonhandicapped. On the positive side, the goal of the aforementioned legislation is to provide adequate assessment and thus educational and remediation services. On the negative side, the central issue to both major pieces of legislation is the determination of the dominant language of the child, a difficult goal to achieve. The determination of language dominance is frequently limited to a cursory estimate of the language proficiency required to function in a particular setting (i.e., school). As a result, it is difficult to ascertain whether the inability of a child to respond adequately to test items is due to (1) lack of linguistic skills in English, (2) unfamiliarity with the required task (e.g., labeling) or stimulus items (e.g., line drawings), (3) dialectal variation in the non-English language, or (4) other sociolinguistic factors that affect language use or (5) a combination of these factors.

If examiners err in ascertaining language dominance and do not recognize that language use (including choice of language) varies with topic and interaction, the following may occur: (1) nonhandicapped children will be placed in classrooms in which the language of instruction is not the one in which they are proficient, (2) handicapped children will be assessed in a language they do not understand, or (3) handicapped children will be placed in regular bilingual classrooms and thus not receive appropriate supportive services. To implement appropriate assessment policies and procedures, several decisions must be made before and during the testing process.

ASSESSMENT DECISIONS

How language is defined dictates how it is measured. If an individual defines language as knowing names of colors, body parts, animals, or shapes or using embedded phrases, wh-questions conjunctions, tense and plural markers, then that is what is measured. If, however, language is defined as communicative competence (Hymes, 1971), which includes more than just linguistic competence (Chomsky, 1957), the measure will be broader in scope. Furthermore, most testing paradigms, according to Troike (1983), "treat testees as purely passive objects, like oranges to be squeezed for juice, rather than as active participants in the testing event, with their own goals, agendas, and strategies, which may differ with individuals, ethnic groups, and social classes" (p. 213). In addition, the assessment tools used by diagnosticians may dictate their theory and philosophy of language and thus their therapeutic approach.

But what if the basic premise, including definitions and tools, is questionable? Perhaps knowing the names of colors and certain syntactic structures is not a guarantee for social and intellectual success in school and life. Furthermore, it may not be possible to measure this complicated, synergistic phenomenon at all, let alone by simplistically sampling some of its characteristics. Can an individual know about the parts (e.g., syntax, vocabulary) and thus make assumptions about the whole (communicative competence) when the whole is never equal to the sum of the parts? Indeed, so-called language measures may not be measures of language at all if we look beyond surface structures. As pointed out by Troike (1983),

> From a theoretical viewpoint . . ., it is essentially impossible ever to fully assess the linguistic competence of an individual through the limited sampling of performance that a test must consist of. This is particularly true since we lack as yet anything like a full description of any language as a basis for constructing testing instruments, or a full account of even one individual's competence as a basis for validating our sampling. (p. 213)

Perhaps we should admit that we are attempting to measure a behavior we do not clearly understand. Then we can decide either not to evaluate it, to evaluate it poorly, or to evaluate it in the best manner possible. Because we will reject the notions of not evaluating (i.e., ignoring the problem) or evaluating poorly (i.e., contributing to the problem), let us pursue the option of evaluating the communication skills of children in the best way possible, recognizing the strengths and weaknesses of both our attempts and our findings.

To a large extent, assessment is a problem solving process for which a series of decisions must be made. This process involves deciding how data will be collected as well as how it will be interpreted. There are several options or decision alternatives professionals must consider when faced with the responsibility of assessing

LEP-NEP individuals. What follows is a guide for communication assessment decision making. We encourage the reader to evaluate each of the various alternatives within the framework of his or her skills, training, and clinical-educational setting. Some decisions will be bound to previous decisions, others will not. All decisions will make a difference in the value of the outcome and thus the life potential of a child.

Decision 1. Should the LEP-NEP child be assessed using discrete-point tests, integrative measures, or ethnographic approaches?

Tests of language or communication ability can be classified according to the theoretical basis on which they are developed. Discrete-point testing is based on the notion that evaluation of the parts will provide an understanding of the whole. Integrative measures attempt to tap the synergistic characteristics of communication, including the interrelationship between syntax, semantics, and phonology. An ethnographic approach focuses on the form and function of language in the naturalistic setting and allows for social and cultural variations according to topic, situation, and speaker. Let us trace the developmental history of these assessment alternatives and evaluate their appropriateness with language-minority children.

Early philosophers and linguists were interested in how verbal messages were communicated and what variables affected their use. In an attempt to understand this process, decades of research dissected the verbal message and focused on the structure. The Chomskian revolution of the 1960s questioned the structuralist theory and proposed a psycholinguistic framework for the understanding of language. It was no longer possible to measure the structure without attempting to understand the psychological processes underlying the linguistic utterances. The question of competence (the underlying process) versus performance (the observable end product) became an important issue.

For those who wished to "measure" language, the simplistic notion of measuring discrete points to understand the whole became less realistic. Furthermore, linguists returned to the original question of the earlier philosophers: why, when, and how do individuals vary their utterances in context? This theoretical shift, which has been occurring, or rather reappearing, during the past decade, ties language structure to communication and context (Bates, 1976). The assessment approaches that parallel this shift in theoretical thinking require little or no manipulation of the child's environment; doing so renders the assessment invalid. In comparison, discrete-point tests reflect their theoretical bias, manipulate the child's environment, and are particularly punitive when used with minority populations. For example, items chosen for testing may primarily sample mainstream articulation and language skills. Language variation may not be considered in item selection during the process of test development and may be ignored in the criteria for scoring. These factors alone are discriminatory with minority children. Discrete-point tests may also penalize children who are knowledgeable about their subculture but lack experience with mainstream society.

In between, discrete-point tests and ethnographic approaches are the integrative measures that attempt to capture the synergy of various linguistic skills, albeit by means of structured or contrived approaches. Integrative testing is based on the notion that language ability cannot be determined by independently measuring the individual components of language as attempted in discrete-point testing approaches. As Oller (1979) states, "If discrete items take language apart, integrative tests put it back together. Whereas discrete items attempt to test knowledge of language one bit at a time, integrative tests attempt to assess a learner's capacity to use many bits all at the same time" (p. 37).

Various methods of integrative testing have been proposed. These approaches include oral and written cloze tests (omission of every *n*th work in a discourse sample), dictation, description, paraphrasing, and oral interviews (Oller, 1979). Language samples may also be evaluated using several integrative criteria. For example, scoring for the Student Oral Language Observation Matrix (California State Department of Education, 1981) uses the following five criteria: comprehension, fluency, vocabulary, pronunciation, and grammar. Each of these areas is rated on a five-point scale ranging from "no competence" to "native-like competence." (See Erickson and Omark, 1981, for a review of assessment approaches.)

An ethnographic approach has a different orientation than the two previously described assessment methods: It acknowledges the relationship between the child and other participants in an interaction. Each participant is affected by the other. Neither the environment nor the child is manipulated because doing so would merely provide information on how the child performs in another situation with other participants. In discrete-point and integrative testing the variables are defined *a priori,* and the child's communication behavior is filtered through these variables. In contrast to this top-down approach, an ethnographic assessment is a bottom-up approach in which the variables are derived through systematic data collection and an analysis process using a variety of ethnographic methods, such as participant observations, informal interviews, and field notes. The typology that is created is then validated. (See Omark, 1981b.) The data that emerge from this approach reflect the interaction between the child's inherent abilities and environmental experiences.

All three assessment approaches — discrete-point testing, integrative measures, and ethnographic methods — have merit as well as the potential for discriminating against and thus misdiagnosing language minority children. Taylor and Payne (1983) describe culturally valid tests as those tests that "do not discriminate unfairly either for or against a client for cultural reasons or because of cultural variations within a culture based on such factors as age, gender, socioeconomic class or dialect" (p. 11). Therefore, thoughtful decisions when selecting assessment approaches must be made. Information that can be gained by one approach may be balanced by a loss of information in another. All three approaches, if done adequately, can be appropriate for evaluating the communicative ability of LEP-NEP children. If done inadequately, biased assessment and subsequent inappropriate remediation will result.

Whether theoretically current or not, discrete-point testing is ingrained in the educational system. Indeed the plethora of discrete-point tests available on the market attests to their viability in spite of changing theoretical currents. Although these tests have traditionally misclassified minority students (Oakland, 1977; Samuda, 1975), they continue to be developed and used. Because they may label normal children as handicapped, despite their expediency and simplicity, the price may be too high to pay. School districts, federal policy, and perhaps tradition encourage their use. Even PL 94–142 mandates that more than one diagnostic test be used, even though two culturally and linguistically biased tests may not be better than one.

Similarly, integrative measures and ethnographic approaches, although based on more contemporary theory, may provide nondiscriminatory information yet not therapeutic direction. For example, what is gained by using terms such as "comprehensibility" (Savignon, 1972) or "quality of reporting and organization" (Bond, Epstein, and Matz, 1977) with integrative measures? Does the test giver have a better understanding of the child's problem and thus of remediation? There is no question that discrete-point tests measure only a limited aspect of a child's linguistic ability, but do global descriptors provide more direction? Furthermore, are non–discrete-point tests feasible in the clinical-educational setting? Integrative and ethnographic approaches are only viable alternatives if the professional is willing to evaluate language samples, use integrative approaches, observe a child in the classroom and other settings, or interview significant others in the life of the child. The professional must then use this information to make an appropriate diagnosis and implement recommendations. In contrast, discrete-point tests are usually easy to administer and score. Unfortunately, the simple assessment approach may solve short-term needs of the professional while creating long-term problems for the child whose linguistic ability is misdiagnosed.

Decision 2. Is the purpose of the assessment to determine the communicative skills the child has mastered or the child's potential for acquiring such skills?

An alternative approach to assessing communication is to evaluate the child's *potential* for acquiring particular skills rather than assessing the skills mastered. This approach to assessment has been advocated by Feuerstein, Rand, and Hoffman (1979). In contrast to theory that suggests that there are maturational prerequisite skills to learning, Feuerstein and colleagues believe that delays in cognitive (and thus linguistic) functioning can be evaluated through a Learning Potential Assessment Device and then remediation can be done through a systematic teaching approach. Because linguistically and culturally diverse students have not had the same opportunities to know the content of IQ tests, it is necessary to provide new learning tasks, observe how the child learns, teach problem solving and principles of learning, and then apply these principles to solving new problems (Baca and Cervantes, 1984). Although this approach penalizes cultural differences in perceptual and learning styles and appears to be based on a deprivation or deficit model, it does attempt to focus on a child's learning potential.

Ethnographic assessment of minority children (Iglesias, 1984) allows for a similar modifiability approach. Rather than measuring static performance, an approach that is dynamic in nature is advocated: The problem is identified, changes are made in the child's environment, and then changes in the child's performance and modifiability are evaluated. This approach is particularly effective when it is necessary to ascertain whether the child's difficulty in communicating is due to (1) differences between the child's culture and the culture from which the standard was derived or (2) the child's inability to learn.

An example of the importance of differentiating between the two alternatives just mentioned is illustrated in the following case. Let us assume that an examiner is attempting to evaluate the discourse skills of an LEP child who has been enrolled in a bilingual class for 3 years and is presently being partially mainstreamed into an English-only class. The examiner asks the child to "talk about something that happened at school" and expects the child to answer in a topic-centered discourse style (Michaels and Cook-Gumperz, 1979) — that is, a single clearly identifiable topic in which the focus is a single event or topic. Rather than being topic-centered, the child's response is topic-associative, a style considered by the English-speaking teacher not to be age appropriate. Furthermore, the child is expected to have acquired this different way of organizing discourse during 3 years of school. It is, however, an appropriate discourse style within the culture of the child. Is the child just using the discourse style of his or her culture or is the child using discourse skills that are below those expected for his or her age or grade level? In this case, the answer cannot be obtained from a static assessment procedure that does not differentiate "differences" from "disorders." A clear differentiation can only be made when the behavior being assessed is observed in both cultural or linguistic groups of the same age or grade level. Clinicians using an ethnographic approach to assessment must be extremely familiar with the characteristics of communication as well as linguistic skills of both the majority and the minority populations to make this differentiation.

Decision 3. Should a norm-referenced or a criterion-referenced assessment tool be used?

Thorndike (1918) observed two somewhat distinct groups of educational measures: one "asks primarily how well a pupil performs a certain uniform task"; the other "asks how hard a task a student can perform with substantial perfection, or with some specified degree of success" (p. 16). In the former, referred to as norm-referenced, the child's performance is viewed in relation to the performance of others. In the latter, referred to as criterion-referenced, the degree to which a child's performance compares to a previously set performance standard is evaluated. Although both approaches sort students, the type of sorting is different. The norm-referenced assessment tools sort children on the basis of their performance in relation to the mean performance score obtained from a standardized sample. The criterion-referenced assessment tool sorts children on the basis of their mastery of specific skills. Both procedures could result in biased assessments if careful consideration is not given to the standardization procedure and interpretation of results.

The two procedures require that a particular standard be specified. In the case of norm-referenced assessment tools, the standard specified is the behavior of the particular population selected on a particular uniform task. For example, the child's performance on the Test for Auditory Comprehension of Language (Fifth Edition; Carrow, 1973) is compared to the performance of a selected sample of (English speaking) middle class Black, Anglo-American and Mexican-American children of ages 3 through 6 years. In the case of criterion-referenced assessment tools, the specific behavioral objectives selected become the performance standards. For example, the child is expected to produce the pronoun "he" in seven of ten mandatory contexts. A binary decision is made for each criterion. The child may either demonstrate or not demonstrate the mastery of each skill assessed.

The notion of a "standard" raises the question "whose standard?" Most norm-referenced assessment tools, whether in English or in another language, are standardized on a population that is often different from the one being assessed (such as the minority child). For example, most commercially available tests that have both English and Spanish versions (e.g., *Compton Speech and Language Screening Evaluation* [Compton, 1983], a *Preschool Language Scale* [Zimmerman, Steiner, and Pond, 1979], or *Expressive One Word Picture Vocabulary Test* [Gardner, 1979]) have been standardized on native English speaking children. The norms presented by the test developers are those obtained for the English speaking population and are incorrectly assumed to be equivalent for the Spanish speaking population. The result is a standard that is biased against language minority children.

The same problem of sampling bias is also encountered in tests specifically designed for and normed on Spanish speaking populations (e.g., Spanish Picture Vocabulary Test [Wiener, Simon, and Weiss, 1978]). These tests have been normed on a limited sample of children from a limited region of the United States. In reality, the norms provided for these tests are more like local norms than national norms. For guidelines in evaluating the technical qualities of tests, see Appendix 1.

The same issue of "whose standards?" can be raised for criterion-referenced tests. Someone must select the specific skills assessed and must specify at what age or grade level these skills are to be mastered. For example, criterion-referenced assessments used in many schools are designed to parallel curriculum objectives. Thus, the individuals responsible for developing the curriculum objectives indirectly set the standards. Since school curricula tend to reflect the values and beliefs of the dominant group within the society, the child's performance is being compared to that group rather than the minority group to which the child belongs.

The use of locally developed norms has often been advocated as a means of ensuring that the performance of the child being assessed is compared with that of children of the same sociocultural background. There are two issues that need to be considered when contemplating developing and using local norms. The first issue is one of logistics. Who is going to do this? The cost, in terms of time and skill required to develop norms for each of the assessment tools, may far exceed the benefit gained from such an endeavor.

The second issue relates to the interpretation of these norms. Let us assume norms are obtained for two adjacent speech communities, each of which is composed of families of a similar cultural and linguistic background. A particular child's performance, according to the norms for community A, is normal; but according to the norms for community B, the child's performance is below average. Perhaps the child moves from community A to community B. Does moving a few blocks or crossing a bridge result in this child's becoming handicapped? Note that regardless of which norms are used, the child is functioning in a community whose standards are different from the child's original community. (For a further discussion of the problems involved in norming tests for minority populations, see Omark, 1981a, and Toronto and Merrill, 1983.)

Decision 4. Should standardized tests be administered in a nonstandard manner?

Another approach to nondiscriminatory assessment is to use standardized tests in a nonstandard manner. With either discrete-point or integrative tests, the tester can use an assessment approach that provides the opportunity for the minority child to perform at a maximum level. A test can first be administered with the standardized approach, after which it can be presented in a nonstandard manner. The written report should include an explanation of how both scores were obtained.

Various authors (e.g., Terrell, 1983; Toliver-Weddington, 1981) have discussed options for nondiscriminatory assessment procedures. In general, these procedures attempt to take into account the child's linguistic, cultural, and academic exposure and focus on *what a child can do.* Following are suggestions from the literature and our experience.

1. Before using a test, examine each item to evaluate whether the child would have had access to the information being tested.

Table 7–4. Nondiscriminatory Testing Examples

Standard Test Item	Child Explanation
Point to parachute	"hot air balloon"
Point to net	"basketball hoop"
Which two go together (or are the same?) (pictures of cat-car-cat)	"The cat and the car 'cause the car hit this cat and the other cat got away."
Donde esta Chica?	"pequeña" (dialect variation)
What's this? (no response to picture of a typewriter)	"Apple computer" (response after encouragement to guess)

2. Reword instructions.
3. Provide additional time for the child to respond.
4. Continue testing beyond the ceiling.
5. Record all responses, particularly when the child changes an answer, explains, comments, or demonstrates.
6. Compare the child's answers to dialect or to first language or second language learning features. Rescore articulation and expressive language samples, giving credit for variation or differences.
7. If the test does not have practice items, develop several so that the process of "taking the test" is established.
8. On picture vocabulary recognition tests, have the child name the picture in addition to pointing to the stimulus item to ascertain the appropriateness of the label for the pictorial representation.
9. Have the child explain why the "incorrect" answer was selected.
10. Have the child identify the actual object, body part, action, photograph, and so forth, particularly if he or she has had limited experience with books, line drawings, or the testing process.

Table 7–4 provides examples from our clinical experience that will clarify how significant information can be obtained about a child's knowledge of the world if we take the time to find out. After standard test administration was completed (column 1) the children's "errors" were explored (column 2) by having the child either name the picture or explain the answer.

Decision 5. In what language (first, second, or both) should the assessment be conducted?

Interest in the assessment of communicatively disordered LEP-NEP children emerged from the desire to decrease the number of LEP-NEP students who had been misclassified as handicapped and placed in special education classes (Mercer, 1973). As a result, laws and policies have focused on procedures that will avoid this error and are based on the belief that testing children in a language other than their most proficient one could result in normal LEP-NEP children being classified as handicapped. Thus, PL 94–142 and several state laws require that the assessment materials and procedures be administered in the language or mode of communication in which the child is most proficient (i.e., the "dominant" language).

Before considering the issue of assessing LEP-NEP children in their most proficient language, let us consider what we would do in an analogous situation: the assessment of a hearing impaired child who uses simultaneous communication (oral and manual). When assessing this child, could we (1) assess the child only in the dominant society's mode of communication, oral; (2) assess the child only in his or her "dominant" or "most proficient" mode; (3) assess the child using one mode and 2 weeks later assess the child in the other mode; or (4) assess the child using both modes (oral and manual) simultaneously. Most speech-language pathologists would have no difficulty in deciding that alternative 4 is the correct answer. Neither assessing the child in only one mode nor assessing two modes separately would provide a true picture of the child's communication proficiency. The same type of logical reasoning used to decide what mode to use in the assessment of the bimodal hearing impaired child should be followed in deciding on what language to assess LEP-NEP children. Unfortunately, rather than relying on logical reasoning, we have allowed well intentioned but illogical legislative mandates to determine what we do.

There is no question that if a child speaks only one language, the child must be assessed in that language. However, the majority of linguistic minority children do not fall at either end of the linguistic continuum. This is especially true of preschool and school-aged children. Thus, assessing these children in one language, even after screening for the so-called "dominant language," provides only a limited sample of their communication abilities. For example, in a recent evaluation a "Spanish dominant child" was administered the Spanish and English versions of the Boehm Test of Basic Concepts (Boehm, 1970). Her performance on both versions was three standard deviations below the mean. However, when the total number of correct responses was calculated, regardless of whether the response was in English or Spanish, her performance was slightly above the mean. This is by no means an isolated case. Our clinical experience with hundreds of minority children indicates that many of these children have a communication system that intertwines features of both cultures and features of two languages.

A related question in deciding which language should be used for assessment is the practice of using translated tests. Taylor and Payne (1983) suggest that to minimize the linguistic bias of discrete-point tests, stimulus items should be changed to forms parallel to those used by the child's speech community. In the case of LEP-NEP children, these changes mean the translation of the test items into the child's language. For example, the *Expressive One Word Picture Vocabulary Test — Spanish Edition* (Gardner, 1979) provides various dialectal alternatives for each stimulus item (e.g., "bús," "ómnibus," "camión," and "guagua" for the picture of a bus).

Although translated tests reduce test bias (for at least the child understands what is being asked), there are some major problems with translated tests. First, the use of a translated form *negates* the use of any of the norms established in English. Second, many aspects of language cannot be translated. Consider the following:

1. Languages vary in their use of markers for gender, time, honorifics, and so forth.
2. Languages vary in the amount of information presented via tonal changes and intonation patterns.
3. Languages vary according to cultural rules, such as who uses what form to whom.
4. Languages vary in areas of semantics due to different cultural views, values, and experiences.
5. Languages vary according to structural rules, such as subject-verb-object (S-V-O) versus subject-object-verb (S-O-V).
6. Languages have dialectal variations primarily in vocabulary usage and pronunciation rules.
7. Languages have rule systems that vary with registers.

Given these variations among languages and cultures, translating test items becomes a dangerous procedure.

Furthermore, monolingual English-speaking clinicians may develop a false sense of security if they think that knowing how to pronounce the particular stimulus items provided in the test manuals is sufficient to conduct a valid assessment in another language. What happens if the child's response is correct linguistically but incorrect according to the test manual? Can the clinician recognize typographical errors (chice for chico), missing alternative responses (cla-cetin but not media), or incompatible complexity of lexical items (zarpa, pata, and garra for paw) of a test such as in the *Expressive One Word Vocabulary Test* (Gardner, 1979)?

Another problem with translated tests is that only those structures deemed important in English are assessed (e.g., a test might assess noun-verb-number agreement but never noun-adjective-gender agreement). Finally, a major problem with the use of translated tests is that the content assessed and the procedure through which this content is assessed might be outside the experience of the child. For example, several of the presently available tests require the child to be familiar with "common objects" and to label those objects with a one-word label. But perhaps the child comes from a culture in which labeling objects is an unfamiliar task or the "common" objects are not "common" in the culture of the child. Although translating test items may be a well-meant approach to assessing LEP-NEP children, it certainly creates as many problems as it solves.

Decision 6. What are the respective roles of bilingual versus mono-lingual speech-language pathologists in the evaluation of LEP-NEP children?

It is obvious that a bilingual bicultural professional trained in communication disorders with language minority children and knowledgeable about the specific dialect of the child is the most appropriate professional to provide services for this population. Competencies for these professionals have been suggested by the Committee on Status of Racial Minorities (American Speech and Hearing Association, 1985). However, just as the definition of bilingualism varies, so do characteristics of bilingual professionals. First, not all bilingual professionals are bicultural. Second, bilingual professionals differ in language proficiency (i.e., literacy, dialect usage, and fluency) as well as when (childhood or postadolescence) and how (environmental or academic learning) they acquired the non-English language.

Although the bilingual bicultural trained professional may be the most appropriate choice for assessing a language minority child, this may not be a realistic option. Therefore, until there is a significant increase in the number of bilingual bicultural professionals in the field of communication disorders, alternative approaches must be considered. There is a danger, however, in even suggesting alternative approaches because some agencies and educational units at the local, state, and federal levels may view the temporary alternatives as permanent solutions to a problem. Indeed, when alternatives are offered, pursuit of excellence in service provision may be ignored or at least impeded. Rationalizations such as "we don't have the funds, the personnel, or the time" may become easy excuses for failure to provide appropriate educational programs. Within this framework, which warns against complacency and a lack of activism toward developing maximum services, we offer the following options and guidelines for monolingual communication specialists who are responsible for the assessment of language minority children.

The primary responsibility of the monolingual English speaking communication specialist is to be a *child advocate* who facilitates appropriate services through referrals, monitoring, cooperation, and coordination of activities. Rather than passively presenting discrete-point test results at an IEP conference on a language minority child, the monolingual communication specialist should present contemporary theory, communication data based on an ethnographic perspective, results of testing in the child's first and second languages, and information on nondiscriminatory test results. The assertive professional will question the validity of discrete-point tests, will ask whether or not the parent conference was conducted in the language in which the parent is most comfortable, will insist that testing be done in both languages in various environments and with various interactors, and will identify linguistic and cultural differences in interpreting results.

The monolingual professional can also provide testing in English, oral peripheral and hearing evaluations, nonverbal assessments, and — with guidance — basic speech and language screening procedures. Furthermore, monolingual professionals should strive to increase their own linguistic and cultural consciousness (see Appendix 2). A monolingual professional may not speak the language *of* the child but can certainly speak *for* the child.

Just as government and social policies regarding bilingualism have been characterized by differing (sometimes polar) opinions, goals, and methods, so has the development of the 1985 ASHA position paper on "clinical management of communicatively handicapped minority language populations." Beginning with the Bilingual Language Learning System (BLLS) ASHA project (1982), followed by several reviewed and revised drafts, and ending with the ASHA position paper, guidelines for bilingual and monolingual professionals have been proposed. Following are suggestions for monolingual professionals based on the position paper, BLLS Manual, and the experiences of the authors of this chapter. These suggestions fall into two categories: (1) specific options and cautions and (2) alternative strategies that can be developed. Also presented are guidelines in the use of interpreters and translators during the assessment and remediation processes.

There are several options for bilingual assistance from which child advocate monolingual professionals may choose as they coordinate efforts to assess the language(s) of an NEP child. Bilingual assistance is a positive step in providing an adequate assessment approach. Mattes and Omark (1984) suggest developing a networking system for bilingual service delivery. However, monolingual professionals must also recognize their limitations and not be lulled into believing that all evaluation results, just because they are conducted by a speaker of the first language (L1) of the child, can be considered reliable and valid. Consider the following strengths and weaknesses in the use of various bilingual assistance resources.

Assistance from a Bilingual Aide, Allied Professional, or Student in Training

This option assumes that in addition to having bilingual skills, the individual has been trained in disorders of communication, knows the relevance of information to be obtained during a parent interview, can administer tests appropriately, and can provide accurate and unbiased information. Aides trained in speech-language pathology may be very helpful so long as guidelines are established and continuing education is provided (Toliver-Weddington and Meyerson, 1983). Although professionals from other fields may have a sensitivity to clinical methodology, they may be limited in information on communication disorders and have a different perspective as to the significance of the disorder. It is always curious to observe that a monolingual speech-language pathologist may question the perspective and recommendations that another professional has on communication disorders of a monolingual English speaking child yet yield to information on an NEP child when it is provided by a bilingual professional from another field. In some geographical areas, it is possible to enlist the assistance of bilingual students in speech-language pathology and audiology. Their levels of training must be considered in addition to their degrees of bilingualism and biculturalism.

Assistance from a Family Member or Friend of the Client

Although this approach appears to be a viable alternative, and sometimes the only obvious alternative, using a bilingual individual from the familial or social environment of the parent or child as an interpreter introduces possible problems. In addition to their lack of training in the field, the personal nature of the questions in a case history may violate cultural values. In addition, the interviewer will be unaware of when to probe for further information or the helpers may insert their own personal interpretations of information, particularly if they are family members. The desire to help the child perform well or to modify or accommodate the evaluation procedures and test items may occur as a result of "being helpful."

Assistance from a Member of the Community

A bilingual community member would appear to be a viable choice to assist in a parent interview or child evaluation. However, the evaluator must be aware of the issues of confidentiality, status of the individual in the community, dialect variations, and language ability, as well as the limited knowledge of speech, language, and hearing disorders on the part of these individuals. In addition, they are often asked, as are interpreters for the deaf, to assist without financial reimbursement for transportation and time, let alone their services.

In sum, the use of translators or interpreters may appear, on the surface, to solve the problem of assessing children in their native language or determining language dominance, but it cannot be used as a panacea or without caution. Further concerns arise when translators or interpreters speak a different dialect than the client. For example, speakers of Spanish may be from Spain, Mexico, South America, Cuba, Puerto Rico, or various areas of the United States and thus have variant phonological rules and vocabulary. Also, social class distinctions affect language use (Saville-Troike, 1984) and may interfere with an evaluation of a child's language ability. For example, an interpreter from an upper or middle class background may evaluate the utterances of a child from a low income group as disordered in L1 when indeed the child may only be using a dialect that is unfamiliar to the interpreter. A similar situation occurs when speakers of a nonstandard dialect of English are evaluated as disordered rather than different by uninformed mainstream professionals (Adler, 1979). At the other extreme, the interpreter may be from a lower socioeconomic status (SES) background and thus unfamiliar with vocabulary and speech patterns of a client from a higher SES group.

Furthermore, a rather simplistic yet obvious problem inherent in a monolingual professional's selection and use of a bilingual interpreter to assist in assessment is that the professional is in no position to evaluate the communicative skills of the interpreter in L1. As indicated earlier with regard to obtaining prevalence data on bilingualism, self-reporting often is not an adequate measure.

Alternative strategies for use of professional personnel have been proposed when communication specialists do not meet the recommended competencies of professionals serving LEP-NEP children. The 1985 ASHA position paper on clinical management of communicatively handicapped minority language populations suggests that if the use of interpreters or translators is the only alternative, the speech-language pathologist or audiologist should take the following steps:

1. Provide extensive training to the assistant on the purposes, procedures, and goals of the tests and therapy methods. The assistant also should be taught to avoid the use of gestures, vocal intonation, and other cues that could inadvertently alert the individual to the correct response during test administration.
2. Preplan for an individual's services to ensure the assistant's understanding of specific clinical procedures to be used.
3. Use the same assistant(s) with a given minority language client rather than using assistants on a random basis.
4. Use patient observation or other nonlinguistic measures as supplements to the translated measures, such as (a) the child's interaction with parents, (b) the child's interaction with peers, (c) pragmatic analysis. (p. 31)

Because bilingual education has been supported legally and implemented subsequently in various forms at the state and local levels, competencies of bilingual education teachers have been delineated both officially (e.g., California) and unofficially. Guidelines rather than requirements for bilingual special education professionals have been suggested (Bergin, 1980). Similarly, the 1985 ASHA position paper only suggests the following general competency guidelines for professionals who treat language minority clients: (1) language proficiency, (2) knowledge of normative processes, assessment, and intervention, and (3) cultural sensitivity.

Until more definitive requirements regarding training and competencies are proposed and implemented, professionals must evaluate their own competencies in this area. Appendix 3 provides a form for evaluation of professional effectiveness of those involved in communication assessment of LEP-NEP children. It should be apparent after assessing oneself (or others) with this form that all monolingual (or bilingual) professionals have skills that can contribute to the assessment of the language minority child. In some areas, however, they may lack skills and thus need to recruit alternative resources.

CONCLUSIONS

Communication assessment of all individuals should (1) be based on contemporary psycholinguistic and sociolinguistic theory, (2) reflect the nature of the communication process in the natural environment, (3) consider linguistic and cultural variations, and (4) be an ongoing process that reflects changing communicative needs (Erickson, 1981). Furthermore, assessment approaches should stress what children *can* do rather than what they *cannot* do, how they *succeed* rather than how they *fail,* and why they should be *appreciated* rather than *penalized* for their cultural and linguistic versatility. And if individuals are indeed diagnosed as communicatively handicapped within their linguistic or cultural milieu, they should receive appropriate therapeutic services. Current issues in assessment procedures for identifying and providing remediation for communication disorders in LEP-NEP children can best be described as Hunt (1966) did two decades ago in reference to early childhood programs for poverty children:

> What perturbs me about our present state of affairs is that our failure to investigate these matters during those decades before they acquired social and political urgency . . . leaves us puny now when we need to be strong in terms of theory and scientific evidence. (p. 140)

The United States appears to have a schizophrenic attitude toward bilingualism, as demonstrated through its reluctance to support bilingual education while paradoxically spending millions of dollars on foreign language instruction in high schools and colleges. The first approach, bilingual education could develop a literate population in numerous languages in addition to English; the second approach attempts to develop bilingual skills at an age when it is less effective. In other words, monolingualism is promoted during the years when bilingualism can be best developed and bilingualism is touted for monolinguals at the age when it is more difficult to acquire. The report of the 1979 President's Commission on Foreign Language and International Studies, according to Grosjean (1982), warns that "the incompetence of Americans in foreign languages is nothing short of scandalous and becoming worse" (p. 66).

As communication specialists, we are challenged by the task to alleviate communication disorders and not confuse them with communication differences. With the language minority child, we must question our own beliefs and biases, strengths and weaknesses, policies and decision making processes. Countries cannot speak to each other, trade with each other, or negotiate peace if there is not a respect for cultural and linguistic differences. We are indeed a part of a bigger picture.

APPENDIX 1

Technical Test Evaluation Checklist*

1. Are all purposes of the test clearly defined and stated?
2. Does the manual outline possible limitations or misuses of the test?
3. What is the most recent revision of the test?
4. Are the standardization populations adequately defined or delineated, including the following?
   a. Number of subjects
   b. Sex of subjects
   c. Ethnicity of subjects
   d. Age or grade of subjects
   e. Region of the country in which the subjects reside
   f. Socioeconomic status of subjects
   g. Specification of special conditions, such as handicaps
5. Are standardization groups for test development, reliability, and validity clearly differentiated from each other and adequately described as in No. 4?
6. Is the child being tested represented by the standardization groups in terms of background, culture, and so forth?
7. Are the theoretical constructs and their relevance to behaviors measured by the test clearly explained?
8. Are the time of administration and method of administration appropriate to the following?
   a. Child's development level
   b. Child's cultural background
   c. Child's dominant language
   d. Child's special limitations (i.e., handicaps)
9. Is there reliability data reflecting the following?
   a. Test-retest reliability
   b. Alternate form reliability
   c. Split-half or internal consistency
10. Is the reliability correlation coefficient of sufficient strength to establish consistency (i.e., .80 or higher)?
11. Does the manual provide standard errors of measurement for the following?
   a. Each subtest and total score
   b. Each age or grade level
   c. Both sexes
   d. Each ethnic group
   e. Any other subpopulation
12. Does the test manual provide validity data for the following?
   a. Each intended use of the test
   b. Each subpopulation in the standardization group
   c. Face validity

---

*From Watson, D. L., Omark, D. R., Grouell, S. L., and Heller, B. (1980). Nondiscriminatory assessment practitioner's handbook (pp. 66–67). San Diego: California State Department of Education. Reprinted with permission.

    d. Criterion validity, including predictive and concurrent
    e. Construct validity
13. Are test contents appropriate for the following?
    a. All subpopulations
    b. Developmental levels of children on whom test will be used
    c. Language skills of children on whom test will be used
    d. Cultural values of children on whom test will be used

APPENDIX 2

Consciousness Raising Activities for Professionals who do not Speak the Language of their Client

1. Evaluate your own cultural and linguistic heritage (e.g., holidays, foods, family endearments) because the process may help you appreciate your uniqueness as well as the heritage of others.
2. Recognize and deal with your ethnocentrism, xenophobia, biases, prejudices, and fears of minorities that have developed because you have not shared their experiences just as they may not have shared yours.
3. Seek experiences that facilitate your understanding of other languages and develop your cultural sensitivity.
4. Remember that with few exceptions, parents from all cultures and socioeconomic groups love their children and want the best for them, although family structures, values, and attitudes toward handicaps may vary from yours.
5. Avoid becoming complacent with the notion that you are "doing the best you can, considering the circumstances"; instead, work for excellence in providing services that are linguistically and culturally appropriate.
6. Consider how your attitudes toward bilingualism as well as other languages, cultures, and SES groups affect your personal and thus professional behavior.

APPENDIX 3

Evaluation of Professional Effectiveness
in Communication Assessment of NEP Children

	Little or No Ability		Very Knowledgeable and Capable		
Trained in second language acquisition and ESL	1	2	3	4	5
Trained in bilingualism and bilingual education	1	2	3	4	5
Trained in disorders of speech and language	1	2	3	4	5
Trained in associated factors (hearing, oral, motor, etc.)	1	2	3	4	5
Competent speaker of L1 of child and family	1	2	3	4	5
Competent speaker of L1 dialect of child	1	2	3	4	5
Competent speaker of L2 of child and family	1	2	3	4	5
Competent speaker of L2 dialect of child	1	2	3	4	5
Skilled in parent interviewing in L1 and knowledgeable about significance of information obtained	1	2	3	4	5
Aware of cultural and linguistic differences in testing procedures and processes	1	2	3	4	5
Aware of cultural and linguistic differences in testing items	1	2	3	4	5
Sensitive to nonverbal communication patterns of the culture	1	2	3	4	5
Trained in assessing form and function of L1	1	2	3	4	5
Trained in assessing form and function of L2	1	2	3	4	5
Aware of family attitudes toward handicapping conditions	1	2	3	4	5
Capable of providing therapeutic services in L1	1	2	3	4	5
Capable of providing therapeutic services in L2	1	2	3	4	5

REFERENCES

Adler, S. (1979). *Poverty children and their language: Implications for teaching and treating.* New York: Grune and Stratton.

American Speech and Hearing Association (1961). Public school and hearing services. *Journal of Speech and Hearing Disorders,* Monograph Supplement 8.

American Speech and Hearing Association (1982). *Bilingual language learning system manual.* Rockville, MD: Author.

American Speech and Hearing Association (1985). Clinical management of communicatively handicapped minority language populations. *ASHA, 27*(6), 29–32.

Baca, L.M., and Cervantes, H.T. (1984). *The bilingual special education interface.* St. Louis: Times Mirror/Mosby.

Bates, E. (1976). *Language and context: The acquisition of pragmatics.* New York: Academic Press.

Bergin, V. (1980). *Special education needs in bilingual education.* Washington, DC: National Clearinghouse for Bilingual Education.

Birdwhistell, R.L. (1970). *Kinesics and context: Essays on body motion communication.* New York: Ballantine.

Bloom, L. (1970). *Language development: Form and function in emerging grammars.* Cambridge, MA: MIT Press.

Boehm, A. (1970). *Boehm test of basic concepts.* New York: The Psychological Corporation.

Bond, J.T., Epstein, A.S., and Matz, R.D. (1977). Methods for assessing the language production of the young child. *Anthropology and Education Quarterly, 8,* 84–86.

California State Department of Education (1981). *Student oral language observation matrix.* Sacramento, CA: Office of Bilingual Bicultural Education, California State Department of Education.

Carrow, E. (1973). *Test for auditory comprehension of language.* Austin, TX: Learning Concepts.

Castellanos, D. (1984). *The best of two worlds: Bilingual-bicultural education in the U.S.* Trenton: New Jersey Department of Education.

Chomsky, N. (1957). *Syntactic structures.* The Hague, Netherlands: Mouton.

Compton, A.J. (1983). *Compton speech and language screening evaluation.* San Francisco: Carousel House.

Dianna v. State Board of Education, Civil Action No. C–70 37 RFP (N.D. Cal Jan 7, 1970 and June 18, 1973).

Erickson, J.G. (1981). Communication assessment of the bilingual bicultural child: An overview. In J.G. Erickson and D.R. Omark (Eds.), *Communication assessment of the bilingual bicultural child: Issues and guidelines* (pp. 1–26). Baltimore: University Park Press.

Erickson, J.G., and Omark, D.R. (1981). *Communication assessment of the bilingual bicultural child: Issues and guidelines.* Baltimore: University Park Press.

Feuerstein, R., Rand, Y., and Hoffman, M.B. (1979). *The dynamic assessment of retarded performances: The learning potential assessment device: Theory, instruments and techniques.* Baltimore: University Park Press.

Gardner, M.F. (1979). *Expressive one word picture vocabulary test.* Novato, CA: Academic Therapy Publications.

Grosjean, F. (1982). *Life with two languages: An introduction to bilingualism.* Cambridge, MA: Harvard University Press.

Healey, W.C., Ackerman, B.L., Chappell, C.R., Perrin, K.L., and Stormer, J. (1981). *The prevalence of communication disorders: A review of the literature.* Rockville, MD: American Speech, Language, and Hearing Association.

Hunt, J. (1966). *The challenge of incompetence and poverty.* Urbana: University of Illinois Press.

Hymes, D. (1971). *On communicative competence.* Philadelphia: University of Pennsylvania Press.

Iglesias, A. (1984). Assessing communicative performances of LEP children in the classroom. *Workshop on communicative disorders and language proficiency: Assessment, intervention, and curriculum implementation.* Los Alamitos, CA: National Center for Bilingual Research.

Lau v. Nichols, 414   U.S.   563; 39L. ED IId 1, 945. Ct. 786 (1974).

Leibowitz, A.H. (1982). *Federal recognition of the rights of minority language groups.* Rosslyn, VA: National Clearinghouse for Bilingual Education.

Mattes, L.J., and Omark, D.R. (1984). *Speech and language assessment for the bilingual handicapped.* San Diego: College-Hill Press.

McLaughlin, B. (1977). Second-language learning in children. *Psychological Bulletin, 84*(3), 438–459.

Mercer, J.R. (1973). *Labeling the mentally retarded.* Berkeley: University of California Press.

Michaels, S., and Cook-Gumperz, J. (1979). A study of sharing time with first grade students: Discourse narratives in the classroom. *Proceedings of the Fifth Annual Meeting of the Berkeley Linguistic Society,* pp. 647–659.

Oakland, T. (1977). *Psychological and educational assessment of minority children.* New York: Brunner/Mazel.

Oller, J.W. (1979). *Language tests at school.* London: Longman.

O'Malley, J.M. (1976). *Language minority students with limited English proficiency.* Rosslyn, VA: National Clearinghouse for Bilingual Education.

Omark, D.R. (1981a). Conceptualizations of bilingual children: Testing the norm. In J.G. Erickson and D.R. Omark (Eds.), *Communication assessment of the bilingual bicultural child: Issues and guidelines* (pp. 99–113). Baltimore: University Park Press.

Omark, D.R. (1981b). Pragmatics and ethological techniques for the observational assessment of children's communicative abilities. In J.G. Erickson and D.R. Omark (Eds.), *Communication assessment of the bilingual bicultural child: Issues and guidelines* (pp. 249–284). Baltimore: University Park Press.

Samuda, R.J. (1975). *Psychological testing of American minorities: Issues and consequences.* New York: Harper and Row.

Savignon, S. (1972). *Communicative competence: An experiment in foreign language testing.* Philadelphia: University of Pennsylvania Center for Curriculum Development.

Saville-Troike, M. (1978). *A guide to culture in the classroom.* Rosslyn, VA: National Clearinghouse for Bilingual Education.

Saville-Troike, M. (1984). *The ethnography of communication: An introduction.* Baltimore: University Park Press.

Schieffelin, B., and Eisenberg, A. (1984). Cultural variations in children's conversations. In R. Schiefelbusch and J. Pickar (Eds.), *The acquisition of communicative competence* (pp. 377–420). Baltimore: University Park Press.

Taylor, O.L., and Payne, K.T. (1983). Culturally valid testing: A proactive approach. *Topics in Language Disorders, 3*(3), 8–20.

Terrell, S.L. (Ed.) (1983). Nonbiased assessment of language differences. *Topics in Language Disorders, 3*(3).

Thorndike, E.L. (1918). The nature, purpose and general methods of measurements of educational products. *Measurement of educational products, seventeenth yearbook of the National Society for the Study of Education,* Part II. Bloomington, IL: Public School Publishing Company, pp. 16–24.

Toliver-Weddington, G. (1981). *Valid assessment of children.* San Jose, CA: San Jose State University.

Toliver-Weddington, G., and Meyerson, M.D. (1983). Training professionals for identification and intervention with communicatively disordered bilinguals. In D.R. Omark and J.G. Erickson (Eds.), *The bilingual exceptional child.* (pp. 379–395). San Diego: College-Hill Press.

Tomblin, J.B., and Liljegreen, S.J. (1985). The identification of socially significant communication needs in older language-impaired children: A case example. In D.N. Ripich and F.M. Spinelli (Eds.), *School discourse problems* (pp. 219–230). San Diego: College-Hill Press.

Toronto, A., and Merrill, S. (1983). Developing local normed assessment instruments. In D.R. Omark and J.G. Erickson (Eds.), *The bilingual exceptional child* (pp. 105–121). San Diego: College-Hill Press.

Travis, L., Johnson, W., and Shover, J. (1937). The relation of bilingualism to stuttering. *Journal of Speech Disabilities, 2,* 185–189.

Troike, R.C. (1983). Can language be tested? *Journal of Education, 165*(2), 209–216.

Tucker, J.A. (1980). Ethnic proportions in classes for the learning disabled: Issues in nonbiased assessment. *Journal of Special Education, 14,* 93–105.

U.S. Commission on Civil Rights (1975). *A better chance to learn: Bilingual bicultural education.* (Publication No. 51.) Washington, DC: National Clearinghouse for Bilingual Education.

U.S. Department of Commerce, Bureau of the Census (1983). *National data books and guide to resources: Statistical abstracts of the U.S., 104th edition.* Washington, DC: U.S. Government Printing Office.

Van Riper, C. (1947). *Speech correction: Principles and methods.* New York: Prentice-Hall.

Watson, D.L., Omark, D.R., Grouell, S.L., and Heller, B. (1980). *Nondiscriminatory assessment practitioner's handbook.* San Diego: California State Department of Education.

Watzlawick, P., Beavin, J.H., and Jackson, D.R. (1967). *Pragmatics of human communication: Study of interactional patterns, pathologies and paradoxes.* New York: Norton.

Wiener, F.D., Simon, A.J., and Weiss, F.L. (1978). *Spanish picture vocabulary test* (unpublished manuscript).

Zangwill, I. (1909). *The melting pot.* New York: Macmillan.

Zimmerman, I.L., Steiner, V.G., and Pond, R.E. (1979). *Preschool language scale, Spanish Version.* Columbus, OH: Charles E. Merrill.

Chapter 8

Barriers to the Delivery of Speech, Language, and Hearing Services to Native Americans*

Gail A. Harris

Many problems confronting American Indians today parallel those faced by the non-Indians who began organizing for the rights and services for the handicapped 20 years ago. The primary goal — equal access to services for all handicapped — is identical. Because of a number of barriers, however, equal access to services is not a reality for the American Indian in the 1980s.

Indian populations employ different cultural, linguistic, and belief systems. Many Native Americans live in reservation communities isolated from major urban centers, which poses unique challenges to rehabilitation professionals and systems that attempt to address their needs. Major obstacles to service delivery include poverty, high unemployment (40 to 80 percent), substandard housing, lack of education, and exclusion from mainstream American life — geographically, politically, economically, and educationally.

Within this chapter, the following barriers to the delivery of speech, language, and hearing services to American Indians are addressed within the context of the needs of the communicatively impaired: the service delivery systems and personnel; and barriers as-

---

*The terms American Indian and Native American are used interchangeably throughout this chapter. "Tribe" refers to the federally recognized groups of American Indians within the United States.

This chapter is adapted from a paper presented at the 1985 National Colloquium on Underserved Populations, American Speech-Language-Hearing Association.

sociated with geographical, jurisdictional, cultural, and linguistic factors. Through an elucidation of the barriers and a discussion of the solutions we gain a better appreciation of the needs of this population and the creative multiagency approaches necessary to arrive at solutions to long-term and complex problems.

SERVICE DELIVERY: SYSTEMS AND PERSONNEL

Educational and medical services to American Indians are provided primarily by two Federal agencies, the Bureau of Indian Affairs (BIA), an agency of the Department of the Interior, and the Indian Health Service (IHS), a division of the U.S. Public Health Service.

The Bureau of Indian Affairs

The Bureau of Indian Affairs provides services to approximately 25 percent of the Indian school-aged children throughout the United States, and is considered a "state" by definition under PL 94–142 (The Education of all Handicapped Children Act of 1975, as amended). The remaining Indian children are enrolled in public, cooperative, tribal, parochial, and private schools.

A 1972 survey by the BIA Office of Indian Education programs estimated that 38 percent of children in BIA schools were classified as handicapped. The most prevalent disabilities among Indian children are communication disorders, learning disabilities, mental retardation, and emotional problems (Rameriz, 1976). The BIA employs 27 speech-language pathologists but no audiologists to serve children in approximately 200 schools, a situation that raises serious concerns regarding the adequacy of services for these children.

The BIA elucidated in its state plan for the fiscal year 1981–83 numerous barriers impeding its progress in providing special education or rehabilitative services. These included the following:

1. Lack of adequately certified, qualified personnel to teach and supervise special education programs;
2. Difficulty in obtaining parental involvement due to language problems in communicating with parents and inaccessibility of the parent because of great distances between the parent's home and the school the child attends; and
3. Difficulty in accurately evaluating children who are linguistically and culturally different. (Bureau of Indian Affairs, 1981, p. 3–1)

These personnel, geographical, and cultural or linguistic barriers stated by the BIA are common to all programs that serve or attempt to serve handicapped American Indians of all ages.

The Indian Health Service

Although the IHS has significantly reduced Indian mortality, morbidity rates, and the prevalence of infectious diseases, attention to rehabilitation has been limited to medical rehabilitation and the establishment of alcoholism treatment and prevention programs. Evidence of comprehensive rehabilitation programs within this agency is lacking. The IHS has no established national guidelines for services to the handicapped and disabled Indian populations. The IHS service units (clinics and hospitals) do not typically maintain a registry of handicapped children, nor do their inpatient-outpatient recording systems provide documentation of disabilities and handicapping conditions. When handicapped individuals do receive services, it is on an *ad hoc* basis. This situation may be a direct result of a lack of policy regarding the handicapped, coupled with limited fiscal resources resulting in a scarcity of rehabilitation professionals within the IHS system.

In a report from the Neurosensory Disabilities Program of the IHS, Stewart (1985) indicated that no IHS area within the nation had comprehensive speech pathology–audiology services available, even on an itinerant basis. Staff composition of speech-language-hearing professionals within the IHS nationwide is limited to 17 audiologists, 2 speech-language pathologists, and 6 audiology technicians. The number of audiologists employed compared to speech-language pathologists may reflect the attention to the surveillance of otitis media, the leading disease of Indian populations.

The IHS Indian Children's Program based in Albuquerque, New Mexico, offers diagnostic and in-service training in speech-language pathology but has only two speech-language pathologists to serve a population of over 200,000 Indians in New Mexico and Arizona. Owing to the lack of communication disorder professionals within the IHS system, it is reported that as many as 74 percent of the communicatively disabled Indians are not receiving services (Toubbeh, 1985).

Indian Headstart

Over 100 Headstart programs currently operate on tribal lands. Of the 1,500 handicapped children enrolled, *speech impaired* is the leading category of disability. Speech-language services for these children, when they are provided, are generally diagnostic in nature and limited further by fiscal and personnel inadequacies of the Indian Headstart programs. Poor roads, absence of public and private transportation, and limited funds further isolate the handicapped Indian preschool child from services when they are available in neighboring communities.

Other Service Providers

Other federal agencies such as the Rehabilitation Services Administration, Office of Special Education and Rehabilitative Services, and the Administration on Aging have not served handicapped and disabled members of Indian populations either in a manner commensurate with their needs or in parity with other citizens of the United States. Lack of appropriate services to American Indians is a result, in part, of unique barriers created by the insularity of these delivery systems, geographical isolation, jurisdictional ambiguities, and cultural and linguistic differences, coupled with a high incidence of communicative disorders among these diverse populations.

The Consortium for Handicapped Indian Children: A Report (1980), states that "the main problem encountered in the present day system of Indian education is the lack of any clear distinction between the responsibilities of the federal government and those of the states" (p. 6), which results in an educational system that frequently falls short of providing even the nonhandicapped children with an appropriate education.

Jurisdictional Barriers

Unlike other minority groups, American Indians have a legal trust relationship with the Federal government and are eligible, therefore, to receive services directly from the federal government as well as from the states. A result of this jurisdictional overlap and ambiguity regarding loci of responsibility has been gaps in services and frequent duplications, specifically with regard to identification of programs and evaluation procedures for the disabled (*Consortium for Handicapped Indian Children, 1980*).

Some states do not provide services to Indian children in the public schools, assuming it is a federal responsibility. Disabled urban Indians are often denied state services (Medicaid and other indigent health care programs and services), including transportation, wheelchairs, orthotics, and prostheses because the states believe that the IHS has this responsibility. The frustration to Indian clients, families, and professionals by jurisdictional confusion has created an attitude of skepticism and mistrust on the part of the Indian people and has contributed to high levels of frustration and perceived ineffectiveness on the part of professional personnel.

Gelfand (1982) reported a reluctance on the part of all minority individuals to utilize services, despite need and impairment, citing cultural attitudes toward institutions. These attitudes are probably the result of historic and continuing negative interactions and experiences between the minority individual and the institution. The perpetuation of jurisdictional ambiguities regarding services to the handicapped has done little to effect a positive change in these attitudes among American Indians.

Geographic Barriers

Remoteness and Isolation. Approximately 50 percent of the Indian population of the United States reside on reservations. These persons have limited access to comprehensive rehabilitation services. Indian reservations comprise 81,000 square miles of land in the United States; 35 percent of this land is located in Arizona, encompassing 22 different reservations.

To gain a perspective of the geographical barriers to service, it helps to conceptualize some reservations in terms of their actual size. The Navajo Nation, equivalent in size to the state of West Virginia, consists of 25,000 square miles spanning the states of Arizona, New Mexico, and Utah; the Papago Reservation, equivalent to the size of the state of Connecticut, comprises 14 separate districts; and the Hopi Reservation is larger than the states of Rhode Island and Delaware combined.

The sizes of these reservations present a unique challenge to health and rehabilitation professionals and to the tribes in the delivery of services to a population that is both remote and generally isolated from major medical and rehabilitation centers. The Rehabilitation Services Administration (RSA) (1982) indicated that Indians are not conveniently located for easy participation in federal and state vocational rehabilitation programs because of their isolation and dispersion in rural areas. The RSA states that "given the cultural and geographic obstacles that confront reservation Indians plus the lack of mobility that characterizes severely disabled persons in general, the extent to which severely disabled Indians avail themselves to services is seriously questioned" (p. 6).

Elderly Indians do not receive services they would otherwise be entitled to receive under the Older Americans Act because of physical, psychological, and logistic barriers. Einisman (1981) high-lighted program inaccessibility for minority elderly persons result-ing from lack of transportation and compounded by deficiencies in outreach, information, and referral programs.

Long-Term Care Facilities. There are nine Indian nursing homes on tribal lands in the United States. The three most common diagno-ses of patients in these nursing homes are diabetes mellitus, alcohol abuse, and stroke. The incidence of institutionization after stroke highlights the need for rehabilitation services, especially in speech-language pathology.

Owing to their geographical locations, none of these facilities has convenient access to speech-language services. Nursing home administrators cite scarcity of qualified personnel and high attrition rates of staff as leading problems in service delivery (Mick, 1983).

Attrition of Professionals. The remoteness of Indian reserva-tions poses an additional barrier to the provision of comprehensive services to the handicapped — namely, recruitment and long-term retention of professionals to provide services on reservations. In some instances, reservation-based housing is unavailable, requiring lengthy commuting to work. For many nonindigenous professionals, the isolation from families, friends, and urban areas with familiar recreational and cultural facilities creates a sense of isolation and loneliness. The high attrition rate of personnel was cited by the BIA as a major problem in establishing special education programs in compliance with PL 94–142. A nationwide recent survey of speech-language pathologists working with Indian populations indicated that 75 percent were in their current positions for 2 years or less (Harris, 1985).

INCIDENCE AND PREVALENCE DATA: COMMUNICATIVE DISORDERS

Delivery of services to Indians is clouded and complicated by a lack of epidemiological data. No previous studies or surveys have an-swered the critical questions of numbers of speech-language im-paired or hearing impaired Indians.

Compilation of information regarding the number of communi-catively impaired Indians, the number receiving services, and the number in need of services is a difficult, if not impossible, task. This difficulty is traceable to (1) the variety of sites and number of agen-cies that provide service, (2) the lack of documentation of disabilities by a major service provider (IHS), and (3) the fact that many states or agencies have not specified the ethnic background of the handicapped individuals they serve. Even taking into account the information on the number of handicapped persons served by the BIA and some states, data are not available on how many persons are in need of service.

Those reports that do exist estimate the prevalence of communicative disorders to be between 5 and 15 percent higher than in the general United States population. The BIA indicated that of the 5,225 children and adolescents aged 3 to 21 years who received special education services within BIA schools during the 1983–84 school year, 24 percent were classified as speech impaired and 53 percent as learning disabled. Certainly these percentages could be challenged due to the absence of culturally and linguistically valid instruments and assessment procedures to evaluate language and cognitive functions in American Indians. On the basis of available data, the leading communication disorder affecting American Indian children is conductive hearing loss (Stewart, 1983).

Much controversy exists in the literature regarding the effects of fluctuating hearing loss on language development and continued learning problems (Downs, 1981; Kaplan, Fleshman, Baum, and Clark, 1973). Given the prevalence of this disease among the American Indian population, it is a question of serious concern.

Several studies have documented that 30 percent or more of infants in American Indian and Alaskan Native communities are affected by otitis media during the first year of life (Brody, Overfield and McAlister, 1965; Goodwin, Shaw, and Feldman, 1980). Otitis media and ear disease were responsible for the highest number of total encounters (patient visits) within the IHS delivery system, and these infections continue to be the highest reportable diseases among this population (Toubbeh, 1985). Despite the high incidence of otitis media there has been a serious reduction in fiscal and personnel resources available for the otitis media programs (Stewart, 1985). (See Chapter 9 for a thorough discussion of otitis media and other ear diseases in American Indians.)

"Language insufficiency" and "inadequate mastery of English" have been repeatedly cited in the educational literature as the most serious educational problems of Indian children today (*Young Native American Children and Their Families: Educational Needs Assessment and Recommendations*, 1976). It is uncertain whether this "inadequate mastery of English" is a question of bilingualism, language learning and use differences, language disorders, or a combination of all three.

LANGUAGE DIFFERENCES

Language Diversity

The language diversity of the Indian population presents a complex barrier to identification, assessment, treatment, and family involvement with respect to communicative disorders. Over 200 different Indian languages are spoken in the United States, with dialectal variations within each. This diversification of languages dashes the hope that an "Indian assessment battery" could be developed that would somehow address the nonbiased assessment issues or the training of "Indians" who could serve the diverse linguistic composition of this ethnic minority group.

The absence of bilingual and bicultural professionals, lack of appropriate normative data regarding language and speech development within these populations (native and English languages) and lack of appropriate assessment tools and techniques to be used with this group create problems similar to those experienced by other ethnic minority groups. However, these barriers are further compounded by (1) the nature and diversity of Native American languages; (2) limited information and professional knowledge regarding characteristics of Indian English; (3) the phonology, semantics, and syntax of Indian languages; and (4) the culturally determined rules of language use, be it English or the native language (Bayles and Harris, 1982).

In addition, there is limited understanding among Indian populations regarding the fields of speech-language pathology and audiology. In a 1981 survey of American Indian awareness of speech-language pathology and audiology, 93 percent of the respondents were unaware of the services available from speech-language pathologists, and 65 percent were unaware of the services provided by audiologists (Harris and Bayles, 1981).

These language issues are complex and cannot be addressed adequately within this chapter. The lack of elaboration herein should not be interpreted, however, as a denigration of their importance. The work of Leap (1973, 1980, 1982), Wolfram, Christian, Leap, and Potter (1979), and others provide professionals with a description of Indian English patterns for certain tribal groups.

Problems presented with translation of English tests into Indian languages are described by DeAvila and Havassy (1974) and Rosenbluth (1976). In addition, discussions of the phonology, semantics, syntax, and pragmatics of certain Indian languages are available in the literature on cultural anthropology and linguistics.

Child-rearing Practices and Language Use

A discussion of the effects of child-rearing practices and cultural determinants of language use is given here. These factors are highlighted for they may affect the majority of Indian individuals regardless of whether they are monolingual English speakers or bilingual in English and the native language, and whether they are reservation residents or urban dwellers. These factors may also determine performance of Indians in an evaluation or observation context.

Culturally determined child-rearing practices will influence an individual's language learning and language use and may persist for members of that group even when the external indices (e.g., dress, location, language spoken) of culture are absent. Miller (1975) reported that the majority of Indian families, regardless of their traditional or urban identity status, fail to use the high degree of child-rearing language practices characteristic of the dominant culture. Familial practices and attitudes regarding language use may affect the child's willingness or unwillingness to speak, average length of utterance, response time, initiation of conversation, and turn-taking behaviors. These differences may result in performance differences on instruments that measure intelligence and language skills. (See Chapter 3 for a discussion of anthropological considerations in communication assessments.

Superior scores on visual-motor tasks and reduced performance on verbal tasks of intelligence and psycholinguistic measures have been attributed to a cultural emphasis on performance rather than on verbal or abstract skills (Browne, 1984; Garber, 1968; Kirk, 1972; Kunske, 1969; Lombardi, 1970).

For example, Indian children are typically present as observers at all tribal events and are expected to assume a quiet, passive role. Their presence is dictated by the culture for it is through these observations that the customs and rituals of the tribe are learned. Silent watching and listening appear to be the manner in which Indian children acquire traditional skills (beadwork, basketmaking, and weaving) within their culture. Use of speech is minimal in both the instructional phase (adult to child) and performance outcome (child to adult).

Maternal expectations regarding language behavior of Navajo and Anglo-American preschool children differ significantly. Although Anglo-American mothers perceived active speech and physical behavior as self-disciplined, exciting to observe, evidence of active learning, and advantageous for the child's development, Navajo mothers interpreted the same behaviors as discourteous, restless, self-centered, and undisciplined (Guilmet, 1979).

Indeed, for certain minority groups in the United States, silence is culturally appropriate and expected in situations that would evoke language in the dominant Anglo-American culture. Among the Western Apache, for example, children are chided for acting like a "white man" if they talk too much or speak English within the village. Within this community, situations that are ambiguous, unfamiliar, or new will call for silence on the part of traditional Apaches. These ambiguous situations may include a change in mood or status of the individual (after a death in the family) or return of an individual to the village after a long absence (such as a child returning from boarding school) (Basso, 1970).

Therefore, a child's reluctance to speak, use of truncated utterances, or refusal to engage in verbal communication with an examiner must not be interpreted immediately as an indication of a communicative or emotional disorder. In some instances, these behaviors are reflective of appropriate cultural patterns for interactions with strangers or adults and denote cultural integrity.

The relationship between speakers determines the grammatical structures used within some minority language groups. The social relationship and status of the individuals within the clan (a subgroup of membership within a tribe) or within the tribe may determine if there is verbal interaction and what form that interaction will take (Blanchard, 1983). Language diversity includes far more than differences in form.

To interface effectively with the American Indian population, clinicians and researchers must examine the early experiences, expectations, and rules that govern communication as a process within the cultural context of the linguistic community.

CULTURAL ATTITUDES TOWARD AND BELIEFS ABOUT HANDICAPS

Perhaps the most important aspect of transcultural interaction and the least attended to is that of attitudes or underlying belief systems of both the dominant and the Indian cultures. Attitudes evolve from an individual's value system and culture — and often a value system becomes so ingrained in a person's mind that his or her values become truth, usually not only for that particular person but also for all humans. Practitioners must acknowledge the potential for differences in perception of the causes and meaning of disabilities, the elements necessary for and differences in the value of rehabilitation, and the differences between their own belief systems and

those of their clients; consequently, they must devise culturally consonant methods of interacting in a transcultural situation.

The terms *disability, impairment, handicap,* and *rehabilitation*
are not easily translatable into Native American conceptual or linguistic terms. These terms are based on cultural perceptions of an
individual, and of his or her role in a society, and are directly related
to the definition of what is "normal" in performance, achievement,
and activity within a specific cultural context.

According to Kleinman, Eisenberg, and Good (1978), illness is
culturally shaped, in the sense that how people perceive, experience,
and cope with disease is based on their explanations, which are specific to the particular social position they occupy and systems of
meaning they employ. This appreciation of cultural attitudes regarding illness and disability is critical to the habilitation and rehabilitation of Indian individuals. Although there is great cultural diversity among the more than 511 American Indian tribes and
communities in the United States, each of which represents uniqueness in language, beliefs, and diagnostic and healing procedures,
there is, nevertheless, a universal thread connecting these tribal entities with one another, which separates them from the belief system
of the modern technological world. There is a shared belief that to be
healthy, humans must rest in delicate balance within themselves
(body, mind, spirit), with other people, and with Mother Earth.
When this delicate balance is disturbed for any number of reasons,
illness, accidents, and handicaps occur. These orientation systems
provide classification schemes separating health from pathology,
normalcy from deviancy, and well-being from disorder. These opposi-
tions are not cross-culturally constant, nor are interpretations of the
phenomena consistent (*Feasibility Study Report,* 1979). These differences must be recognized, accepted, and attended to by the professional if cooperation with and involvement in the rehabilitation
process is to transpire.

Dukepoo (1980) reported that a lack of awareness, respect, and
tolerance of culturally different practices and beliefs on the part of
many non-Indian staff members not only precludes the delivery of
quality care to the Indian patient, it also serves as primary deter-
rents to seeking necessary health care services by individual
Indians.

Some Indian people accept a handicapped child as a special gift
from the Great Spirit. Others believe that the handicapped individual had a choice in his or her state or that the handicap results from
a moral transgression or witchcraft. For rehabilitation personnel
this may necessitate alterations in the manner, method, and se-

quence of rehabilitation practices. For example, prior to a surgical procedure (e.g., repair of a cleft lip or palate) or the initiation of therapeutic intervention, it might be appropriate that a medicine person be consulted. This is the prerogative and responsibility of the family, but acknowledging that the surgical or rehabilitation process could be delayed pending the family's interaction with traditional medicine people indicates respect of these practices and a willingness to work within the cultural schema of the community.

Special attention must be given to the family's explanation of the cause of the handicap. For example, this author discussed her thoughts with an Indian medicine woman regarding a hypothetical situation of a child born with multiple disabilities as a result of rubella. The author's position was that by counseling the family that the child's condition was due to a disease and not "cosmic order," she could relieve a burden of guilt from the family, for they would then know there was no wrongdoing on their part and that other causal factors were not involved.

This medicine woman explained that within her tribe this child would be accepted as *special* and that the family was given a unique opportunity to learn to love and care for a special individual. To explain that this difference was caused by a germ, she said, would deny the family the traditional rationale for loving, accepting, and providing for the child.

In summary, attitudes toward handicapped individuals vary greatly among Indian people. In some Indian cultures, there is greater acceptance of the handicapped individual, acceptance based on the belief that each person, regardless of limitations imposed by his or her disability, has a viable role to play within the tribal community. As traditional tribal roles and community cohesiveness have eroded for some Indian tribes, so too has the acceptance of the disabled. These changes are not unlike the varying attitudes within other cultures. Some American Indian groups view the responsibility of caring for the disabled as a tribal one, others see it as an individual family responsibility, and still others look to state and federal systems for support.

It would be erroneous to believe that there are specific beliefs or attitudes that cut across tribal boundaries. Perceptions regarding handicaps vary greatly. What appears similar is that explanations that do exist may range from beliefs that the handicap is a punishment, a blessing, evidence of a transgression, a choice of the individual, due to witchcraft, or due to bad thoughts.

The critical point is that speech, language, and hearing professionals must become familiar with the attitudes and beliefs of the group they serve in order to guide their case history queries, understand the family's willingness or reluctance to provide care, and become personally involved in the rehabilitation process. Inquiries regarding traditional beliefs must be made in a careful and respectful way with the clear purpose of gaining understanding and securing and sharing information so that the best care possible can be provided for the individual.

Responses to requests for information will be carefully considered by the medicine person or informant, and the individual requesting the information may have to be very patient, for the response may be withheld until a level of trust is established.

SOLUTIONS

The barriers presented by the American Indian population to the delivery of appropriate speech-language-hearing services are many and not easily resolvable. The complexity and difficulty of these barriers, however, do not absolve agencies or associations from addressing them. In fact, owing to the lack of information and advocacy within Indian populations, it becomes their responsibility.

This section presents possible solutions that are a compilation of recommendations of various groups, from various sources, and which, sadly, have been suggested (but have not been well implemented) for many years.

Service Delivery: Systems and Personnel

1. A policy regarding the handicapped American Indian must be articulated by the Indian Health Service, and this policy should be communicated to Indian tribes and service providers.
2. The Indian Health Service should undertake a revamping of its encounter form and data tracking system to provide information on the incidence, prevalence, and extent of disabling conditions among Indians to determine the program and personnel needs.
3. The Indian Health Service should establish a national handicapped child registry to reduce the delay in identification and discontinuity of services, and to alert the Headstart and Indian educational systems of the need for special education services.
4. The Indian Health Service should establish an office of the handicapped (similar to the Office of Special Education of the BIA) to act as a coordinating agent for all actions relating to disabled Indians.

5. The lack of adequately trained personnel to serve within the BIA and IHS should be addressed in a number of different ways.

    a. University-based training programs should recruit and retain American Indian trainees within the fields of speech pathology and audiology to increase the cadre of professionally trained bilingual and bicultural Indian personnel, which will lead to a reduction in the attrition rate of professionals in reservation settings.

    b. Training programs should prepare individuals to provide services to culturally and linguistically different populations in a realistic manner. This training must include the discussion of culture, cultural differences, and "culture shock" and also elucidate the professional satisfaction of solving problems and working within a cultural environment in which, if the personnel are receptive, they can learn a great deal not only about the American Indian but also from them. This training should occur in degree-oriented programs for preprofessionals and through continuing education opportunities for practicing professionals.

    c. The realities of the inadequacies and inappropriateness of the current delivery system must be examined. New ways of providing services by using paraprofessionals and native speakers must be set into motion.

    d. Cultural orientation to tribal communities should be provided by the Indian associations and tribes for educational and medical personnel.

6. Information regarding the prevention and amelioration of handicapping conditions must be presented to Indian people in a manner that is respectful of their cultural perspective and appropriate for their living situations.

7. The Indian Headstart programs should be adequately funded to provide professional services to the handicapped preschool children enrolled.

8. Adequate funding should be reestablished for the IHS Otitis Media program.

9. A focus on the handicapped American Indian at agency levels and sensitization of service providers at local levels can generate needs related to manpower development (indigenous), research, and demonstration programs, as well as consideration by Federal and state agencies of reallocation of funds.

10. The IHS should increase its number and type of rehabilitation personnel.

Jurisdictional Barriers

1. The concept of comprehensive care for the handicapped and chronically disabled must incorporate both medical and habilitation or rehabilitation services. An understanding of the concept by first line providers of health care can ensure appropriate movement of patients or clients from one stage of care to another.
2. The legislative mandates of the Indian Health Service and the Bureau of Indian Affairs should be communicated to federal and state agencies with specific responsibilities toward handicapped Indians. Likewise, the federal and state agencies should make every effort to communicate their respective mandates to the IHS and BIA. Tribal involvement in this communication process is mandatory.
3. Clarification of agency responsibility for providing services to citizens who are members of American Indian tribes must be clearly articulated within the agencies, to field-based personnel and to the potential recipients of these services.

Geographic Barriers

1. The remoteness and isolation of Indian reservations must be accepted as a challenge to serving this population, not viewed as an excuse for ignoring it.
2. Realistic expectations regarding the cultural differences and cultural isolation an individual may experience in living and working on a reservation must be provided.
3. Realistic expectations on the part of the employing agency (federal, tribal, or state) regarding case-load size, territory to cover, and number of miles to drive must be established to prevent or delay professional burnout.

Incidence and Prevalence Data: Communicative Disorders

1. Prevention and adequate surveillance programs should be continued to address otitis media and fetal alcohol syndrome.
2. An appropriate data recording system must be developed to determine the actual incidence or prevailance for this population.
3. Information regarding language acquisition facilitation techniques should be communicated to Indian families.

Language Diversity

1. The extensive diversity of the linguistic composition of Indian communities must be realized and addressed by empowering native speakers to serve in professional and paraprofessional roles in the identification and treatment of communicative disorders.
2. An understanding of the cultural relevance of Indian languages and dialects must be shared with educators; in addition, the educational and economic benefits of knowing the standard English dialect should be elucidated.
3. Professionals must rely on their clinical skills as well as information about the typical language performance of the community in order to make clinical judgments regarding communication disorders in Indian individuals.
4. Clinicians must enlist the assistance of native speakers to act as interpreters and developers of assessment tools in the assessment procedures of bilingual Indian children.

Cultural Attitudes and Beliefs Toward Handicaps

1. Professionals must become aware of attitudes and belief systems of the population with whom they are working and attempt to incorporate these attitudes and beliefs into their case history and interviewing techniques, assessment procedures, and counseling techniques.
2. Professionals should seek out information regarding attitudes toward handicapping conditions from informants within the community in which they work.
3. Training programs should address the diversity of attitudes and beliefs regarding handicapping conditions as they prepare students to counsel families and provide therapeutic intervention.

ACKNOWLEDGMENTS

Preparation of this chapter was funded by the Native American Research and Training Center, University of Arizona, National Institute of Handicapped Research, Cooperative Agreement No. G0083C0094.

REFERENCES

Basso, K. (1970). *Portraits of "the whiteman": Linguistic plan and cultural symbols among the Western Apache.* London: Cambridge University Press.

Bayles, K., and Harris, G. (1982). Evaluating speech-language skills in Papago Indian children. *Journal of American Indian Education, 21*(2), 11–20.

Blanchard, E. (1983). The growth and development of American Indian children and Alaskan Native children. In G. Powell (Ed.), *The psychological development of minority group children.* New York: Brunner/Mazel.

Brody, J., Overfield, T., and McAlister, R. (1965). Draining ears and deafness among Alaskan Eskimos. *Archives of Otolaryngology, 81*, 29–33.

Browne, D.B. (1984). WISC-R scoring patterns among Native Americans of Northern Plains. *White Cloud Journal, 3*(2), 3–16.

Bureau of Indian Affairs (1981). *Fiscal year 1981–1983 state plan for part B of the Education of the Handicapped Act as amended by Public Law 94–142.* Washington, DC: Author.

The Consortium for handicapped Indian children: A report. (1980). Prepared by the National Association of State Boards of Education and Indian Education Training.

DeAvila, E.A., and Havassy, B. (1974). The testing of minority children — a neo-Piagetian approach. *Today's Education, 63*, 72–75.

Downs, M. (1981). Contribution of mild hearing loss to auditory language learning problems. In R. Roesser and M. Downs (Eds.), *Auditory disorders in school children.* New York: Thieme-Stratton.

Dukepoo, F. (1980). *The elderly American Indian.* San Diego: San Diego State University, University Center on Aging.

Einisman, V. (1981). Long-term care and minority elderly. In E.P. Stanford and S.A. Lockery (Eds.), *Trends and status of minority aging.* San Diego: San Diego State University, University Center on Aging.

Feasibility study report: Proposed research and training center for habilitation/rehabilitation of Native Americans with neurosensory disabilities (1979). Lawrence, KS: Native American Research Associates.

Garber, M. (1968). *Ethnicity and measures of educability: Differences among Navajo, Pueblo, and rural Spanish-American first graders on measures of learning style, hearing, vocabulary, entry skills, motivation, and home environment processes.* Unpublished doctoral dissertation, University of Southern California, Los Angeles.

Gelfand, D. (1982). *Aging: The ethnic factor.* Boston: Little, Brown.

Guilmet, G. (1979, Spring). Maternal perceptions of urban Navajo and Caucasian children's classroom behavior. *Human Organization, 38*(1), 87–91.

Goodwin, M., Shaw, J., and Feldman, C. (1980). Distribution of otitis media among four Indian populations in Arizona. *Public Health Reports, 95*(6), 589–594.

Harris, G. (1985). *A survey of speech-language pathologists serving Native American populations.* Tucson: Native American Research and Training Center, University of Arizona.

Harris, G., and Bayles, K. (1981). *Speech-language pathology and audiology: Native American perspective.* Poster session presented to the Convention of the American Speech-Language-Hearing Association, Los Angeles.

Kaplan, G., Fleshman, T., Baum, C., and Clark, P. (1973). Long-term effects of otitis media: A ten year cohort study of Alaskan Eskimo children. *Pediatrics, 52*, 577–585.

Kirk, S.A. (1972, October). Ethnic differences in Psycholinguistic Abilities. *Exceptional Children*, 112–118.

Kleinman, A., Eisenberg, L., and Good, B. (1978). Culture, illness and care:

Clinical lessons from anthropological and cross cultural research. *Annals of Internal Medicine, 99*(2), 251–258.

Kuske, I. (1969). *Psycholinguistic abilities of Sioux Indian children.* Unpublished doctoral dissertation, University of South Dakota, Rapid City.

Leap, W. (1973). On grammaticality in Native American English: The evidence from Isleta. *International Journal of the Sociology of Language, 2,* 79–84.

Leap, W. (1980). Cleft and pseudo cleft in Tewa English. In E. Brandt and F. Barkin (Eds.), *Speaking, singing and teaching: A multidisciplinary approach to language variation.* (Anthropological Research Papers, No. 20). Tempe: Arizona State University.

Leap, W. (1982). Semilingualism as a form of linguistic proficiency. In R. St. Clair and W. Leap (Eds.), *Language renewal among American Indian tribes.* Rosslyn, VA: National Clearinghouse for Bilingual Education.

Lombardi, T. (1970). Psycholinguistic abilities of Papago Indian school children. *Exceptional Children, 36,* 485–493.

Mick, C. (1983). *A profile of American Indian nursing homes.* Tucson: Long Term Care Gerontology Center, University of Arizona.

Miller, D. (1975). Native American families in the city. In G. Powell, J. Yamamoto, A. Romero, and A. Morales (Eds.), *The psychosocial development of minority group children.* New York: Brunner/Mazel.

Rameriz, B. (1976). *Background paper on American Indian exceptional children.* Prepared for the National Advisory Council on Special Education.

Rehabilitation Services Administration (1982). *Characteristics of persons rehabilitated, summary by race of clients FY 1981.* Washington, DC: Author.

Rosenbluth, A. (1976, March). The feasibility of test translation between unrelated languages English to Navajo. *TESCL Quarterly.*

Stewart, J. (1983). Communication disorders in American Indian populations. In D. Omark and J. Erickson (Eds.), *The bilingual exceptional child.* San Diego: College-Hill Press.

Stewart, J. (1985). *Summary of communication disorders unit sensory disabilities program.* Unpublished manuscript, Albuquerque, NM.

Toubbeh, J. (1985, January-February-March). Handicapping and disabling conditions in Native American populations. *American Rehabilitation,* pp. 3–9.

Wolfram, W., Christian, D., Leap, W.L., and Potter, L. (1979). *Variability in the English of two Indian communities and its impact on reading and writing* (Final report, NIE Grant No. NIE-G-77-0006). Arlington, VA: Center for Applied Linguistics.

Young Native American children and their families: Educational needs assessment and recommendations (1976). U.S. Bureau of Indian Affairs, Office of Indian Education Programs.

Chapter 9

Hearing Disorders Among the Indigenous Peoples of North America and the Pacific Basin

Joseph Stewart

Studies and reports on hearing disorders and their prevalence in the United States have generally been derived from the predominant culture — that is, white, English speaking, largely urban, and generally accessible. As a result, generalizations from such reports to other, but comparatively small populations have limited or no validity. In this chapter, the problems of hearing disabilities among those indigenous peoples of the United States, some of its possessions and territories, and some adjacent areas are explored from the viewpoint of the effects of cultural, genetic, and other variables that affect the distribution of hearing disorders, their recognition, and the provision of remedial services for them.

THE POPULATION

The culturally diverse populations covered in this chapter are largely the non-European, indigenous peoples who are descendents of the original inhabitants of areas now controlled by the United States (as in the case of Guam, Samoa, Micronesia, and the Polynesians of Hawaii); peoples who reside in lands adjacent to such territories (such as the aborigines of Australia); and the original inhabitants of North America (as in the case of the Native Americans of this continent, termed American Indians for the purpose of this chapter). Although the cultural diversity of these groups is as evident as their racial differences, the common bond uniting them for present purposes is the fact that all are generally isolated from the prevailing American society by virtue of geography, socioeconomic status, level of education, and poor access to health care.

The last point, lack of access to health care, is of particular significance in that little information dealing with hearing disorders in these populations has focused on ear diseases and their sequelae. Moreover, research on nonmedical effects of hearing loss has typically received much less attention than medically related concerns, which has traditionally placed health above education on the apparent assumption that with good health the potential for good education would follow.

The Pacific Basin

The peoples of the Pacific islands have but one common and tenuous bond — all are of Asiatic origin. Within this broad category, immense individual variations abound. The Maoris of New Zealand, for example, are Polynesian and much more closely related to native Hawaiians and Samoans than to their nearest neighbors, the aborigines of Australia, who are in turn close relatives of the natives of New Guinea. The residents of Guam are a mixture of many racial strains, including Chamorro, Filipino, Spanish, and Japanese. Although they are also multiracial, their neighbors in other islands in Micronesia do not reflect such an extensive infusion of racial strains. While such mixing is probably secondary to other variables in analyzing hearing disorders in these groups, the extent and severity of hearing disorders do seem to vary as a function of racial differences. These differences must be acknowledged and explained wherever possible.

United States and Canada

Indians of North America. Generally thought to be a much more homogeneous group of people than the groups occupying the Pacific islands, American Indians defined for our purposes also reflect a complex physiological and cultural mosaic. The Asiatic origins of the American Indian appear to have been geographically extensive and diffuse, with common cultural traits assimilated from one group to another over the thousands of years the Indians were isolated on the North American continent. Definitions of what constitutes an "Indian" are many, with no common genetic, cultural, or political terms being commonly accepted by all. For our purposes, these are comparatively inconsequential except for those variables that are race dependent and capable of control.

Data on the prevalence and nature of hearing disorders in this population almost exclusively pertain to those Indians who are counted as such by the Department of the Interior and live on or near a reservation or in a native village. This group numbers approximately 800,000 persons. All have access to Indian Health Service (IHS) facilities. An approximately equal number of Indians reside in urban areas and are lost to data bases as they receive health services from a wide variety of sources, not all of which make ethnic identification data available.

EXTENT OF THE PROBLEM

True incidence and prevalence data on the extent of hearing disorders in these culturally diverse populations do not exist. However, the information presented in the following discussion is sufficiently broad, if viewed in the context of the time when it was collected, to allow incidence and prevalence inferences to be drawn.

Australia

In a report of a meeting on aboriginal health care in Australia, Vincent (1979) stated that the numbers of severely deaf persons in that population did not constitute a major problem. Yet in this same book, Rao (1979) compared the rates of hearing impairment in the non-aboriginal Australian (16 per 1,000) with those in the aboriginal Australian (157 per 1,000) and observed that 95 percent of these problems were secondary to otitis media (OM). Vercoe (1979) reported that neurosensory hearing loss was high in only one locale in Australia, the Yalata area of South Australia, but this observation is qualified by the stated need for surveys to determine its accuracy. The Australian literature is overwhelmingly concerned with the various forms of OM affecting aborigines from all areas of the Australian continent. Brown (1979) states that the first description of the disease appeared in the literature in 1882, with little in the way of subsequent observations until the 1960s and 1970s. Moran, Waterford, Hollows, and Jones (1979) report that the aborigines have one of the highest rates of middle ear disease in the world and that prevalence has increased over the past 40 to 50 years.

Clements (1968) reported on a survey of children at Allawah Grove, which indicated that both OM and resultant hearing losses were high, but he did not presume that these findings would extend to other Western aborigines. The preliminary study by Lewis, Barry, and Stuart (1976) conducted at Cherbourg, Australia, revealed a high incidence of both ear and hearing disorders, a finding confirming results obtained 2 years earlier by Lewis (1974), who conservatively estimated that 60 percent of all the children of at least partial aboriginal descent have either active or quiescent ear disorders.

Brown's pilot study (1972) from the Northern Territory indicated that 10 percent of the aboriginal children there had hearing impairment sufficient to be educationally handicapping, whereas 62 percent showed evidence of past or present middle ear disease. In a sample of 59 adults, three had active middle ear disease, five had socially inadequate hearing, and seven had a hearing loss of 25 dB or more in the better ear. For Australia generally, Willis (1979) noted that at that time the incidence of OM in children was 20 percent with a reliable estimate that 15 percent of all aboriginal children under 15 years of age would have hearing loss of sufficient degree to be termed a disability.

Brown (1979) has also reviewed recent findings by various investigators in Australia, including Kirke's reports of 1969 and 1970, in which incidences in children were reported to be 29 percent for chronic ear disease and 24 percent for significant hearing impairment. Urban, in 1972 (personal communication), reported respective incidences of 40 percent and 31 percent in schoolchildren in larger rural centers.

Sunderman (1979) conducted a survey in Western Australia in which only 14.1 percent of the ears examined were normal; foreign bodies were found in 1.7 percent, debris or wax (or both) in 9.8 percent, dry perforations in 8.9 percent, wet perforations in 10 percent, and opaque, retracted, or scarred ear drums in 55.6 percent. Mild hearing loss (less than 20 dB) was reported in 24 percent, moderate loss (20 to 30 dB) in 7 percent, and severe loss (more than 30 dB) in 8.1 percent of the subjects. The range of incidence was thought to be related to such factors as standard of living and nutrition.

Middleton and Francis (1976) reported the results of a survey of 73 children below 39 months of age on a settlement in the Northwest Territory, where they found infected or damaged ears to be the fourth most commonly reported problem, affecting 38.4 percent of the sample. Infected ears was the fourth most common reason for a hospital visit (5.4 percent).

Although OM is generally recognized around the world as a nearly universal childhood disease, for the Australian aborigine (1) the disease rate is excessive compared to the nonnative population;

(2) the rate of hearing loss resulting form OM reflects the severity of disease episodes, which results from (3) insufficient or natural healing capability, which allows the development of such severe sequelae.

Pacific Basin

Hawaii. As noted previously, the native Polynesian population is a small minority in Hawaii. The literature on hearing disorders in this population is also very small. A thesis by Watson (1966) appears to be the closest approximation of possible prevalence of hearing disorders among Hawaiian Polynesians. Watson conducted his research in Nanakuli, a rural area on the island of Oahu. This island was selected because of a suspected high incidence of ear disease and hearing loss. The community of approximately 9,000 people was socioeconomically depressed and of a complex racial mixture. Approximately 5,000 residents were at least partially of native Hawaiian extraction. A sample of 114 children were followed over the first 4 years of life. Only *two* children were found to have normal tympanic membranes throughout this period. Screening audiometry was performed on 64 percent of the children at age 4 years, and 26 percent of the number tested failed two frequencies at 20 dB and were referred for diagnostic testing.

American Samoa. According to the American Samoa Health Coordinating Council (1978), chronic ear infection has been a major health problem for many years. In 1976, it was determined that 50 percent of all pediatric outpatients were suffering from OM even though this was not the primary reason for clinic visits. This report also cited a 1971 survey which determined that 9 percent of a sample of 675 children had discharging ears and another 3 percent dry perforations. One year later, a sample of 998 first grade children showed 5 percent with OM and another 5 percent with perforations. By 1976, a sample of children from 6 to 8 years showed 3.5 percent with active OM and 1.3 percent with chronic OM (COM) with perforation.

In the project evaluation of the American Samoa Hearing Screening Project for 1977–78, McCuddin (1978) reported that 8 percent of the population of children had a hearing loss, with middle ear infection or wax impaction being a chief cause in over 90 percent of the cases. This finding is not consistent with the survey of hospital records by Harding (1978), in which only 24 children were reported in the patient population as being either significantly or severely deaf. This discrepancy may be related to a Samoan cultural tendency to be intolerant of disabilities. This tendency contributes to concealment, rather than to reporting, of such problems. Thus, an exact number of children in American Samoa with hearing disorders may be difficult to obtain.

Harding (1978) has also reported that among elementary school children (ages 6 to 13) in American Samoa during 1974-75, OM occurred in 3.8 percent of the children examined, with hearing problems occurring in 0.16 percent and deaf mutism in 0.08 percent. These data were obtained from a total of 2,426 students examined. Data from 1976 obtained from 1,205 students between 6 and 8 years old showed 3.48 percent with OM and 1.32 percent with COM with perforation. The discrepancy between McCuddin's and Harding's findings (8 percent versus 0.16 percent hearing loss) cannot be resolved from reading the two reports.

Micronesia. Micronesia consists of the Trust Territories, a combination of six Pacific island groups, plus Guam. This widely dispersed territory of over 2,000 islands covers an area approximately the size of the continental United States. About one half of the 200,000 residents of the area are Guamanian, the only islanders holding United States citizenship. The peoples of the other five districts of Micronesia are eligible for the same benefits as United States citizens. The available data on hearing impairment in these groups come from two areas only, Guam and Palau (Belau). Their various political futures are presently being determined.

The earliest data from Guam were published in 1970 by Eldridge, Brody, and Wetmore and revealed that in a sample of 1,541 school-aged children, 16.8 percent had a loss of hearing (more than 20 dB), primarily associated with OM. Of 157 children failing audiometric testing who were then examined otoscopically, 50.3 percent had active OM, 8.3 percent had a perforation, another 19.7 percent had wax obstruction, and only 21.7 percent showed no pathological findings. Severity of hearing loss was directly related to perforation. These rates are among the highest ever reported for these conditions. More recently, Stewart (unpublished data, 1977) reported a 16 percent COM rate with about 25 to 35 percent of schoolchildren showing evidence of middle ear disease. Deafness resulting from a previous rubella epidemic affected some 125 children and left another eight deaf and blind.

Headstart screening on Palau in 1982 (Stewart, unpublished data, 1982) revealed that 43 children (39 percent) had middle ear disease, 18 (16 percent) had tympanic membrane perforations, and 46 (29 percent) had obstructing cerumen. Headstart audiometric data the following year showed that 77 (65 percent) of the children who were screened failed the test.

More recently, Olkeriil (1982) reported a survey of 292 residents of Koror, capital of Palau, 59.6 percent of whom were under 10 years of age. Following otoscopic examination, 18.2 percent were referred to ENT clinics. Eleven of those referred had perforated tympanic membranes, 11 had excessive cerumen, 12 had fluid in the canal, 4 had drainage from the canal, 1 had a congenital ear defect, and 1 had a foreign body on the ear. Of the 309 ears tested by tympanometry, only one third were normal. Type B tympanograms constituted 21.7 percent of the total. Audiometric screening resulted in failure rates of 42.3 percent for the very young and 40 percent for adults. Because of ambient noise level, these findings were believed not to be indicative of the hearing status of Palauans generally. Because all the subjects between the ages of 54 and 84 years failed, however, investigation of the hearing of the older population was judged to be warranted.

Although Micronesia is geographically distant from Australia, the similarities in disease patterns between the aborigines and the peoples of the Pacific Basin is clearly evident. OM and hearing loss account for a disproportionately high number of hospital visits and hearing screening failures with (1) highly persistent disease patterns followed by (2) excessive disease chronicity, resulting in (3) unresolved hearing deficiency and related sequelae.

American Indian. There have probably been more reports published on ear diseases and hearing disorders among American Indians than on any other peoples discussed in this chapter. Numerous summaries of these findings have been published relatively recently (e.g., Stewart, 1983; Wiet, DeBlanc, Stewart, and Wieder, 1980). A summary of the research on hearing disorders among American Indians is presented in Table 9–1. Many of the studies in this table must be viewed in the context of variations in ages of subjects, dates, time of year of data collection, different audiometric and otological standards, and such additionally complicating factors as tribal (ethnic) identity and blood quantum.

As can be seen from careful examination of Table 9–1, there is a marked variability in reported ear diseases among American Indians, ranging from 0.2 percent (McCandless and Parkin, 1976) to 48 percent (Kaplan et al., 1973) for COM, and from 12.7 percent (Doyle and Morwood, 1976) to 33 percent for overall ear pathology in children under the age of 2 years (Brody, Overfield, and McAlister, 1965).

Text continued on page 254

Table 9–1. Hearing Disorders Among American Indians: Summary of Selected Articles

Author, Date	Population and Site	Purpose	Major Findings
R.F. Baske (1968)	Indian students, K through 12 (N-348) at Hays, Mission, and Lodgepole, Montana, schools	Screening for ear disease, using audiometry and Otoscopy	26.2% had some form of ear disease, 13.8% with current disease (including serous otitis media, which accounted for 60.5% of "current disease"). Otoscopic examination normal in 72% with abnormal audiograms; 22.5% with normal audiograms had abnormal otoscopic.
J.D. Baxter and D. Ling (1972)	Eskimo from Baffin Zone, Canada	Preliminary hearing survey of population of Baffin Zone	"Otoscopic examination revealed a generally high prevalence of ear disease with considerable variation in the extent of the problem from one settlement to another. . . . Tympanometry did not prove to be useful as a screening technique."
J.D. Baxter and D. Ling (1974)	Eskimo from Baffin Zone, Canada	Survey of amount of hearing loss and ear disease	"Most chronic otitis media and conductive hearing loss is found among children in the southern settlements, where from 13 to 19% of the school population suffers from the disease."
J.D. Baxter et al. (1979)	Inuit Eskimo, elementary school children, Canada	Evaluation of modalities local medical treatment of COM (3½ years)	"All modalities of local medical treatment applied, including simple cleaning of the external canal alone, led to significant amelioration of the suppurative ear disease in these children."
J.D. Baxter (1981)	Inuit Eskimo, Canada	Study of factors associated with otitis media	High incidence attributed to socioeconomic factors such as overcrowded housing and bottle feeding.
J.D. Baxter (1982)	Inuit Eskimo, Canada	Observations on evolution of chronic otitis media in the Inuit of Baffin Zone	During 8 year interval between two surveys, ⅓ of Inuit with COM underwent spontaneous healing. "The prevalence. . . did not decrease as others acquired the disease during the period under discussion."

Q.C. Beery et al. (1980)	White Mountain (AZ) Apaches, 25 subjects with history of OM, 3 to 36 years of age	Study of Eustachian tube function	". . . the ET of the American Indian was functionally different from that of Caucasians previously studied and was characterized by comparatively abnormal, low passive tubal resistance which may be considered to facilitate ventilatory function and to impair protective function. The difference may account for the high prevalence of OM with perforation and the low incidence of cholesteatoma in this population."
D.E. Berg et al. (1971)	Indian children in Omaha, NE	Study of association between serum and secretory immunoglobulins in COM in Indian children	"All three serum classes of immunoglobulins were significantly increased over that of the normal white populations."
J.A. Brody et al. (1965)	Alaska Eskimos, Aleuts, and Caucasians	Study of relationship of draining ears and deafness	Ear pathology established in 1/3 of Eskimo population by 2 years of age, probably the population that eventually has severe hearing loss. Those who had no draining ear before the age of 2 not likely to develop ear problems.
K. Cambon et al. (1965)	British Columbia Indians, Canada	Otologic-audiologic survey	16% of 504 subjects found to have current middle ear pathology. 45% known to have had previous disease. Disease related to poor social conditions, family history, and presence of nasal discharge.
P.J. Doyle and D. Morwood (1976)	British Columbia Indian children, Canada	Study incidence of ear disease and evaluate screening methods	1109 Indian children showed 12.7% middle ear disease, namely, serous otitis, perforation, or cholesteatoma. Pure-tone and impedance audiometry, both unsatisfactory, could not be performed on children from birth to 4 years old.

Table continued on following page

Table 9–1. Hearing Disorders Among American Indians: Summary of Selected Articles (continued)

Author, Date	Population and Site	Purpose	Major Findings
W.J. Doyle (1977)	Osteologic study on specimens from Caucasian, Indian, and Black subjects, Pittsburgh	Study of Eustachian tube function, otitis media, and related conditions on various parameters	Appears that Eskimo and Indian population have ET systems that are less efficient than those of Caucasians and Blacks
M.D. Graham (1975)	Indians of coastal British Columbia, Canada	Survey of ear disease prevalence and availability of medical facilities	"A high prevalence of middle ear disease was found in all age groups and in all sites surveyed. . . (except). . . where general living conditions were more favorable, i.e., the residential schools, and where medical supervision was present."
J.B. Gregg et al. (1965)	Osteologic study of prehistoric temporal bones of Indians of South Dakota	Study altered mastoid development suggestive of presence of infections during period of growth	"The findings suggest that the people represented by these skulls must have had a significant amount of infectious middle ear disease during the period of the development of their mastoids."
J.B. Gregg et al. (1970)	Indian school children, South Dakota	Study of ear disease	Otolaryngologic and radiographic data show 24% of 385 subjects, age 6 to 16 years, with past evidence of significant ear disease but sufficient only to cause hearing impairment in small fraction of study sample.
W.K. Ickes and D. Keel (1982)	Headstart Indian and non-Indian children in Anadarko, OK	Investigate validity of presumed high prevalence of otitis media among Indian children	Comparison of Indians and "mixed ethnic" children for middle ear disease showed no statistically significant differences.
B.F. Jaffe (1969)	Navajo Indian Reservation (NM, UT, AZ)	Determine incidence of ear disease	CSOM at 3 large boarding schools show 4.2% perforation rate; 30% of subjects had suppuration at time of examination. Bilateral perforations found in 17% of students with perforations.

B.F. Jaffe et al. (1970)	Navajo Indian Reservation (NM, UT, AZ)	Study tympanic membrane mobility in newborns	18 of 101 newborns showed poor mobility of TM during first or second day of life. At end of 6 weeks, 11 of 18 still had poor mobility. Four of these later developed AOM with suppurative drainage by 5 months of age. Six developed AOM, and 1 had persistent SOM during 7 months of life.
R.L. Johnson (1967)	Navajo Indian school children (NM, UT, AZ)	Otoscopic survey of COM incidence	In sample of over 3000 children, 7% found with current or past evidence of COM, a rate 15 times greater than for the population at large. One quarter of these were bilateral.
S.C. Johonnott (1973)	Eskimo children, Alaska	Compare COM rates of urban and rural residents	Of 136 urban children, 1 with active COM and 5 with inactive COM (4.4%). Of 300 rural children, 17 had active COM and 38 had inactive COM (18.3%). More rural children had family history of ear disease.
G.J. Kaplan et al. (1973)	Eskimo children, Alaska	Ten year cohort study of long term effects of otitis media	76% subjects had one or more OM episodes since birth, 78% of these during first 2 years of life. Perforations and scars were present in 48%. Hearing loss of +26 dB in 16%. Those with history prior to age 2 years with hearing loss of +26 dB, statistically significantly lower scores in verbal ability, reading, total math, and language.
D. Ling et al. (1969)	Eskimo children, Cape Dorset, Canada	Medical-audiologic examinations to determine incidence of middle ear disease and hearing impairment	"Significant hearing impairments occurred very rarely, as compared with middle ear disease, which affected 30% of the population aged 0-9 years. Investigation of older children in the Cape Dorset school population suggested that disease and hearing loss were among the factors contributing to educational retardation."

Table continued on following page

Table 9–1. Hearing Disorders Among American Indians: Summary of Selected Articles (continued)

Author, Date	Population and Site	Purpose	Major Findings
A.J. Lupin (1976)	Northern native populations, literature review	Review of otitis media in these populations, effects and causative factors	"Suggestions are made for improved follow-up and a plea is made for improved home conditions for the native populations."
J. Maynard (1969)	Review of health statistics, Native Alaska infants	Determine epidemiology of disease in this population	Records of 322 infants, 1960–1962, showed 18% incidence of otitis media, closely related to frequency of upper respiratory infections.
G. McCandless (1973)	Arapahoe, Shoshone Indians (WY), children and young adults	Screening for otitis media; comparing pure-tone audiometry, impedance, and otoscopy as middle ear disease detectors	Average failure rate = 13.6%, less than 5% for adhesive chronic or purulent OM; 61% agreement between otoscopy and pure-tone screening and 93% agreement between otoscopy and impedance.
G. McCandless and J.L. Parkin (1976)	Selected IHS Service Units in five states	Obtain baseline data on otitis media	Site / % Perforation / % Overall ear problems: Florida 1.9 — 29.2 Idaho 5.0 — 23.8 Nevada .2 — 5.2 South Dakota 2.5 — 16.7 Utah 2.0 — 28.7
D. McShane (1979)	Research summary Ojibwa Indian children	Middle ear disease and effects on hearing, learning	"The possible relationships between recurrent otitis media and language and educational deficits. . . have been virtually ignored in regard to Indian children."

Reference	Population	Study	Findings
S.M. Nelson and R.I. Berry (1984)	School children, Navajo Reservation	Audiometric-otologic screening	Examined 15,890 Navajo school children between 1978 and 1980 for ear disease and hearing loss. ". . . Prevalence data and correlations of hearing level with ear disease are presented. 4% of the children had ear disease perforations, 2.3% middle ear effusions, 1.9% TM atelectasis, and 0.4% had sensorineural hearing loss. Microtia was found in 1:935. . . . Cholesteatoma was rare."
G. Perkins and G. Church (1960)	Wind River (WY) Reservation children	Pediatric evaluations of 214 children	37 children between birth and 3 years with otitis media, the most common disease requiring follow-up.
P. Ratnesar (1976)	Eskimo, Algonkin Indians, and Caucasians in Labrador and Newfoundland	Study of incidence of chronic ear disease among groups living in same environmental conditions	"The variation in the disease pattern in the different ethnic groups was shown to be related to the aeration of the middle ear cleft."
D. Reed and W. Dunn (1970)	Eskimo children, Alaska	Study of occurrence of otitis media in six villages	Initial surveys showed history of one or more episodes of OM for 63% of 641 children. Nearly all with history showed TM abnormalities, compared with 11% without history. Hearing loss of +25 dB in 27% of children over 3 years; 43% had new episodes during the year of study, with highest incidence below 2 years.
D. Reed et al. (1967)	Eskimo children, Alaska	Study of relationship between otitis media and hearing loss	Cohort study of 378 children from birth to 4 years showed 65% of children with one or more episodes of otorrhea before first birthday; 89% before second birthday; 31% had hearing loss of +26 dB.

Table continued on following page

Table 9-1.   Hearing Disorders Among American Indians: Summary of Selected Articles (continued)

Author, Date	Population and Site	Purpose	Major Findings
K. R. Reinhard et al. (1970)	Native children, Alaska	Bacteriological study of 130 cases of purulent, perforating otitis media	More than 40 species, of 18 genera, of bacteria found to be etiological agents of bacterial OM, the majority of which are commonly found in the pharyngeal flora of the population studied. "The bacteriological factors alone do not fully explain the extremely high prevalence . . .".
M. E. Roberts (1976)	Indian children, British Columbia, Canada	Survey of 1,109 subjects to determine incidence of middle ear disease and to compare pure-tone audiometry and impedance	12% of subjects had middle ear disease requiring treatment; 19% showed abnormal audiograms, 30% abnormal impedance results.
O. Schaefer (1971)	Eskimos, Canada	Study relationships of bottle feeding and otitis media	"Analysis of otoscopic findings and infant nutrition histories of 536 Eskimos . . . shows an inverse relation of incidence of chronic middle ear disease and duration of lactation enjoyed in infancy with a minimum incidence of otitis in individuals breast fed more than 12 months."
J. R. Shaw et al. (1981)	Indian communities (AZ)	Study of relationships of environmental and behavioral factors with otitis media	"The contrasting rates of occurrence among children living under apparently similar environmental conditions suggest that factors, as yet unidentified, characterize those at high risk of repeated infections."

J. R. Shaw et al. (1982)	Indian communities (AZ)	Longitudinal study of otitis media in community settings	"Comparison of various attributes of severity and persistence of otitis media showed that more high-risk children had attacks after age 2 years than children not at high risk. Significant differences were evident, however, between children who had contrasting experience with occurrence of otitis after age 2. Prevalence of hearing loss and impedance abnormalities were significantly higher among children who had 3 or more attacks of otitis after age 2 than among children with fewer than 3 attacks."
G. H. Spivey and N. Hirschhorn (1977)	Adopted Apache children	Study of illness incidence of Reservation and urban adopted Apache children	Adopted Apache children had more illness, including OM, than their non-Apache siblings but less than Reservation Apache children
L. L. Titche et al. (1981)	Osteologic study of prehistoric Arizona Indian skulls	Determine prehistoric mastoiditis prevalence	"The infection rate was much lower than that which had been found in two previous studies of skulls from the Northern Plains of the United States."
E. A. Tower (1979)	Alaska Natives	Historical review of otitis media literature 1954–1979	Cites surgical success rates and calls for a more conservative approach to surgery. Stresses medical treatment, citing 50% spontaneous healing rate as a result.
B. S. Watrous et al. (1980)	Indian, Hispanic, and Caucasian institutionalized population, New Mexico	Study of otitis media prevalence in three racial groups	Examination of ears and search of medical records showed high prevalence for TM abnormalities in all 3 groups (52.5%, N = 120). Indian group showed the highest proportion of TM abnormalities, followed by Hispanic, then Caucasian. Within Indian group, the Navajo showed much higher prevalence than Pueblo Indians.

Table continued on following page

Table 9–1. Hearing Disorders Among American Indians: Summary of Selected Articles (continued)

Author, Date	Population and Site	Purpose	Major Findings
E. A. Weymuller and D. G. Reed (1972)	Alaska Natives	Report on otologic problems of Alaska Natives at Mt. Edgecumbe School	Found incidence of OM and complications = 13%. Since dry ear is of utmost importance, modified radical and classical radical mastoidectomies most frequently performed. "Type IV and V tympanoplasties are not considered feasible."
R. J. Wiet (1979)	Arizona Indians	Report on patterns of ear disease	Origin of high prevalence of OM in Indians multifaceted. Unusually high prevalence of related disorders — oral clefts, facial paralysis in diabetics and absence of otosclerosis ". . . suggest racial inheritance as predominant factor for pattern of ear disease."
R. J. Wiet et al. (1980)	American Indians and Alaska Natives	Review of natural history of OM in Native American population	"American natives are prone to otitis media at an early age and represent a group which is at risk to develop the disease. Acute suppurative disease reaches its peak prior to the age of two years. If untreated, it may resolve or become a persistent effusion of the middle ear, but more likely will go on to permanent perforation. Otitis media with effusion accounts for about 20% of all childhood ear disease in the American native. Causes for otitis media in American natives are multifaceted, but remain heavily genetic with subgroups more prone to the disease than others. Anatomic factors involving poor eustachian tube function are especially prevalent in this population."

| R. D. Zonis (1968a) | White Mountain Apache, Arizona | Survey of COM in one community | Prevalence of COM = 8.3% with an additional 13% showing healed perforation or tympanosclerosis. "The relative freedom from complications seems to attest to the benign nature of this condition in the southwestern Indians." |
| R. D. Zonis (1968b) | White Mountain Apache, Arizona | Study of immunologic factors in this population | "Serum immunoelectophoresis on 42 American Indians with chronic otitis media and 25 without evidence of ear infection revealed four people with reduced or absent immunoglobulin A, all of whom were in the otitis media group . . . compared with a prior study which showed that only 0.2% of a normal population showed such a deficiency or delayed synthesis of secretory IgA might be a major factor in the etiology of chronic otitis media in the southwestern Indian." |

The relationships between acute otitis media (AOM) rates and those for COM are not always clearly definable from available data. In one report (Goinz, 1984), the overall prevalence of AOM based on health records for Indians in Michigan, Minnesota, and Wisconsin (1980 data) was 12.5 percent. A screening program for children in those same states indicated a COM rate of less than 1 percent. A similar, but much earlier, report (Corkery, 1973) of declining COM unrelated to AOM rates from a single reservation in Wyoming indicated a 39.7 per 1,000 perforation rate among patients 15 years of age and older, dropping progressively to 9.3 per 1,000 at the less than 1 year to 4 year age range. Although still alarmingly high, the lower rate was attributed to a change in the course of middle ear disease during the preceding 15 years. This change was assumed to be a reflection of increased use of antibiotics, changes in the reservation environment, increased community awareness of the need for services, and changes in the percentage of Indian blood.

The hazards of making inferences from any given data base are increased when comparative data from two sources are used. These hazards were evidenced in a recent research project on the Navajo reservation (Stewart, 1984), where an analysis of hospital records indicated a COM rate of 2.1 percent for two successive years, 1980 and 1981. During this same time, a survey of nearly 16,000 school-aged Navajo children (Nelson and Berry, 1984) reported 4 percent of the children had perforated tympanic membranes. An additional 2.3 percent were found to have middle ear effusions and 0.4 percent had a sensorineural hearing loss. The results of the two sets of data are not contradictory, but they do show the need for great specificity in describing the group on which the data are based, the definition of disease being used, and the time when the data were collected. Stewart also found that AOM rates varied from 6.2 to 19.3 percent of all hospital visits, whereas COM rates varied from 4.7 to 22.5 percent of all visits, depending upon location of the treatment facility.

Epidemiological data on hearing loss are even less reliable and, as mentioned previously, have not been given the attention that middle ear disease has received. Although the overwhelming number of patients with hearing loss have the conductive type, some information on sensorineural hearing loss is available.

In the McCandless and Parkin study (1976), patients from five widely differing service facilities (in Florida, South Dakota, Idaho, Nevada, and Utah) were tested, with an overall result of 20.9 percent being found to have a hearing loss from any cause, including impacted cerumen. Of this number, 10.6 percent had conductive losses secondary to OM. Another 2.2 percent were found to have conductive losses not related to OM. Children below 3 years of age had a 27.5 percent incidence of conductive hearing loss; the incidence in older children stayed at 20 percent until age 10 years. With some fluctuation, the conductive hearing loss incidence declined beyond this age. Sensorineural hearing loss became evident in the 18 to 21 year group in 4.4 percent, and it gradually increased (as expected) with age after 40 years. In the 70 to 80 year age range, 40.6 percent were found to have sensorineural losses, as did 54.5 percent in the 80 to 90 year range.

Canterbury and his associates (1981) have found that hearing impairment in Alaska was greater there than in many other parts of the United States, owing in part to the excessively high OM rate among the native population (Indian, Eskimo, and Aleut) of that state, as reflected in the reports in Table 9–1. In one study, between 9 and 17 percent of native Alaskans entering high school had some degree of sensorineural hearing loss. In comparison with the population at large, native Alaskans had (1) a higher failure rate on hearing screening tests, (2) a higher occurrence of conductive loss and abnormal impedance findings at younger and older ages, (3) a higher proportion of mixed and sensorineural losses, (4) more hearing losses of every type, and (5) a substantially higher frequency of severe hearing loss after age 20 years. Similar findings hold for the American Indian population outside Alaska as well.

VARIABLES ASSOCIATED WITH HEARING DISORDERS

Racial, Anatomic, Familial

Although not amenable to extensive direct investigation, the issues of racial and anatomical differences in ear disease prevalence have been addressed.

Eldridge and colleagues (1970) observed on Guam that although a low frequency of ear disease episodes were reported, the rate of hearing loss associated with it was alarmingly high and speculated that each infection might be more damaging owing to a "structural abnormality" of the ear. Although no such factor was known to exist among Guamanians, "the study of temporal bone anatomy and genetic evaluation of kindreds would be useful."

A native Samoan, Dr. Faifeta'i Sailua, Director of the ENT Clinic in Pago Pago, reported to Harding (1978) that it was his perception that Samoan skulls are broader than Caucasian skulls, resulting in a more horizontally placed eustachian tube, a finding also made for various American Indians and cited in Table 9–1.

In Australia, Brown (1979) disputed an observation by Ratnesar that attributed anatomical factors relating to the eustachian tube as significant in the causation of COM among Labrador Eskimos. At the same time, Gray (1979) stated that it was his clinical impression that part-blooded aborigines are much less prone to ear pathology than full-blooded American Indians.

A similar observation to Gray's, among American Indians, has been made by Corkery (1973), whose review of 162 patient charts found that incidence of perforations for full-blooded persons was 10 times greater than for patients who were one half or less Indian, with half-blooded persons having a perforation rate seven times that of Indian patients who were less than one half Indian. Corkery noted that it was impossible to separate blood quantum as a factor from environmental factors and patient care receptiveness.

Zonis (1968b) observed that even with the variable of weather controlled, Apache and Navajo Indians seem to be particularly susceptible to OM. Watrous, Garcia, Brown, and Wasylenki (1980) have also found definite differences in OM states in an institutionalized population for whom all environmental conditions were identical. OM was most severe for Navajos and Apaches, less severe for Pueblo Indians, even less severe for Hispanics, and least severe for Caucasians. Doyle's (1977) osteological studies have shown distinct racial differences in skull structures related to eustachian tube function, and Beery, Doyle, Bluestone, Cantekin, and Wiet (1980) have studied the effects measured by tests of eustachian tube function on Apache Indians. The more horizontal placement of the eustachian tube in Apache (and other) Indians results in a less efficient aeration of the middle ear cleft. This, in turn, improves the condition under which the pathogens responsible for the disease can proliferate, increasing the probability of earlier, and more severe, disease.

A number of investigators have observed a familial relationship to OM in the Indian population. Family history and comparisons of siblings' medical histories (Cambon, Galbraith, and Kong, 1965; McCandless and Parkin, 1976; Spivey and Hirschhorn, 1977) all address this finding. On the basis of a current research project, Indian Health Service clinical records also confirm familial clustering of disease. In Australia, Kirke (cited in Brown, 1979) has also associated family size and overcrowding resulting in increased and prolonged exposure to disease and higher OM.

Age

OM is documented as an extremely early onset disease in many of the locales under consideration. In Australia, Willis (1979) claims that most authors agree that onset is soon after birth. Rao (1979) reported that nearly every infant on Bathurst Island had OM before the age of 3 or 4 months, with 50 percent of the children below age 10 years having a perforation. Moran and colleagues (1979) found the peak prevalence throughout Australia to be at 3 years of age. Clements (1968) observed a sharp drop in incidence by age 5 years. In Hawaii, Watson (1966) found an incidence of 44 percent OM during the first 4 years of life, highest during the first year. No comparable data are available from Micronesia and American Samoa.

In the American Indian population, the pervasiveness of OM among the very young is widely recognized (Baske, 1968; Baxter, 1981; Baxter and Ling, 1974; Baxter, Katsarkas, Ling, and Carson, 1979; Beery et al., 1980; Berg, Larsen, and Yarrington, 1971; Brody et al., 1965; Cambon et al., 1965; Doyle and Morwood, 1976; Jaffe, 1969; Jaffe, Hurtado, and Hurtado, 1970; Johonnott, 1973; Johnson, 1967; Kaplan et al., 1973; Ling, McCoy, and Levinson, 1969; Spivey and Hirschhorn, 1977; Stewart, unpublished data, 1982; Stewart, 1983, 1984; Stuart, 1979; Sunderman, 1979; Timmerman and Gersen, 1980; Titche, Coulthard, Wachter, Thies, and Harris, 1981; Toubbeh, 1984; Tower, 1979; Ventry, 1980; Vercoe, 1979; Vincent, 1979; Watrous et al., 1980; Weymuller and Reed, 1972; Wiet, 1979; Wiet et al., 1980. Stewart (1984) found for the Navajo that 60 percent of patient visits for AOM occurred before age 5 years.

Toubbeh (1984) found similar age patterns of perforation among Indians living in Alaska, Montana, Wyoming, and Southern Arizona with the peak number of perforations reported at approximately 18 months, declining in numbers from Alaska south.

Although OM is predominantly a disease of the very young, IHS records show that it is a problem affecting Indians at all ages, with a prevalence in one instance of 1 percent of all Navajos 65 years of age and older (Stewart, 1984). In most populations, OM is rarely seen in adult life. The Navajos whose cases were reported all exhibited current active disease with histories of reported occurrences from childhood.

Paradise (1980), reviewing the overall literature on OM, notes that the disease is most common during the first 2 years of life and relates this to a number of factors: (1) The greater susceptibility of the young, particularly to upper respiratory infections (an association repeatedly noted in the literature); (2) abundance of nasopharyngeal lymphoid tissue, which may predispose the child to recurrent chronic local infection and obstruct the eustachian tube; and (3) the questionable (because of possible socioeconomic confounding factors) association of bottle versus breast feeding, discussed in detail later in this chapter; (4) positional factors in feeding, also discussed later; and (5) less competent eustachian tube function in the very young. The relationship of nonanatomical factors, such as inadequate health care, substandard nutrition, and related social conditions, was not pursued by Paradise but is worthy of consideration, as these factors interact with other variables discussed in this chapter.

Sex

Paradise (1980) states that OM is more common among males, with about 59 to 72 percent being males, a finding not found in literature pertaining to the groups here, in which sex is rarely mentioned as a variable. Canterbury and associates (1981) reported that 56 percent of the clients seen in Alaska were male, whereas Stewart (1984) found that when sex was adjusted to the ratio found in the population (48 percent male, 52 percent female), slightly more females than males were OM patients except for the under 1 year old group, of which 46 percent were female and 54 percent were male. At the two major hospitals on the Navajo reservation in Arizona and New Mexico, age of first episode was earlier for males, and the mean number of episodes the first year of life were one more for males (5 females and 6 males). Nelson and Berry's survey (1984) of school-aged Navajo children found appreciably more males (53.1 percent) failed the test compared with 46.9 percent of females.

The sex ratio in the Toubbeh research (1984) showed 53 percent female and 47 percent male, with 42 percent of the males and 37 percent of the females having bilateral involvement, whereas on Guam, Eldridge and colleagues (1970) reported that although boys constituted 53.3 percent of the total children screened, they represented 67.5 percent of those with hearing loss. In the absence of any other mention of a sex difference, it may be assumed that this variable is not pronounced in the populations reported.

Immune System

Brown (1979) states that, in Australia, although a number of writers contend that acquired or inherent immunological deficiency plays a significant part in the disease prevalence in the aboriginal population, persistently high levels of serum immunoglobulins may be a reflection of frequent infection as opposed to an increased or normal immunity. Stuart (1979) found that in Cherbourg, Australia, aboriginal children maintained higher levels of IgG, IgA, and IgM, which he attributed to overstimulation of the immune system from frequent early infections.

Two studies on American Indians are of interest in this regard. Berg and colleagues (1971) found blood levels of the same three classes of immunoglobulins significantly to be higher in his sample of Sioux children than would be found in the white population. Zonis (1968b) speculated that the delayed or deficient IgA synthesis he found in the Apaches studied might be assumed to be a major factor in southwestern Indian COM incidence.

Anatomical and genetic variables associated with the common racial backgrounds of the peoples of the North American continent and the Pacific would appear to greatly influence the occurrence of OM and hearing loss. The significant variables at this time appear to include (1) Asiatic origin, with the concomitant of (2) eustachian tube placement and insufficient middle ear aeration, (3) sex, for which both incidence and severity appear to be sex-linked to some extend, (4) relative inefficiency of the immune system, and (5) age, with both extremes of the lifespan continuum disproportionately affected.

Geography and Climate

The peoples of the Pacific Basin, Australia, New Zealand, and North America can be primarily considered rural dwellers who, in the case of those for whom reservations were established, were generally consigned to geographical areas of little use to the new colonizers of their countries. In some cases, these areas coincided with the aboriginal land area occupied or traveled upon. In other cases, notably among the Indians, the lands were foreign and largely valueless at the time. In the case of the Pacific peoples, no geographical relocation was undertaken, but significant impacts on the cultures resulted form the colonists' insistence upon having their own cultures prevail. The results were devastating to native economic systems, religions, and overall lifestyles.

Insofar as hearing disorders are concerned, geography, climate, and place of residence appear to play rather individualized roles with respect to disease prevalence. The temperatures and humidity of Alaska, for instance, are extensively different from those in Samoa, but OM prevalence in both areas has been nearly identical. It may be that distance from a treatment facility may be a more critical geographical variable than climate conditions or geographical environment. In those relatively few studies comparing urban with rural Indians (Johonnot, 1973; Spivey and Hirschhorn, 1977), urban dwellers were found to have a lower OM rate, but it was still above that for non-Indians.

Paradise (1980) observes that OM prevalence is higher in cold weather and related to upper respiratory infection. He states that it is reasonable to assume that there would be a greater prevalence and severity in colder than in warmer climates but cautions that studies on the question have apparently not been reported.

The findings reported by Brody (1964) that 14 percent of Alaskan Caucasians and 34 percent of Alaskan Eskimos showed that hearing loss attributed to OM reflects the effects of both climate and genetic factors on the disease and its sequelae.

Lewis (1974) reports seasonal variations in disease prevalence in Australia. Rao (1979) maintains, contrary to expectations, that ear problems in Australia are aggravated by heat and humidity, in contrast to the claims made that communities with dry, cold climates are associated with high OM prevalence. Rao cites Bathurst Island as a case in point.

Humidity and temperature variations are insignificant in American Samoa, Hawaii, and Micronesia. Patient visits reported in American Samoa by Harding (1978) over the three years 1973 to 1975 revealed the following months as peak months for OM: December (1973); March, June, and July (1974); and June and August (1975).

As McShane (1982) notes from the literature on Indian susceptibility to OM secondary to mucopurulent rhinitis — a condition also found in Australia (Jose, 1979) — and upper respiratory disease, there are seasons, from midwinter through early spring, during which OM is more prevalent. For example, Zonis (1968a) has observed that Apaches in Arizona were particularly susceptible to OM whether the reservation they lived on had a cold or warm climate.

One difference that may be climate related is inferred from the literature. Two of the Australian reports (Jose, 1979; Willis, 1979) point out that pain does not seem to be a prominent symptom of OM in the aboriginal population, and Eldridge and colleagues (1970) speculate that Guamanian children may have a high rate of asymptomatic middle ear inflammation. As pain is an almost universal symptom of OM in the Indian population, the climatic variable may be one meriting further investigation.

The association of OM with upper respiratory infections is seen to have a direct relationship to disease rate variations during the year. The highly variable weather conditions in the various locales under consideration do not support climate and geographical location as primary considerations in susceptibility of the people to the disease.

Infant Nutrition, Feeding Position, and Diet

In Australia, Jose (1979) reports that among the aborigines, breast feeding appears to confer some protection against chronic rhinitis, a precursor to OM. A report from American Samoa, cited by Harding (1978), has stated that OM on these islands results partially from horizontal feeding with a bottle rather than almost vertical feeding as is common during breast feeding.

A number of studies have been reported in the literature on this subject form the vantage point of the American Indians. Schaefer (1971), for example, in accounting for more OM when there is a higher standard of living, argued that the trend toward bottle feeding and shorter lactation periods in more acculturated Eskimo families may be an important variable in this phenomenon. Citing a lack of protective features in cow's milk, he observed substantially more disease of greater severity in the bottle-fed children.

Ellestad-Sayed and colleagues (1979) studied the feeding issue in Manitoba (Canada) Indian communities and found that fully bottle fed infants were hospitalized 10 times more often, and spent 10 times more time in the hospital, than did breast fed children. The infections were primarily in the lower respiratory and gastrointestinal tracts, with disease patterns found to be independent of family size, overcrowding, parental income, and education.

Specific to OM, Timmermans and Gerson (1980) studied 315 children in Labrador, Canada, 47 of whom were non-native, and found that the prevalence of OM was inversely related to the age when bottle feeding started. They suggested that OM was a result of a process leading to chronic foreign body granuloma formed by milk forced into the relatively short and straight eustachian tube by the intraoral pressures necessary in bottle feeding. Beauregard (1971) has given several reasons why position is a significant variable in this regard: (1) In breast feeding, the infant is almost always held in a more upright position, (2) breast feeding does not require generation of as strong a negative pressure, and (3) the infant has to adapt sucking technique for the bottle, whereas the breast adapts itself to the infant's sucking.

One of the more detailed analyses of dietary effects on OM among Australian aborigines is that of Stuart (1979), who cited research indicating that children were dependent on the mother's diet. He recommended ascorbic acid supplements for the children, as well as for the mothers.

Sunderman (1979) commented on dietary effects from a more

conventional viewpoint. He observed that dietary changes accompanying acculturation, with coincidental extended contact with white people, is accompanied by discharging ears.

For a number of years, until very recently, breast feeding was associated to a large extent with lower income families. Such a preconception would further obscure the interaction of variables associated with the effect of feeding on OM. It now appears that although breast feeding may help prevent OM, the variable is confounded by (1) feeding position — breast feeding while the infant is supine offers no advantage over bottle propping, (2) adequacy of the mother's diet, and (3) the time the nursing infant is given supplementary solid food and its nutritional composition.

Other Environmental Factors

Vincent (1979) cited poor housing, poor sanitation, overcrowding, and poor water as common denominators in OM among the aborigines. Brown (1979) indicated that socioeconomic depression, associated with gross overcrowding, poor living conditions, and inadequate hygiene, is a key obstacle to prevention in this population.

In Hawaii, Watson (1966) described the area of his study as characterized by high proportions of low income families, dilapidated housing, and high unemployment while Olkeriil (1982), speaking for Palau, cited limited health services, unsanitary urban living conditions, polluted environment, and hot, humid climate as factors contributing to overall health problems in Koror and other sites in the Trust Territories.

Many of the authors of articles pertaining to the Indians suggest a major role is played by these variables in the prevalence of OM in this population. Reinhard, Huntley, Becker, Philip, and Jackson (1960) stated that bacterial infections alone could not account for the excessive rates of OM, and various socioeconomic variables have been reported in many of the studies cited in Table 9–1.

Shaw, Todd, Goodwin, and Feldman (1981), in research conducted over several years, found no environmental or behavioral factor to be strongly or consistently associated with the incidence of acute suppurative otitis media (ASOM) or the frequency of disease attacks. Neither overall rates of ASOM nor high rates of ASOM (three or more attacks during the first year of life) were found to be associated with presence or absence of adverse environmental conditions.

A broader scope of environmental and related conditions, as specified by Paradise (1980), is perhaps more inclusive of the following factors: Crowding, poor nutrition, inadequate hygiene, relative insensitivity and lack of attention to symptoms, lack of access to high quality health care, and limited compliance with prescribed medical regimens. Paradise concludes, on the basis of the number of studies implicating these factors, that they must be provisionally considered real.

As substandard living conditions are routinely associated with OM prevalence in these populations it is easy to assume a cause-and-effect relationship. The limited research evidence presented, however, requires that such an assumption, although having some validity, must be kept in perspective. The racial variations in disease prevalence, cited previously, when living conditions and other factors are highly similar, is of particular significance in this regard.

Service Delivery Systems

Although they evolved separately, the medical-audiological service delivery systems for the indigenous peoples of Australia, Micronesia, and North America show many common characteristics — for example, they are government operated, thinly distributed, and underfunded. More local autonomy, improvements in living conditions and facilities, recognition of the problem, and emphasis on public education and professional training of local persons are keys to improved service delivery.

In Australia, otolaryngological services are provided largely by private practitioners through regional health offices operated by the government. Services under direct governmental control tend to stress the pediatric population. At the present time, OM detection and treatment programs are often operated in conjunction with trachoma control programs. A recent trend is for the aborigines to be trained to provide services to their own people.

American Samoa and Micronesia are considered as "states" for purposes of health planning and United States government funding. There is one medical center in American Samoa, the Lyndon B. Johnson Tropical Medical Center, which is staffed by both Caucasian and Samoan professionals. In common with most of the other programs in Australia and North America, the hearing program consists primarily of nurse operated screenings on children for hearing and vision problems.

Facilities in Guam, owing to its location and status as a United States possession for over 80 years, has the highest level of medical care in Micronesia. It has a moderately sized and staffed hospital operated by the government of Guam, several private medical clinics, and a large naval hospital whose services are available to Guama-

nians affiliated with the armed services. Audiological and ENT services have been available since 1968 and, owing to a particularly competent and dynamic staff, services have been expanded to include
programs for the speech handicapped, deaf-blind, learning disabled,
developmentally disabled, and others. Finally, the University of
Guam has initiated a bachelor's level training program in speech
and hearing for all of Micronesia.

In the Republic of Palau, the only hospital (in Koror) is a government facility. Dispensaries staffed by a nurse or nurse's aide provide
services in the outer islands. Patients having major problems are
sent to Guam or Honolulu for further treatment.

In common with other indigenous people in the areas discussed
in this chapter, there is a very strong movement for self-
determination among various geopolitical factions. Their future status has either recently been decided or is currently under consideration at the local level.

The service delivery systems for North America have certain
similarities in first having been established by the respective gov-
ernments of Canada and the United States. Even though assimilation and movement of Native Americans into cities has changed the
systems considerably, the Indians of each country tend to identify
health care providers with the government system rather than with
the private sector.

Services in the United States are provided through regionalized
programs to all federally recognized tribes throughout the country.
Administrative supervision is provided by an Area Office, which
oversees the locally based health facilities.

Specific programs for hearing disabilities for North American Indians were first established in 1970 with the primary focus on OM
remediation and control. Depending upon the Area and the success
in meeting the original program objectives, these services have expanded to include speech therapy, maxillofacial anomalies clinics,
cleft palate services, and developmental disabilities programs. In addition to early detection and intervention programs for a wide range
of hearing impaired children, a full range of audiological and otological services, including the dispensing of hearing aids, is also
provided.

Owing to individual program variations in local needs, funding
base, local governmental and tribal interest, and accessibility of necessary personnel, no given program can be termed typical of the
overall system. Personnel shortages in such medical specialties as
ENT, for example, necessitate the use of private practitioners whose
availability is not consistent. As is the case for programs in Austra-

lia and the Pacific Basin, each Area uses indigenous paraprofessionals in varying degrees, ranging from fully qualified operating room technicians who are capable of performing otoscopy, audiometry and impedance tests to persons with minimal experience in puretone screening audiometry only. Other health care providers in the field are responsible for patient contact at home, providing parent counseling, overseeing treatment regimens, and similar tasks which may or may not require the use of instruments. Hearing aid followup presents particular problems, especially for the elderly user, who may live alone. Local paraprofessionals in varying locations perform these functions in the absence of any nearby hospital or clinic.

Throughout the United States there is a concerted effort to see that Indians have access to all services and systems to which they are entitled as citizens. Programs such as Medicaid and Medicare are now being integrated more fully into the service delivery system, and many states have for years been primary providers of services, such as hearing screening, so that there has not been much overlap of programs. As more Indians enter the mainstream workforce, they take greater advantage of hospital and medical insurance plans to provide for their needs.

The major unmet needs of Indians with hearing impairment generally are related to (1) the lack of comprehensive hearing health care in any given Area; (2) the competition for scarce funds with higher priority, life-threatening conditions; and (3) low public awareness of the need for and availability of programs to prevent, identify, treat, and rehabilitate hearing disorders and ear diseases.

Income

In general, the residents of the Pacific islands, Australia, Indian reservations, and Alaskan villages have recent histories with much in common; all were small bands of people, many of them nomadic, and dependent upon their immediate environments for their survival. The advent, and eventual dominance, of the Europeans into their homelands resulted in their exposure to and dependence upon lifestyles that were completely foreign to them. Without the educational skills and shared cultural values, such as the necessity to compete, the indigenous peoples were suddenly put into the lowest stratum of the new society with little hope of ever rising. With some racial intermingling, new social strata have evolved, with those of mixed ancestry able to ascent higher and faster within the prevailing non-native culture. These people generally then have more educational opportunities of which they are better equipped to take advantage without the strong bonds of the native culture impeding their course.

In one recent instance, the withdrawal of the foreign influence has had even more dramatic effects on local lifestyles. During World War II, the remote islands of the Pacific were rapidly inundated with Caucasians with different motivations for occupying the territory. Much has been written of the destructive effects that the withdrawal of armed forces following that war had on the economy and culture of Micronesia, when the major economic base of the islands, and the people who were responsible for it, were suddenly withdrawn. Having been given responsibility for most of Micronesia following the war, United States support for the islanders caused it to develop into a near welfare state with high unemployment — because of no industries and no business base — that retained the American lifestyle, which largely overtook the native way of life.

In Palau, about half the population of 14,000 lives in Koror, largely owing to a decline of the native farming economy (Olkeriil, 1982) and a migration to the capital in pursuit of government jobs, the greatest source of employment. The Guamanian economy, by virtue of the island's status and location, is much more stable in the urban area but, again, it is largely dependent on the United States military presence and a fluctuating tourist industry.

Although it was not as directly affected by wartime activities as Micronesia, American Samoa has undergone drastic changes in its economy during the postwar years. There are two industries in Samoa besides tourism, tuna canning and the export of copra. Although the people are citizens of the United States and have voting rights, their political impact is minimal. Except for the Guamanians, the remainder of the Pacific islanders have even less influence on political decisions that affect their lives. Their small numbers, their distance from the mainland United States, and their lack of control over their own destinies make these people among the most disenfranchised under the American sphere of influence.

American Indians are traditionally at the lowest rung of the economic ladder, with unemployment on some reservations currently running at 80 percent. Although there are numerous family industries among American Indians, ranging from ivory carving in Alaska to basket making in Florida, with few significant exceptions these industries have not provided a substantial economic base in the community. Many reservations have developed mineral resources, such as coal, gas, uranium, and oil, and these industries have provided employment, but their impact upon the overall economy likewise has been minimal. Attempts to locate small industries on reservations have met with mixed success, and current efforts at establishing bingo games and tax-free sales of tobacco and liquor on tribal property have had varied impact, but at best provide only minimal work opportunities. In some locales, Indian tribes have developed a tourist industry with motels, recreational facilities, and hunting and fishing opportunities.

The largest employer of Indians is the federal government, primarily through the IHS and Bureau of Indian Affairs (BIA). The skills necessary for government employment have necessitated increased awareness and opportunity for education. With relatively recent legislation mandating that qualified Indians be given job preference in these two agencies, more young Indian people have work opportunities in both city and reservation settings. A number of federal and tribal scholarship programs are encouraging Indian youth to pursue the course of advanced education, largely with the aim of furthering self-determination. Service delivery systems, income, and political power are closely interrelated and, in the case of the peoples described, work to the detriment of this care. In each of these small populations service delivery is hindered by (1) geography — miles of tundra, desert, and ocean separate the groups into even smaller groups, (2) lack of resources to provide for transportation of professionals and patients to adequate facilities for their care, and (3) the shortage of professional personnel willing and able to live in the places where they are needed.

Adequate service delivery systems to address these problems would seem to depend on (1) an adequate economic base for the consumers of these services and the taxes that would accrue from it, (2) a substantial number of voting citizens who could then exert the political influence necessary to effect desirable changes in the system, which in turn could (3) draw upon local talent to develop the professional cadre to provide these services. None of the populations under consideration in this chapter have any one of these key factors.

Cultural Factors

Any culture that does not recognize the existence of a health problem, or that cannot provide treatment, must have the problem resolved by neglect or, if serious enough, by death. Although all the peoples described in this chapter have native medical practitioners, very little information is available from most of them regarding the recognition of hearing disease and impairment. For example, there is evidence that in Micronesia the very high prevalence of otorrhea has led to its being considered a normal occurrence (Olkeriil, 1982).

A similar situation reportedly existed in Alaska until a few years ago. Welch (personal communication, 1978) reports that the director of maternal and child health services indicated that mothers in American Samoa typically gave no more thought in the past to ear discharges than to a running nose.

Relatively extensive literature exists pertaining to the treatment of ear disorders affecting American Indians. In addition to the use of native medicines obtained from plants, heated animal fat has been placed in the ear canal by practitioners from many Indian tribes. Eagle down (which is also treated spiritually) and seal or whale blubber have also been used in the ear canal (Bedwell, 1978). One tribe in New Mexico, the Zuni, admonishes children that their grandmothers live in the ear, and putting anything in the canal may harm grandmother; this may help prevent ear disorders.

Socioeducational Implications

The severity of socioeducational factors in the life of the child with hearing deficiency is undisputed and has been the subject of research, discussion, and planning for a number of years. Without adequate hearing a child will not fully develop those life skills upon which his or her entire life depends — speech, language, full educational potential, and vocational choice. The effects of hearing impairment acquired in later life have received less attention, clearly, but still point to the necessity of adequate hearing as the cornerstone of adequate communication skills, which are critical to all aspects of living and quality of life.

Over the past 15 years, the greatest amount of discussion, investigation, and controversy has been over the effects of OM — whose pervasiveness has been seen throughout this chapter to be overwhelming in some groups — on the languages and learning skills of the affected child. More and more of the published reports, which have included research on aborigines (Lewis, 1976) and Alaska natives (Kaplan et al., 1973), have concentrated on the effects of mild, intermittent bouts of OM on these skills.

Two recent articles (Paradise, 1981; Ventry, 1980) have been devoted to critical reviews of the evidence to date and have reached the following conclusions. First, the research to that time was not sufficient to give an unequivocal answer to the questions and that research must continue. Second, there is no overwhelming and conclusive evidence that hearing disorders can result from single or lasting episodes of ear disease in early life, provided that the episodes subside without leaving residual hearing impairment.

More recently, Kirkwood and Kirkwood (1983) have responded to these conclusions with the observations that no single definitive study has showed a causal relationship between relatively mild OM and learning disabilities. Yet the weight of the evidence of the large number of studies, on highly differing populations, meets the criterion of biological plausibility (among others), so that a strong suggestion of relationship can be made.

If this latter conclusion has validity, findings from other unpublished research reports on American Indian children may be of interest. McShane (1982), citing his own research on Ojibwa children using the Wechsler Intelligence Scales and the Illinois Test of Psycholinguistic Abilities (ITPA), found differences between a group with a history of OM (more than four episodes) compared with a group of children with fewer than four episodes. Children with histories of OM scored lower on auditory-verbal subtests than on the visual subtests, although this difference was not observed in the group of children with fewer episodes.

These results compare favorably with results reported by Stewart (1980) on the verbal skills of Zuni Indian Headstart and elementary school children in which children with histories of repeated episodes of OM prior to the age 2 years were compared with children having no such history. Even in the absence of an OM history, the children largely scored below the norm for those tests requiring auditory skills, although the OM children scored appreciably lower. There was a tendency, also, for children with and without OM histories to score higher on the visual tests. As there has been speculation that Indian children generally appear to be more visually than auditorily oriented, it may be that this variable is confounding the results. Using the criteria of Kirkwood and Kirkwood (1983), however, the evidence for an OM effect on language and learning in Indian children is supportable.

The statement that culture determines behavior is aphoristic. That behavior affects culture is perhaps a less widely held notion, but unless people accept culturally determined beliefs and values on the need for adequate hearing, for example, those beliefs and values and their manifestations, such as the availability of native medical practitioners, will not survive.

For indigenous peoples to accept less well-established values, such as the need for formal education, as we in the United States define it, as well as the need for fully functioning sensory systems to achieve educationally, socially, and vocationally as being of value for its own sake (and not just at the behest of the prevailing Caucasian culture), requires a process of evolution. This process requires that these values be viewed as desirable within the context of the native culture.

That this evolutionary process may be going on may be inferred from the (1) coexistence of traditional and modern medicine, (2) the increasing numbers of Pacific islanders, American Indians, and Australian aborigines entering institutions of higher learning, and (3) the resultant integration of these persons in health, education, legal, and other fields, many of whom are returning to their own locales to practice their professions.

The peoples described in this chapter are often considered among the more culturally diverse in the world. Their problems of prevalence of hearing disability, the cultural recognition of hearing disability as a problem to be met, and barriers to delivery of services have been discussed in detail. The same anthropological techniques used in many of the foregoing reports have equal validity when this problem is addressed in urban and rural predominantly black communities, white Appalachia, or suburban America. Although it is not a regularly addressed aspect of the contemporary curriculum, acquaintance with and appreciation for this body of knowledge is essential for more rigorous research and more effective clinical practice.

The indigenous peoples of North America and the Pacific Basin occupy a geographical area of tremendous expanse, from mountains to oceans and from ice caps to tropics. Variations in temperature range from arctic cold to equatorial heat and humidity and from the dryness of the desert to the wetness of a rain forest. Similar variations are seen in diet, religious beliefs, occupations, and overall lifestyles.

At the same time, these peoples share many similarities. All are of Asian descent, and most live outside the mainstream in small communities, retain those elements of their cultures that have the most value for them, and have stubbornly resisted all efforts to convert them into people that they are not. They also share a number of common problems, including disease susceptibilities, many of which are related to who they are and where they came from.

The European settlers of these aboriginal territories brought with them religious, social, educational, and vocational values that were largely foreign to the original inhabitants. They also brought with them diseases that either were previously unknown or had been treated by traditional medical-religious means by local practitioners. Preexisting conditions for which there were no or insufficient remedies were accounted for by other means. Otitis media, although not an imported problem, was one for which most indigenous people either had treatments or accepted. The use of warmed animal fat in the infected ear was a common example of the first instance; the example of Indian mothers equating a draining ear with the loss of deciduous teeth as an expected consequence of child growth is an example of the second.

The pattern of colonialism in all these areas followed rather similar lines, from "benign neglect" on the one hand to acceptance of responsibility for the welfare of the conquered people on the other. Finding that the problems still would not go away, the governing bodies of these newly conquered territories accepted the responsibility for the care of this new body of citizens. With this responsibility came the need to determine the extent of problems needing resolution, and one of the foremost health problems affecting all of these societies is otitis media and resultant hearing loss.

The peoples of the Pacific islands and North America share the problem of having the highest prevalence of OM and related hearing disorders in the world. Although the reasons for the extent of this problem are not entirely clear, evidence at hand indicates a number of variables at work, all of which not only contribute to the extent of the problem but also work against its solution.

All of the peoples under consideration are of Asiatic origin and a common anatomical skull structure has been implicated as a causative factor. The age at which the disease first strikes and its severity are likely related to anatomy but also, in some instances, to immune system deficiency in infants and feeding practices during infancy. Sex differences appear to be significant in some cases, but this finding by itself is difficult to relate to prevalence. Although geography, climate, and other environmental factors play a role, their individual contributions to the extent of the problem are unclear.

Other environmental conditions, such as housing, nutrition, and economic status, are also thought to contribute to disease prevalence, but, once again, how these variables impact on the problem is not sufficiently established.

Preventing the acute stage of the disease seems as feasible as preventing the common cold. Preventing the chronic stage of the disease depends on an efficient and comprehensive medical service delivery system. The costs of such a system, the need to staff the facilities necessary, and the geographical and climatic obstacles have not, to date, allowed systems to develop that can be truly said to have achieved this prevention potential. Habilitation and rehabilitation programs for the hearing impaired face the same obstacles as programs in primary medical care.

Service delivery problems are further confounded by the fact that the recipients of these services by virtue of their location, numbers and limited participation in the political process, have not developed their political strengths sufficiently to assure improvement.

Dealing with issues so complex as management of otitis media and hearing loss in these populations requires not only technical and professional skills but also the sensitivity to work with and for people whose values and beliefs are not your own, who do not share your own concepts of time, possession, or importance of the problems at hand. The rewards are achieved by the satisfaction that comes with knowing that the problems, although large, are not entirely insurmountable and that each day spent has resulted in tangible benefits to those being served.

REFERENCES

American Samoa Health Coordinating Council. (1978). *American Samoa plan for health, 1978–83*, p. 49.

Baske, R. F. (1968). Ear screening program at the Hays, Mission, and Lodgepole schools. *Indian Health* (USPHS), *1*, 8.

Baxter, J. D. (1981). The evolving attitude in Canada toward the management of chronic otitis media in the Inuit population. *Journal of Otolaryngology, 10*, 81.

Baxter, J. D. (1982). Observations on the evolution of chronic otitis media in the Inuit of the Baffin Zone, NWT. *Journal of Otolaryngology, 11*, 161.

Baxter, J. D., and Ling, D. (1972). Hearing loss among Baffin Zone Eskimos — a preliminary report. *Canadian Journal of Otolaryngology, 1*, 337.

Baxter, J. D., and Ling, D. (1974). Ear disease and hearing loss among the Eskimo population of the Baffin Zone. *Canadian Journal of Otolaryngology, 3*, 110.

Baxter, J. D., Karsarkas, A., Ling, D., and Carson, R. (1979). The conservative treatment of chronic otitis media in Inuit elementary school children. *Journal of Otolaryngology, 8*, 201.

Beauregard, W. G. (1971). Positional otitis media. *Journal of Pediatrics, 79* (2), 94.

Bedwell, K. L. (1978, November). American Indian Medicine Man and the treatment of ear disorders. Paper presented at ASHA Convention, San Francisco.

Beery, Q. C., Doyle, W. J., Bluestone, C. D., Cantekin, E. I., and Wiet, R. J. (1980). Eustachian tube function in the American Indian population. *Annals of Otology, Rhinology, and Laryngology, 89*, 28.

Berg, D. E., Larsen, A. E., and Yarrington, C. T., Jr. (1971). Association between serum and secretory immunoglobulins and chronic otitis media in Indian children. *Annals of Otology, Rhinology, and Otolaryngology, 80*, 766.

Brody, J. A. (1964). Notes on the epidemiology of draining ears and hearing loss in Alaska with comments on future studies and control measures. *Alaska Medicine, 6*, 1.

Brody, J. A., Overfield, T., and McAlister, R. (1965). Draining ears and deafness among Alaskan Eskimos. *Archives of Otolaryngology, 81*, 29.

Brown, M. W. (1972). The extent of ENT disease in the Aboriginal popula-
tion of the Northern Territory. *Journal of the Otolaryngologic Society of
Australia, 3,* 327.
Brown, M. (1979). Otitis media in aborigines: Identification and manage-
ment: 1688–1970. In M. Brown (Ed.), *Ear disease in aboriginal children,*
Melbourne: Otolaryngological Society of Australia.
Cambon, K., Galbraith, J. D., and Kong, G. (1965). Middle-ear disease in In-
dians of the Mount Currie Reservation, British Columbia. *Canadian
Medical Association Journal, 93,* 1301.
Canterbury, D. R., Dixon, C. L., Gish, K. D., Kimball, B. D., Lopez, M. B., Mc-
Carty, M. A., and Bryant, P. (1981). Hearing loss in Alaska.
Clements, D. A. (1968). Otitis media and hearing loss in a small Aboriginal
community. *Medical Journal of Australia, 16,* 665.
Corkery, L. (1973). The natural history of tympanic membrane perforation
on the Wind River Reservation. Report to the Billings Area Indian
Health Service.
Doyle, P. J., and Morwood, D. (1976). Middle ear disease in native Indian
children in British Columbia. Incidence of disease and an evaluation of
screening methods. *Journal of Otolaryngology, 5,* 103.
Doyle, W. J. (1977). *A functional-anatomic description of Eustachian tube vec-
tor relations in four ethnic populations — an osteologic study.* Unpublished doctoral dissertation, University of Pittsburgh.
Eldridge, R., Brody, J. A., and Wetmore, N. (1970). Hearing loss and otitis
media on Guam. *Archives of Otolaryngology, 91,* 148.
Ellestad-Sayed, J., Coobin, F.J., and Dilling, L. (1979). Breast feeding pro-
tects against infection in Indian infants. *Canadian Medical Association
Journal, 120,* 295.
Goinz, J. (in press). Incidence of otitis media among pre-school and school
age children in the States of Michigan, Minnesota, and Wisconsin. *Hearing Instruments.*
Graham, M. D. (1975). Prevalence of middle ear disease among the Indian
population of coastal British Columbia. *Hearing Instruments, 26,* 26.
Gray, L. P. (1979). The aboriginal problem: A western Australian assess-
ment. In Brown, M. (Ed.), *Ear Disease in Aboriginal Children.* Mel-
bourne: Otolaryngological Society of Australia.
Gregg, J. B., Steele, J. P., and Holzhueter, A. (1965). Roentgenographic evalu-
ation of temporal bones from South Dakota Indian burials. *American
Journal of Physical Anthropology, 23,* 51.
Gregg, J. B., Steele, J. P., Clifford, S., and Werthman, H. E. (1970). A multi-
disciplinary study of ear disease in South Dakota Indian Children.
South Dakota Medical Journal, 23, 1.
Harding, J. R. (1978). Otitis media and trachoma prevalence in American
Samoa. Unpublished final report, contract number HEW 7-200789, In-
dian Health Service.
Ickes, W. K., and Keel, D. (1982). High prevalence of otitis media among In-
dian children: Fact or myth. *Hearing Instruments, 33,* 22.
Jaffe, B. F. (1969). The incidence of ear diseases in the Navajo Indians. *La-
ryngoscope, 79,* 2126.
Jaffe, B. F., Hurtado, F., and Hurtado, E. (1970). Tympanic membrane mobil-
ity in the newborn (with seven months' follow-up). *Laryngoscope, 80,* 36.
Johnson, R. L. (1967). Chronic otitis media in school age Navajo Indians. *Laryngoscope, 77,* 1990.

Johonnot, S. C. (1973). Differences in chronic otitis media between rural and urban Eskimo children. *Clinical Pediatrics, 23,* 415.

Jose, D. (1979). Nutritional and immunological factors in otitis media in Aboriginal children. In Brown, M. (Ed.). *Ear disease in aboriginal children.* Melbourne: Otolaryngological Society of Australia.

Kaplan, G. J., Fleshman, J. K., Bender, T. R., Baum, C., and Clark, P. S. (1973). Long-term effects of otitis media: A ten-year cohort study of Alaska Eskimo children. *Pediatrics, 52,* 577.

Kirke, D. (1969). Growth rates of aboriginal children in central Australia. *Medical Journal of Australia, 2,* 1005.

Kirke, D. (1970). *Aboriginal infant and toddler mortality in Central Australia 1965-1969.* Doctoral thesis, University of Adelaide, South Australia.

Kirkwood, C. R., and Kirkwood, M. E. (1983). Otitis media and learning disabilities: The case for a causal relationship. *Journal of Family Practice, 17,* 219.

Lewis, A. N., Barry, M., and Stuart, J. E. (1976). Screening procedures for the identification of hearing and ear disorders in Australian aboriginal children. *Journal of Laryngology and Otology, 88* (4), 335.

Lewis, N. (1974). Otitis media and linguistic incompetence. *Archives of Otolaryngology, 102,* 387.

Ling, D., McCoy, R. H., and Levinson, E. D. (1969). The incidence of middle ear disease and its educational implications among Baffin Island Eskimo children. *Canadian Journal of Public Health, 60,* 385.

Lupin, A. J. (1976). Ear disease in Western Canadian natives with a note on treatment by tympanoplasty. *Journal of Otolaryngology, 5,* 116.

Maynard, J. C. (1969). Otitis media in Alaskan Eskimo children. *Alaska Medicine, 11,* 93.

McCandless, G. A. (1973). Screening for middle ear disease on Wind River Reservation. Final Report, University of Utah Contract, Indian Health Service.

McCandless, G. A., and Parkin, J. L. (1976). Otitis media among various Indian populations. Final Report, University of Utah Contract, Indian Health Service.

McCuddin, C. R. (1978). Project evaluation — American Samoa hearing screening project. Grant No. 09-H-001291-01-0.

McShane, D. (1979). Middle ear disease, hearing loss, and language and educational delay in American Indian children. Unpublished manuscript.

McShane, D. (1982). Otitis media and American Indians: Prevalence, etiology, psycho-educational consequences, prevention and intervention. In Manson, S. (Ed.), *New directions in prevention in American Indian and Alaska Native communities.* Portland: Oregon Health Sciences University Press.

Middleton, M. R., and Francis, S. H. (1976). *Yuendumu and its children — life and health on an aboriginal settlement.* Canberra: Australian Government Publishing Service.

Moran, D. J., Waterford, J. E., Hollows, F., and Jones, D. L. (1979). Ear disease in rural Australia. *Medical Journal of Australia, 2,* 210.

Nelson, S. M., and Berry, R. I. (1984). Ear disease and hearing loss among Navajo children — a mass survey. *Laryngoscope, 94*(3), 316.

Olkeriil, D. (1982). Otoscopic, tympanometric and audiometric survey in

Koror. Unpublished project report, Department of Speech Pathology and Audiology, University of Hawaii — Manoa.

Paradise, J. L. (1980). Otitis media in infants and children. *Pediatrics, 65,* 917.

Paradise, J. L. (1981). Otitis media during early life: How hazardous to development? A critical review of the evidence. *Pediatrics, 68,* 869.

Perkins, G., and Church, G. (1960). Report of pediatric evaluations on a sample of Indian children — Wind River Indian Reservation. *American Journal of Public Health, 50,* 181.

Rao, A. B. N. (1979). Northwest Territory presentation. In Brown, M. (Ed.), *Ear disease in aboriginal children.* Melbourne: Otolaryngological Society of Australia.

Ratnesar, P. (1976). Chronic ear disease along the coasts of Labrador and Northern Newfoundland. *Journal of Otolaryngology, 5,* 122.

Reed, D., and Dunn, W. (1970). Epidemiologic studies of otitis media among Eskimo children. *Public Health Reports, 85,* 699.

Reed, D., Struve, S., and Maynard, J. E. (1967). Otitis media and hearing deficiency among Eskimo children: a cohort study. *American Journal of Public Health, 57,* 1657.

Reinhard, K. R., Huntley, B. E., Becker, R. A., Philip, R. N., and Jackson, H. (1970). Bacteriological studies on exudative otitis media occurring in six communities of Alaskan natives. *Acta Otolaryngologica, Supplementum 260,* 1.

Roberts, M. E. (1976). Comparative study of pure-tone impedance, and otoscopic hearing screening methods. *Archives of Otolaryngology, Supplement 260,* 1.

Schaefer, O. (1971). Otitis media and bottle feeding: An epidemiological study of infant feeding habits and incidence of recurrent and chronic middle ear disease in Canadian Eskimos. *Canadian Journal of Public Health, 62,* 478.

Shaw, J. R., Todd, N. W., Goodwin, M. H., and Feldman, C. M. (1981). Observations on the relation of environmental and behavioral factors to the occurrence of otitis media among Indian children. *Public Health Reports, 96,* 342.

Shaw, J. R., Goodwin, M. H., and Feldman, C. M. (1982). Otitis media project annual report. Phoenix Area Indian Health Service.

Spivey, G. H., and Hirschhorn, N. (1977). A migrant study of adopted Apache children. *Johns Hopkins Medical Journal, 140,* 43.

Stewart, J. L. (1980). *Zuni otitis media research report.* Unpublished internal report, Indian Health Service, Department of Health and Human Services, Rockville, MD.

Stewart, J. L. (1983). Communication disorders in the American Indian population. In Omark, D. R., and Erickson, J. G. (Eds.), *The bilingual exceptional child.* San Diego, College-Hill Press.

Stewart, J. L. (1984). Otitis media among American Indians: Navajo. Unpublished manuscript.

Stuart, J. (1979). Some paediatric aspects of ear disease in aboriginal children. In Brown, M. (Ed.), *Ear disease in aboriginal children.* Melbourne: Otolaryngological Society of Australia.

Sunderman, J. (1979). The management of deafness in children of the Western Australian Outback. In Brown, M. (Ed.), *Ear disease in aboriginal children.* Melbourne: Otolaryngological Society of Australia.

Timmermans, F. J. W., and Gerson, S. (1980). Chronic granulomatous otitis media in bottle fed Inuit children. *Canada Medical Association Journal, 122,* 545.

Titche, L. L., Coulthard, S. W., Wachter, R. D., Thies, A. C., and Harris, L. L. (1981). *American Journal of Physical Anthropology, 56,* 269.

Toubbeh, J. (in preparation). Measurement of effects: Evaluation of the IHS otitis media program.

Tower, E. A. (1979). Chronic otitis media in the Alaskan natives. *Alaska Medicine, 21,* 48.

Ventry, I. M. (1980). Effects of conductive hearing loss: Fact or fiction. *Journal of Speech and Hearing Disorders, 56,* 143.

Vercoe, G. (1979). South Australian presentation: Survey of aboriginal E.N.T disease in the Yalata-Ceduna area. In Brown, M. (Ed.), *Ear disease in aboriginal children.* Melbourne: Otolaryngological Society of Australia.

Vincent, G. K. (1979). New South Wales presentation. In Brown, M. (Ed.), *Ear disease in aboriginal children.* Melbourne: Otolaryngological Society of Australia.

Watrous, B. S., Garcia, C. Z., Brown, G. W., and Wasylenki, E. (1980). *Otitis media in three racial groups in an institutionalized mentally retarded population.* Unpublished manuscript, Indian Health Service, 1980.

Watson, J. (1966, September). *The Nanakuli special project.* Unpublished candidate's thesis. Council of the American Laryngological, Rhinological, and Otological Society.

Weymuller, E. A., and Reed, D. G. (1972). Otological problems of the Alaska native population. *Laryngoscope, 82,* 1793.

Wiet, R. J. (1979). Patterns of ear disease in the Southwestern American Indian. *Archives of Otolaryngology, 105,* 381.

Wiet, R. J., DeBlanc, G. B., Stewart, J. L., and Weider, D. J. (1980). Natural history of otitis media in the American Native. *Annals of Otology, Rhinology, and Laryngology, 89,* 14.

Willis, R. (1979). Deafness in aboriginal children. In Brown, M. (Ed.), *Ear disease in aboriginal children.* Melbourne: Otolaryngological Society of Australia.

Zonis, R. D. (1968a). Chronic otitis media in the Southwestern American Indian, I. Prevalence. *Archives of Otolaryngology, 88,* 40.

Zonis, R. D. (1968b). Chronic otitis media in the Southwestern American Indian, II. Immunological factors. *Archives of Otolaryngology, 88,* 46.

Postscript:

Where Do We Go from Here?

In this book, we have addressed background issues pertaining to anthropological and linguistic considerations associated with the study of communication disorders in culturally and linguistically diverse populations. Following these discussions we have proceeded to present an analysis of normal communicative behavior in a select group of culturally and linguistically diverse populations in the United States. Finally, we have summarized the literature on the prevalence and nature of several cultural and linguistic groups.

So, where do we go from here? First, we must conduct more research, particularly on populations given little attention in this book (e.g., Asians) on the various topics we have explored. Only in this way can we ever hope to acquire a comprehensive view of the diverse and complex nature of culture and of normal and pathological cognition, language and communication as it exists among the populations of the United States.

Second, it is suggested that the reader proceed from this introductory exploration of the nature of communication disorders in culturally and linguistically diverse populations to an examination of appropriate diagnostic and treatment considerations and procedures for these populations. These subjects are covered in our companion volume, *Treatment of Communication Disorders in Culturally and Linguistically Diverse Populations.*

Appendix A

Position of the American Speech-Language-Hearing Association on Social Dialects*

The English language is comprised of many linguistic varieties, such as Black English,* standard English, Appalachian English, southern English, New York dialect, and Spanish influenced English. The features of social dialects are systematic and highly regular and cross all linguistic parameters, i.e., phonology, morphology, syntax, semantics, lexicon, pragmatics, suprasegmental features, and kinesics. Although each dialect of English has distinguishing characteristics, the majority of linguistic features of the English language are common to each of the varieties of English. The existence of these varieties is the result of historical and social factors. For example, due to historical factors, the majority of Black English speakers are Black. However, due to social factors, not all Black individuals are Black English speakers.

The issue of social dialects for the field of speech-language pathology is extremely complex as indicated by the continuous controversy across the nation over the past two decades. There has been confusion among professionals regarding the role of the speech-language pathologist with reference to speakers of social dialects. There has been no consistent philosophy regarding the approach of service delivery to speakers of social dialects. As a result, some speech-language pathologists have denied clinical services to speakers of social dialects who have requested services. Other speech-language pathologists have treated social dialects as though they were communicative disorders.

It is the position of the American Speech-Language-Hearing Association (ASHA) that no dialectal variety of English is a disorder or a pathological form of speech or language. Each social dialect is adequate as a functional and effective variety of English. Each serves a communication function as well as a social solidarity function. It maintains the communica-

---

*Some Black professionals prefer to use the terms Ebonics instead of the more popularly used term Black English. Derived from the words *ebony* and *phonics,* the term Ebonics is intended to avoid the focus on race and emphasize the ethnolinguistic origin and evolution of this variety of the English language.

tion network and the social construct of the community of speakers who use it. Furthermore, each is a symbolic representation of the historical, social, and cultural background of the speakers. For example, there is strong evidence that many of the features of Black English represent linguistic Africanisms.

However, society has adopted the linguistic idealization model that standard English is the linguistic archetype. Standard English is the linguistic variety used by government, the mass media, business, education, science, and the arts. Therefore, there may be nonstandard English speakers who find it advantageous to have access to the use of standard English.

The traditional role of the speech-language pathologist has been to provide clinical services to the communicatively handicapped. It is indeed possible for dialect speakers to have linguistic disorders within the dialect. An essential step toward making accurate assessments of communicative disorders is to distinguish between those aspects of linguistic variation that represent the diversity of the English language from those that represent speech, language, and hearing disorders. The speech-language pathologist must have certain competencies to distinguish between dialectal differences and communicative disorders. These competencies include knowledge of the particular dialect as a rule-governed linguistic system, knowledge of the phonological and grammatical features of the dialect, and knowledge of nondiscriminatory testing procedures. Once the difference-disorder distinctions have been made, it is the role of the speech-language pathologist to treat only those features or characteristics that are true errors and not attributable to the dialect.

Aside from the traditionally recognized role, the speech-language pathologist may also be available to provide *elective* clinical services to nonstandard English speakers who do not present a disorder. The role of the speech-language pathologist for these individuals is to provide the desired competency in standard English without jeopardizing the integrity of the individual's first dialect. The approach must be functional and based on context-specific appropriateness of the given dialect.

Provision of elective services to nonstandard English speakers requires sensitivity and competency in at least three areas: linguistic features of the dialect, linguistic contrastive analysis procedures, and the effects of attitudes toward dialects. It is prerequisite for the speech-language pathologist to have a thorough understanding and appreciation for the community and culture of the nonstandard English speaker. Further, it is a requirement that the speech-language pathologist have thorough knowledge of the linguistic rules of the particular dialect.

It remains the priority of the speech-language pathologist to continue to serve the truly communicatively handicapped. However, for nonstandard English speakers who seek elective clinical services, the speech-language pathologist may also serve in a consultative role to assist educators in utilizing the features of the nonstandard dialect to facilitate the learning of reading and writing in standard English. Just as competencies are assumed and necessary in the treatment of communicative disorders, competencies are also necessary in the provision of elective clinical services to nonstandard English speakers.

From ASHA, September 1983, pp. 23–25.

Appendix B

Standards for Effective Oral Communication Programs

Prepared by

American Speech-Language-Hearing Association
and
Speech Communication Association

Adequate oral communication frequently determines an individual's educational, social, and vocational success. Yet, American education has typically neglected formal instruction in the basic skills of speaking and listening. It is important that state and local education agencies implement the most effective oral communication programs possible.

The following standards for oral communication were developed by representatives of the Speech Communication Association and the American Speech-Language-Hearing Association.

If effective oral communication programs are going to be developed, all components of the recommended standards must be considered. Implementation of these standards will facilitate development of adequate and appropriate oral communication necessary for educational, social, and vocational success.

DEFINITION

Oral Communication: The process of interacting through heard and spoken messages in a variety of situations.

Effective oral communication is a learned behavior, involving the following processes:

1. Speaking in a variety of educational and social situations: Speaking involves, but is not limited to, arranging and producing messages through the use of voice, articulation, vocabulary, syntax, and nonverbal cues (e.g., gesture, facial expression, vocal cues) appropriate to the speaker and listeners.
2. Listening in a variety of educational and social situations: Listening involves, but is not limited to, hearing, perceiving, discriminating, interpreting, synthesizing, evaluating, organizing, and remembering information from verbal and nonverbal messages.

BASIC ASSUMPTIONS

1. Oral communication behaviors of students can be improved through direct instruction.
2. Oral communication instruction emphasizes the interactive nature of speaking and listening.
3. Oral communication instruction addresses the everyday communication needs of students and includes emphasis on the classroom as a practical communication environment.
4. There is a wide range of communication competence among speakers of the same language.
5. Communication competence is not dependent upon use of a particular form of language.
6. A primary goal of oral communication instruction is to increase the students' repertoire and use of effective speaking and listening behaviors.
7. Oral communication programs provide instruction based on a coordinated developmental continuum of skills, preschool through adult.
8. Oral communication skills can be enhanced by using parents, supportive personnel, and appropriate instructional technology.

AN EFFECTIVE COMMUNICATION PROGRAM HAS THE FOLLOWING CHARACTERISTICS

Teaching, Learning

1. The oral communication program is based on current theory and research in speech and language development, psycholinguistics, rhetorical and communication theory, communication disorders, speech science, and related fields of study.
2. Oral communication instruction is a clearly identifiable part of the curriculum.
3. Oral communication instruction is systematically related to reading and writing instruction and to instruction in the various content areas.
4. The relevant academic, personal, and social experiences of students provide core subject matter for the oral communication program.
5. Oral communication instruction provides a wide range of speaking and listening experience, in order to develop effective communication skills appropriate to:
   a. a range of situations; e.g., informal to formal, interpersonal to mass communication.
   b. a range of purposes; e.g., informing, learning, persuading, evaluating messages, facilitating social interaction, sharing feelings, imaginative and creative expression.
   c. a range of audiences; e.g., classmates, teachers, peers, employers, family, community.
   d. a range of communication forms; e.g., conversation, group discussion, interview, drama, debate, public speaking, oral interpretation.
   e. a range of speaking styles; impromptu, extemporaneous, and reading from manuscript.

6. The oral communication program provides class time for systematic instruction in oral communication skills, e.g., critical listening, selecting, arranging and presenting messages, giving and receiving constructive feedback, non-verbal communication, etc.
7. The oral communication program includes development of adequate and appropriate language, articulation, voice, fluency, and listening skills necessary for success in educational, career, and social situations through regular classroom instruction, cocurricular activities, and speech-language pathology and audiology services.
8. Oral communication program instruction encourages and provides appropriate opportunities for the reticent student (e.g., one who is excessively fearful in speaking situations) to participate more effectively in oral communication.

SUPPORT

1. Oral communication instruction is provided by individuals adequately trained in oral communication or communication disorders, as evidenced by appropriate certification.
2. Individuals responsible for oral communication instruction receive continuing education on theories, research, and instruction relevant to communication.
3. Individuals responsible for oral communication instruction participate actively in conventions, meetings, publications, and other activities of communication professionals.
4. The oral communication program includes a system for training classroom teachers to identify and refer students who do not have adequate listening and speaking skills, or are reticent, to those qualified individuals who can best meet the needs of the student through further assessment or instruction, or both.
5. Teachers in all curriculum areas receive information on appropriate methods for: (a) using oral communication to facilitate instruction, and (b) using the subject matter to improve students' oral communication skills.
6. Parent and community groups are informed about and provided with appropriate materials for effective involvement in the oral communication program.
7. The oral communication program is facilitated by availability and use of appropriate instructional materials, equipment, and facilities.

ASSESSMENT AND EVALUATION

1. The oral communication program is based on a schoolwide assessment of the speaking and listening needs of students.
2. Speaking and listening needs of students will be determined by qualified personnel utilizing appropriate evaluation tools for the skills to be assessed and educational levels of students being assessed.

3. Evaluation of student progress in oral communication is based upon a variety of data, including observations, self-evaluations, listeners' responses to messages, and formal tests.
4. Evaluation of students' oral communication encourages, rather than discourages, students' desires to communicate by emphasizing those behaviors that students can improve, thus enhancing their ability to do so.
5. Evaluation of the total communication program is based on achievement of acceptable levels of oral communication skill determined by continuous monitoring of student progress in speaking and listening, use of standardized and criterion-referenced tests, audience-based rating scales, and other appropriate instruments.

Appendix C

Clinical Management of Communicatively Handicapped Minority Language Populations

Prepared by

American Speech-Language-Hearing Association

STATEMENT OF NEED

The special needs of minority language populations (native speakers of languages other than English) were the source of national controversy even before the Bilingual Education Act was enacted nearly two decades ago. Professionals in bilingual education, regular education, special education, linguistics, sociology, second language instruction, psychology, learning disabilities, as well as speech-language pathology and audiology, have debated innumerable issues, approaches, theories, and philosophical positions regarding minority language populations. As a result of this wide-spread controversy, there has been considerable confusion among these various professionals concerning this population.

According to the 1980 Census, 34.6 million or 15 percent of the U.S. population is composed of native speakers of various minority languages. It is estimated by ASHA that approximately 3.5 million of these speakers have speech, language, or hearing disorders that are unrelated to the use of a minority language. Researchers and clinicians are only beginning to amass a knowledge base on the characteristics of normal language development in various minority languages, bilingual language learning, second language acquisition, dominance testing, bilingual assessment and remediation of communicative disorders, and the applications of emerging computer technology for use with minority language groups. Therefore, it would be premature to propose in this paper optimum strategies for identification, assessment, and intervention.

However, it *is* firmly established that most ASHA members are aware of their limitations in language proficiency and in their knowledge of diverse cultures which restrict their competence to serve minority language populations. According to the 1982 ASHA Self Study Survey, 77 percent of the certified speech-language pathologists indicated a need for more knowledge and skill to serve bilingual-bicultural populations. Given that the minority language population is ever increasing, there is an immediate need for professionals to either upgrade their own levels of competence or to employ alternative strategies to address the needs of the communicatively handicapped among the various minority language populations. Thus, it is the purpose of this paper to recommend competencies for assessment and remediation of communicative disorders of minority language speakers and to describe alternative strategies that can be utilized when those competencies are not met.

It is obvious that assessment and remediation of some disorders of communication are not hampered by the client's use of a minority language. For example, assessment of pure tone hearing thresholds, auditory brainstem response, acoustic reflexes, and other similar services may not necessitate much communicative exchange between the examiner and the client. Likewise, assessment of the physical support for speech, assessment of anomalies affecting speech such as cleft lip and palate, palatal insufficiency, oral malocclusion, etc., also may be conducted without proficiency in the minority language. These examples are by no means exhaustive, but are provided to emphasize that there are clinical services that can be provided appropriately by a monolingual English professional to a minority language speaker. However, because the effectiveness of the professional is dependent on interpersonal skill in addition to technical skill the overall professional client relationship is affected when communication is limited.

For many other aspects of speech, language, and hearing, assessment and remediation are much more complicated by the client's use of a minority language. For example, the phonemic, allophonic, syntactic, morphological, semantic, lexical, and pragmatic characteristics of a minority language cannot be adequately assessed or remediated without knowledge of that language. Further, auditory discrimination and speech reception thresholds may be difficult to assess without the ability to test in the minority language.

Voice qualities, such as harshness, breathiness, loudness, pitch, and the production of clicks and glottal stops, vary across languages. These factors may make it difficult to rule out vocal pathology when the examiner is unfamiliar with the vocal characteristics common to a given language.

Hesitations, false starts, filled and silent pauses, and other dysfluent behavior may be exhibited by a bilingual speaker due to lack of familiarity with English. Thus, differential diagnosis of true stuttering from normal dysfluency may be difficult if the examiner is unfamiliar with the client's use of the minority language.

Identification of prosodic or suprasegmental problems is extremely difficult if the examiner is not familiar with the prosodic characteristics of the minority language. Even when the examiner is familiar with the given language, dialect differences *within* that language may be a confounding variable in assessment.

There are also cultural variables that may influence how speech-language pathology and audiology services are accepted by minority language populations. Differences between minority cultures and the general population in traditions, customs, values, beliefs, and practices may affect service delivery. Thus, speech-language pathologists and audiologists must provide services with consideration of such cultural variables, in addition to consideration of language differences.

Thus, it is apparent that the assessment and remediation of many aspects of speech, language, and hearing of minority language speakers require specific background and skills. This is not only logical and sound clinical practice, but it is the consensus set forth by federal mandates such as The Education for All Handicapped Children Act of 1975 (PL 94-142) and The Bilingual Education Act of 1976 (PL 95-561: Title VII of the Elementary and Secondary Education Act of 1965); legal decisions such as Dianna v. Board of Education (1973), Lau v. Nichols (1974), Larry P. v. Riles (1977) and the Martin Luther King Junior Elementary School Children v. Ann Arbor School District Board (1979); and the policies and practices of many professional agencies and organizations such as the National Association for Bilingual Education, the National Center for Bilingual Research, the Center for Applied Linguistics, and the National Hispanic Psychological Association.

Even state regulations are being developed to acknowledge the need for specific competencies to serve minority language populations. In California, for example, school districts are being encouraged by the State Education Agency to require resource specialists, speech-language pathologists and school psychologists to pass a state administered oral and written examination on Hispanic culture, Spanish language, and assessment methodology before they conduct assessments for Spanish-speaking children with limited English proficiency. Other states and U.S. territories with education legislation which addresses the special needs of minority language populations include Alaska, American Samoa, Arizona, Colorado, Connecticut, Indiana, Iowa, Kansas, Maine, Massachusetts, Michigan, Minnesota, New Hampshire, New Jersey, New Mexico, Oregon, Puerto Rico, South Dakota, Tennessee, Texas, Territory of the Pacific Islands, Utah, Vermont, Washington, Wisconsin, and Wyoming (American Speech-Language-Hearing Association, 1982).

CONTINUUM OF LANGUAGE PROFICIENCY

There are scores of different minority languages spoken in the United States. But within each group of minority language speakers there is also a continuum of proficiency in English. In provision of services to minority language speakers with communicative disorders, the continuum is particularly relevant. The continuum includes speakers who are:
- Bilingual English Proficient,
- Limited English Proficient,
- Limited in both English and the Minority language.

Depending on the client's English language proficiency on the continuum, recommended competencies for the professional are:

Competencies

Bilingual English Proficient

There are bilingual individuals who are fluent in English. Those who have greater control of English than the minority language individuals can be regarded as bilingual English proficient.

For individuals who are bilingual English proficient and evidence a communicative disorder in English, it is *not* essential that the speech-language pathologist or audiologist be proficient in the minority language to provide assessment and remediation in *English*. However, the speech-language pathologist must attain certain competencies to distinguish between dialectal differences (due to interaction from the minority language) and communicative disorders. These competencies include understanding the minority language as a rule-governed system, knowledge of the correct phonological, grammatical, semantic, and pragmatic features of the minority language, and knowledge of nondiscriminatory procedures (refer to "Social Dialects: A Position Paper," *ASHA*, September 1983).

Limited English Proficient

Some bilingual individuals and monolingual individuals are proficient in their native language but not in English. Assessment and intervention of speech and language disorders of limited English proficient speakers should be conducted in the client's primary language. This is consistent with federal mandates (PL 94-142 and Title VII of PL 95-561), legal decisions (such as *Dianna v. Board of Education, Lau v. Nichols,* and *Larry P. v. Riles*), and the education regulations of many states.

To provide assessment and remediation services *in the minority language,* it is recommended that the speech-language pathologist or audiologist possess the following competencies:

Language Proficiency: Native or near native fluency in both the minority language and the English language.

Normative Processes. Ability to describe the process of normal speech and language acquisition for both bilingual and monolingual individuals; and how those processes are manifested in oral and written language.

Assessment: Ability to administer and interpret formal and informal assessment procedures to distinguish between communication difference and communication disorders.

Intervention: Ability to apply intervention strategies for treatment of communicative disorders in the minority language.

Cultural Sensitivity: Ability to recognize cultural factors which affect the delivery of speech-language pathology and audiology services to minority language speaking community.

Limited in Both Languages

There are bilingual individuals who are truly communicatively handicapped, possessing limited communicative competence in both languages. For such individuals, speech and language should be assessed in both languages to determine language dominance. Thus, the same competencies listed for limited English proficient speakers are recommended for assessment for this group of speakers. The most appropriate language for intervention would be determined from the assessment.

If the most appropriate language for intervention is the minority language, then the competencies recommended for serving limited English proficient speakers should be met to provide therapy. If the most appropriate language for intervention is English, proficiency in the minority language may not be necessary to provide therapy.

It is important to note that the determination of bilingual dominance in communicatively handicapped individuals may be particularly difficult. It is stressed that both objectives and subjective measures should be utilized to determine if the client's dominant language is either English or the minority language.

Alternative Strategies for Use of Professional Personnel

It is recognized that not all speech-language pathologists and audiologists possess the recommended competencies to serve limited English proficient speakers. Following are some strategies for procuring speech-language pathologists who do meet the aforementioned competencies when there are none on staff.

1. **Establish Contacts.** Bilingual speech-language pathologists or audiologists can be hired by school districts and other clinical programs as consultants to evaluate and remediate minority language speakers on an as needed basis.
2. **Establish Cooperative.** A clinical cooperative can be developed to allow a group of school districts or clinical programs to hire an itinerant bilingual speech-language pathologist or audiologist whose primary responsibility is to serve a specific minority language population.
3. **Establish Networks.** Strong ties could be established between professional work settings and university programs that have bilingual speech-language pathology or audiology programs so that there can be an interchange of existing resources. Once such a liaison is established, it can facilitate recruitment of speech-language pathologists or audiologists who are competent to serve minority language populations after they graduate.
4. **Establish CFY and Graduate Practicum Sites.** Graduate students or recent graduates from bilingual communicative disorders programs, under the direct supervision of a bilingual speech-language pathologist or audiologist, could be used to assist personnel in schools and other clinical facilities in assessment and intervention of limited English-proficient individuals.

5. **Establish Interdisciplinary Teams.** A team approach can be implemented which includes the monolingual speech-language pathologist or audiologist and a bilingual professional equal (e.g., psychologist, special education teacher, etc.) who is knowledgeable of non-biased assessment procedures and language development of the particular minority language.

An agency contracting the services of a speech-language pathologist or audiologist to serve limited English-proficient speakers may not be in a position to evaluate the professional's competencies. Therefore, when employing the preceding alternative strategies, efforts should be made to assure that the speech-language pathologist or audiologist is competent to serve a given minority language population.

Use of Interpreters or Translators

Interpreters or translators could be used with minority language speakers when the following circumstances exist: (a) when the certified speech-language pathologist or audiologist on the staff does not meet the recommended competencies to provide services to limited-English proficient speakers; (b) when an individual who needs services speaks a language which is uncommon for that local area; and (c) when there are no trained professionals readily available with proficiency in that language that would permit the use of one of the previously described alternative strategies. Individuals who could serve as interpreters or translators can include (1) professional interpreters from language banks or professional interpreting services, (2) bilingual professional staff from a health or education discipline other than communicative disorders, or (3) a family member or friend of the client.

If the use of interpreters or translators is the only alternative, the speech-language pathologist or audiologist should:

1. Provide extensive training to the assistant on the purposes, procedures and goals of the tests and therapy methods. The assistant also should be taught to avoid the use of gestures, vocal intonation, and other cues that could inadvertently alert the individual to the correct response during test administration.
2. Pre-plan for an individual's services to insure the assistant's understanding of specific clinical procedures to be used.
3. Use the same assistant(s) with a given minority language client rather than using assistants on a random basis.

4. Use patient observation or other non-linguistic measures as supplements to the translated measures, such as (1) child's interaction with parents, (2) child's interaction with peers, (3) pragmatic analysis.

It is recommended that the speech-language pathologist and audiologist state in their written evaluations that a translator was used and the validity of the results may be affected.

FUTURE DIRECTIONS

It is stressed that the competencies and alternative strategies delineated herein are interim in an effort to address the crisis that presently exists in the delivery of services to minority language populations. Therefore, these competencies and alternative strategies may be subject to revision or expansion as our professional knowledge base continues to increase. In addition to promoting the continued advancement of knowledge, it should be the ultimate goal of the profession to increase the percentage of speech-language pathologists and audiologists who are competent to serve minority language populations. This can be accomplished by 1) stimulating bilingual student recruitment efforts, 2) promoting relevant continuing education activities and, 3) promoting the topic of minority language populations within professional education.

The establishment of competencies in the area of service delivery to minority language populations is not intended to impose prohibitions or a hands-off philosophy for those who do not meet those competencies. But it is the professional responsibility of the speech-language pathologist and audiologist to judge their own minority language proficiency, clinical knowledge base, and cultural sensitivity in terms of the competencies delineated in this paper. Where there are deficiencies that can be reversed, it is incumbent on professionals to upgrade their level of competence through professional and continuing education programs, independent study of the growing literature on minority language populations, and ongoing involvement within the community of minority language speakers. Otherwise alternative strategies should be implemented to serve minority language speakers.

Because the competencies and alternative strategies discussed in this paper are interim, multicultural research and continued development of techniques and materials for assessment and intervention need to be priorities of professionals who provide service to these populations. Professionals also should stimulate further development and implementation of creative alternatives in order to provide appropriate and effective speech-language pathology and audiology services to minority language speakers.

REFERENCES

American Speech-Language-Hearing Association (1982). *Urban and ethnic perspectives,* October, 9–10.

Dianna v. State Board of Education, C.A. 70 RFT (N.D. Cal., Feb. 3, 1970).

Larry P. v. Riles, Civil Action No. 0-71-2270, 343 F. Supp. 1306 (N.D. Cal., 1972).

Lau v. Nichols, 411 U.S. 563 (1974).

Martin Luther King Junior Elementary School Children, et al. v. Ann Arbor School District Board, Civil Action No. 7-71861, 451 F. Supp. 1324 (1978), 463 F. Supp. 1027 (1978) and 473 F. Supp. 1371 (1979) (Detroit, Michigan, July 12, 1979).

Social dialects: A position paper (1983). *ASHA, 25(9),* 23–24.

Public Law 94-142, The Education of All Handicapped Children Act (Nov. 29, 1975).

Public Law 95-561, The Bilingual Education Act (Title VII of the Elementary and Secondary Education Act of 1965).

Appendix D

A Sample Lesson For Teaching Standard English as a Second Dialect Which Utilizes Bilingual Education Approach*

INSTRUCTIONAL FOCUS: Possessives (Morpheme -s with nouns)

OBJECTIVE: Given structured drill and practice contrasting *the use of possessive nouns*, the students will be able to differentiate between standard and nonstandard usage and to formulate sentences using the standard form in response to statements or questions.

LEVEL: Teacher Judgement

MATERIAL: A. Pair of multiple response cards labeled same and different for each student.

               B. Pair of multiple response cards labeled standard and nonstandard.

PROCEDURES:

1. To assess the students' abilities in auditory discrimination, the teacher will lead the students in the following drill. Students will respond by displaying a *same* or *different* response card.

DISCRIMINATION DRILL:

Teacher Stimulus	*Student Response*
• This is Joes car. This is Joe's car.	• different
• That is Steve's house. That is Steve's house.	• same

---

*From Standard English Program, Oakland (CA) Unified School District (1984).

- This is Monika's jump rope.   • different
  This is Monika jump rope.

- Where is Jim's skateboard?   • same
  Where is Jim's skateboard?

- Is that Doug's football?   • same
  Is that Doug's football?

- There is Pam's school.   • different
  There is Pam school.

2. The teacher will explain and model the standard form and have students repeat several examples giving additional help where needed.

3. The teacher will lead the students in the following drill. Students will respond by displaying standard or nonstandard response cards.

IDENTIFICATION DRILL:

• Mary brother is little.	Nonstandard
• Bill store is closed.	Nonstandard
• Tom's truck is red.	Standard
• Ted frog jumps high.	Nonstandard
• Jerome's cat is gray.	Standard
• Terry bicycle goes fast.	Nonstandard
• Jackie's coat is blue.	Standard
• Kevin lunch box is black.	Nonstandard

4. To check for understanding the teacher will call on individual students to respond to questions and statements similar to those in the following drill. Students will respond in complete sentences using the standard form. Students should be instructed to listen for only one nonstandard feature and to respond in complete sentences. Contractions are acceptable.

TRANSLATION DRILL:

Teacher Stimulus	*Student Response*
• Jesse truck is red.	• Jesse's truck is red.
• Monica school is large.	• Monica's school is large
• Larry jacket is black and brown.	• Larry's jacket is black and brown.
• Brian mother is ill.	• Brian's mother is ill

5. In the following drill the students will generate their own sentences in response to the teacher stimulus. The student responses listed here are but examples.

Students should be instructed to respond in complete sentences, although sometimes in everyday speech we do not. Contractions are acceptable.

RESPONSE DRILLS:

Teacher Stimulus	Student Response
• Is that Jessie house?	• Yes, that is Jessie's house.
• Is that John mother?	• No, that is not John's mother.
• Are those Monica skates?	• Yes, those are Monica's skates.
• That is Tobby milk.	• No, that is not Tobby's milk.
• Where are Jerry shoes?	• Here are Jerry's shoes.
• Where is Cassandra coat?	• Cassandra's coat is hanging on the hook.

EXPANSION ACTIVITY (General):

A. Guide students in reading the narrative from the life of Richard Drew (see attached). Discuss content.

B. Direct attention to the italicized phrases. Elicit oral translation phrases. Elicit oral translations of these phrases into possessive form. Example:

The dream of Charles Drew would be *Charles Drew's dream*

C. After working through the entire story orally with students, provide independent practice by having them rewrite the story, translating all the phrases to the standard possessive form. Papers may be exchanged and read for peer evaluation.

EXPANSION: (Upper Grades) — Science/Health/Careers/Black History:

A. Have students research and report on the career of Daniel Hale Williams. How was his career similar to that of Charles Drew?

B. Study the circulatory system for a better understanding of the contributions of both these men to the medical profession.

C. List various medical professions and do research to find out more about them. This may be done through student interviews or by inviting persons from medical professions to speak to the class.

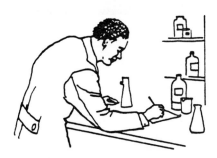

CHARLES RICHARD DREW

The dream of Charles Drew was to become a doctor. He attended Amherst College, but *the courses at this school* did not prepare him to become a doctor. Charles taught for two years to earn money for medical school.

As a doctor, *the interests of this young man* were in blood and blood transfusions. A transfusion is the passing of blood *from the veins of one person to the veins of another.* Dr. Drew discovered a way to change plasma, *the liquid part of the* blood, to powder. This way it could be stored and sent long distances. During World War II, the *wounds of injured soldiers* were treated with this powder. It saved *the lives of many men.* Dr. Drew also learned that *the skin of a person* had nothing to do with blood. All people are alike under the skin.

Because of *the interests of Dr. Drew* in blood, he got the idea of starting a blood bank. Here people could borrow blood when needed. *This idea, spun by Dr. Charles Drew,* caused him to be known as "Father of the Blood Bank."

Author Index

Subject Index

COLLEGE-HILL PRESS

ISBN 0-88744-185-8